CHRONIC PAIN

Volume I

Chronic Pain

Volume I

edited by

Thomas W. Miller, Ph.D., A.B.P.P.

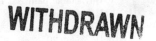

INTERNATIONAL UNIVERSITIES PRESS, INC.
Madison   **Connecticut**

Library of Congress Cataloging in Publication Data

Chronic pain / edited by Thomas W. Miller.
     p.   cm.
    Includes bibliographical references.
ISBN 0-8236-0850-6 (v. 1) —ISBN 0-8236-0851-4 (v. 2)
    1. Intractable pain.   I. Miller, Thomas W., 1943–
[DNLM: 1. Chronic Disease. 2. Pain. WL 704 C55691]
  RB 127.C4753   1990
  616′.0472—dc20
  DNLM/DLC
  for Library of Congress   90-4262
                                                   CIP

Manufactured in the United States of America

Table of Contents for Volume I

II DIAGNOSTIC ISSUES IN CHRONIC PAIN

EDITORIAL INTRODUCTION

Table of Contents for Volume II

IV PERSPECTIVES ON CHRONIC PAIN

EDITORIAL INTRODUCTION

Contributors

FRANK ANDRASIK, PH.D., Professor, Department of Psychology, University of West Florida, Pensacola, Florida

RICHARD T. BECK, PH.D., Associate Professor, Department of Rehabilitation Counseling, Mankato State University, Mankato, Minnesota

CYNTHIA D. BELAR, PH.D., Chief Psychologist and Clinical Director, Behavioral Medicine, Kaiser-Permanente Medical Program, Los Angeles, California

DANIEL BLAZER, M.D., Professor, Department of Psychiatry, Duke University Medical School, Durham, North Carolina

STEVEN F. BRENA, M.D., Professor and Director, Pain Control and Rehabilitation Institute of Georgia, and Clinical Professor, Rehabilitation Medicine, Emory University, Atlanta, Georgia

DOROTHY BROCKOPP, PH.D., Associate Professor, College of Nursing and Markey Cancer Center, University of Kentucky, Lexington, Kentucky

GENE BROCKOPP, PH.D., Associate Professor, Department of Anesthesiology, College of Medicine, University of Kentucky, Lexington, Kentucky

JOSEPH P. BUSH, PH.D., Professor, Department of Psychology, Virginia Commonwealth University, Richmond, Virginia

ERIC J. CASSEL, M.D., Professor, Department of Public Health, Cornell University Medical College, New York City

ERLING ENG, PH.D., Clinical Professor, Department of Psychiatry, VA and University of Kentucky Medical Centers, Lexington, Kentucky

RANDAL D. FRANCE, M.D., Psychiatrist, Private Practice, Salt Lake City, Utah

EDITH W. M. HERMAN, PH.D., Assistant Professor, Department of Medicine, McMaster University, Hamilton, Ontario, Canada

FRANK W. ISELE, PH.D., Psychologist, Private Practice, Glens Falls, New York

LOUIS L. JAY, R.PH., Consulting Pharmacist and Graduate, University of Buffalo, Buffalo, New York

KAY RANGA RAMA KRISHNAN, M.D., Department of Psychiatry, Duke University Medical School, Durham, North Carolina

WOLFGANG F. KUHN, M.D., Professor, Department of Psychiatry and Behavioral Sciences, University of Louisville, Louisville, Kentucky

ROBERT LAKOFF, M.D., F.R.C.P. (C), Associate Professor of Psychiatry, University of Alberta, Canada

PAUL LUSTIG, PH.D., Clinical Psychologist, Private Practice, Madison, Wisconsin

GUIDO MAGNI, M.D., Visiting Professor, Department of Psychiatry, University of Western Ontario, London, Ontario and Department of Psychiatry, Institute of Clinical Psychiatry, Padua, Italy

ROBERT D. MARCIANI, D.M.D., Professor, Department of Oral and Maxillofacial Surgery, University of Kentucky Medical Center, Lexington, Kentucky

H. MERSKEY, D.M., F.R.C.P., F.R.C. Psych., Professor, Department of Psychiatry, University of Western Ontario and Director of Education and Research, London Psychiatry Hospital, London, Ontario, Canada

THOMAS W. MILLER, PH.D., A.B.P.P., Professor and Chief, Psychology Service, VA and University of Kentucky Medical Centers, Lexington, Kentucky

NANCI I. MOORE, PH.D., Clinical Associate Professor and Chief, Psychology Service, Veterans Administration Medical Center and University of Louisville, Louisville, Kentucky

JAMES C. NORTON, PH.D., A.B.P.P., Associate Professor of Psychiatry and Neurology and Associate Program Administrator, Area Health Education Center Program, University of Kentucky, College of Medicine, Lexington, Kentucky

STEWART PAGE, PH.D., Professor, Department of Psychology, University of Windsor, Windsor, Ontario, Canada

MARGARET A. RANKIN, R.N., D.S.M., M.A., Professor, College of Nursing, University of Iowa, Iowa City, Iowa

VICKIE J. REID, M.A., Department of Psychology, Virginia Commonwealth University, Richmond, Virginia

RANJAN ROY, ADV. DIP. S.W., Professor, School of Social Work, the University of Manitoba, Manitoba, Canada

STEVEN SANDERS, PH.D., Executive Director, Pain Control and Rehabilitation Institute of Georgia and Clinical Associate Professor of Rehabilitation Medicine, Emory University, Atlanta, Georgia

DOUGLAS K. SNYDER, PH.D., Professor of Psychology, Department of Psychology, Texas A&M University, College Station, Texas

CRAIG WAGGONER, PH.D., Clinical Psychologist, Thomas Rehabilitation Hospital, Ashville, North Carolina

MARK B. WEISBERG, PH.D., Metropolitan Clinic, Brooklyn Centre, Minnesota

WILLARD WHITEHEAD, III, M.D., Department of Psychiatry and Behavioral Sciences, University of Louisville, Louisville, Kentucky

JOHN F. WILSON, PH.D., Associate Professor, Department of Behavioral Sciences, University of Kentucky, College of Medicine, Lexington, Kentucky

Preface

In writing this two-volume work, the goal has been to bring together a multidisciplinary perspective and to make available to all professionals in the health care delivery system an overview of theory, diagnostic, and treatment issues and a multiplicity of therapeutic perspectives in addressing the diagnostic entity of chronic pain. It is hoped that this unique contribution will provide both conceptual clarity and scholarly direction. This book presents an area of inquiry which has emerged quite recently and is designed to inform the reader, clinician, and scientist, to stimulate new hypotheses, and to generate innovations in both research and clinical intervention in this growing area of study.

This two-volume compendium of empirically based observations is intended for readers who include students, as well as professionals, interested in understanding and helping a broad spectrum of patients who experience chronic pain. The work has four sections. The first section, The Nature of Pain, deals with the nature of pain from both a medical and psychological perspective. Included in this discourse are issues related to the neurosis of pain, economic, ethical and psychosocial considerations, ethnic factors, and the impact of compensation and litigation.

In Section II, Diagnostic Issues in Chronic Pain, is a conjoint effort from both the medical and psychological communities and provides a broad spectrum of approaches to the assessment and diagnostic considerations in addressing the chronic pain patient.

Section III, The Multiple Strategies in the Treatment of Chronic Pain, includes chapters by some of the most well-respected multidisciplinary leaders from the United States, Canada, and Europe. It attempts to address a wide variety of clinical issues regarding the treatment of pain patients, including patient motivation, treatment compliance, and specialized individual and group techniques that represent a multifaceted approach to the management of chronic pain.

Section IV, Perspectives on Chronic Pain represents a unique effort to bring together multidisciplinary perspectives in understanding the diagnosis, treatment, and impact of chronic pain across the life span.

In an effort to understand the nature and consequences of chronic pain for the individual, the family, and the professional practitioner, it is the intention in both of these volumes to address the following specific objectives:

1. To clearly define and provide a framework for understanding the nature and impact of chronic pain.
2. To explicate the critical concepts and variables associated with understanding chronic pain.
3. To identify the essential areas of research interests that converge on our state-of-the-art understanding of diagnostic and therapeutic issues faced by the chronic pain patient.
4. To elaborate on the most effective strategies for intervention by professionals, recognizing the important contributions from the variety of disciplines that have committed themselves to understanding and effectively treating the chronic pain patient.

I am indeed indebted and grateful to the number of people, agencies, publishers, and scientific societies who have provided their support over the years in compiling the collection of clinical and research expertise contained in these two volumes. While there is considerable enthusiasm for the material herein presented, my most sincere intention is to provide a provocative and hypothesis-generating compendium of expert opinion that allows the reader, the practitioner, and the clinical

researcher to entertain new hypotheses, experiment with innovation, and encourage productive exchanges that will benefit
all of humankind in our quest to relieve a condition known as
chronic pain.

Dedication

This compendium on chronic pain is dedicated to all of human-kind who have experienced chronic pain and who have come to know, understand, and adapt to this condition. It is also dedicated to the patients who have been diagnosed and treated through chronic pain programs in the Veterans Administration Health Delivery System, and finally, to my wife Jean, son David, and daughter Jeanine.

Introduction:
The Nature of Suffering
and the Goals of Medicine

Eric J. Cassel, M.D.

The obligation of physicians to relieve human suffering stretches back into antiquity. Despite this fact, little explicit attention, in either medical education, research, or practice, is given to the problem of suffering. I will begin by focusing on a modern paradox: Even in the best settings and with the best physicians, it is not uncommon for suffering to occur not only during the course of the disease but also as a result of its treatment. To understand this paradox and its resolution requires an understanding of what suffering is and how it relates to medical care.

Consider this case: a thirty-five-year-old sculptor with metastatic disease of the breast was treated by competent physicians employing advanced knowledge and technology and acting out of kindness and true concern. At every stage, the treatment as well as the disease was a source of suffering to her.

I am indebted to Rabbi Jack Bemporad, to Drs. Joan Cassell, Peter Dineen, Nancy McKenzie, and Richard Zaner, to Ms. Dawn McGuire, to the members of the Research Group on Death, Suffering, and Well-Being of the Hastings Center for their advice and assistance, and to the Arthur Vining Davis Foundations for support of the research group.

She was uncertain and frightened about her future, but she could get little information from her physicians, and what she was told was not always the truth. She had been unaware, for example, that the irradiated breast would be so disfigured. After an oophorectomy and a regimen of medications, she became hirsute, obese, and devoid of libido. With tumor in the supraclavicular fossa, she lost strength in the hand that she used in sculpturing, and she became profoundly depressed. She had a pathologic fracture of the femur, and treatment was delayed while her physicians openly disagreed about pinning her hip.

Each time her disease responded to therapy and her hope was rekindled, a new manifestation would appear. Thus, when a new course of chemotherapy was started, she was torn between a desire to live and the fear that allowing hope to emerge again would merely expose her to misery if the treatment failed. The nausea and vomiting from the chemotherapy were distressing, but no more so than the anticipation of hair loss. She feared the future. Each tomorrow was seen as heralding increased sickness, pain, or disability, never as the beginning of better times. She felt isolated because she was no longer like other people and could not do what other people did. She feared that her friends would stop visiting her. She was sure that she would die.

This young woman had severe pain and other physical symptoms that caused her suffering. But she also suffered from some threats that were social and from others that were personal and private. She suffered from the effects of the disease and its treatment on her appearance and abilities. She also suffered unremittingly from her perception of the future.

What can this case tell us about the ends of medicine and the relief of suffering? Three facts stand out: The first is that this woman's suffering was not confined to her physical symptoms. The second is that she suffered not only from her disease but also from its treatment. The third is that one could not anticipate what she would describe as a source of suffering; like other patients, she had to be asked. Some features of her condition she would call painful, upsetting, uncomfortable, and distressing, but not a source of suffering. In these characteristics her case was ordinary.

In discussing the matter of suffering with lay persons, I learned that they were shocked to discover that the problem of suffering was not directly addressed in medical education. My colleagues of a contemplative nature were surprised at how little they knew of the problem and how little thought they had given it, whereas medical students tended to be unsure of the relevance of the issue to their work.

The relief of suffering, it would appear, is considered one of the primary ends of medicine by patients and lay persons, but not by the medical profession. As in the care of the dying, patients and their friends and families do not make a distinction between physical and nonphysical sources of suffering in the same way that doctors do (Cassell, 1972).

A search of the medical and social science literature did not help me in understanding what suffering is; the word *suffering* was most often coupled with the word *pain* as in "pain and suffering." (The data bases used were *Psychological Abstracts*, the *Citation Index*, and the *Index Medicus*.)

This phenomenon reflects a historically constrained and currently inadequate view of the ends of medicine. Medicine's traditional, primary concern, for the body and for physical disease, is well known, as are the widespread effects of the mind–body dichotomy on medical theory and practice. I believe that this dichotomy itself is a source of the paradoxical situation in which doctors cause suffering in their care of the sick. Today, as ideas about the separation of mind and body are called into question, physicians are concerning themselves with new aspects of the human condition. The profession of medicine is being pushed and pulled into new areas, both by its technology and by the demands of its patients. Attempting to understand what suffering is, and how physicians might truly be devoted to its relief, will require that medicine and its critics overcome the dichotomy between mind and body and the associated dichotomies between subjective and objective and between person and object.

In the remainder of this chapter I am going to make three points. The first is that suffering is experienced by persons. In the separation between mind and body, the concept of the person, or personhood, has been associated with that of mind, spirit, and the subjective. However, as I will show, a person is not merely mind, merely spiritual, or only subjectively knowable. Personhood has many facets, and it is ignorance of them that actively contributes to patients' suffering. The understanding of the place of the person in human illness requires a rejection of the historical dualism of mind and body.

The second point derives from my interpretation of clinical observations: Suffering occurs when an impending destruction of the person is perceived; it continues until the threat of disintegration has passed or until the integrity of the person can be restored in some other manner. It follows, then, that although suffering often occurs in the presence of acute pain, shortness of breath, or other bodily symptoms, suffering extends beyond the physical. Most generally, suffering can be defined as the state of severe distress associated with events that threaten the intactness of the person.

The third point is that suffering can occur in relation to any aspect of the person, whether it is in the realm of social roles, group identification, the relation with self, body, or family, or the relation with a transpersonal, transcendent source of meaning. Below is a simplified description or "topology" of the constituents of personhood.

"PERSON" IS NOT "MIND"

The split between mind and body that has so deeply influenced our approach to medical care was proposed by Descartes to resolve certain philosophical issues. Moreover, Cartesian dualism made it possible for science to escape the control of the church by assigning the noncorporeal, spiritual realm to the church, leaving the physical world as the domain of science. In that religious age, "person" synonymous with "mind," was necessarily off-limits to science.

Changes in the meaning of concepts like that of personhood occur with changes in society, while the word for the concept remains the same. This fact tends to obscure the depth of the transformations that have occurred between the seventeenth century and today. People simply are *persons* in this time, as in past times, and they have difficulty imagining that the term described something quite different in an earlier period when the concept was more constrained.

If the mind–body dichotomy results in assigning the body to medicine, and the person is not in that category, then the only remaining place for the person is in the category of mind. Where the mind is problematic (not identifiable in objective terms), its very reality diminishes for science, and so, too, does that of the person. Therefore, so long as the mind–body dichotomy is accepted, suffering is either subjective and thus not truly "real"—not within medicine's domain—or identified exclusively with bodily pain. Not only is such an identification misleading and distorting, for it depersonalizes the sick patient, but it is itself a source of suffering. It is not possible to treat sickness as something that happens solely to the body without thereby risking damage to the person. An anachronistic division of the human condition into what is medical (having to do with the body) and what is nonmedical (the remainder) has given medicine too narrow a notion of its calling. Because of this division, physicians may, in concentrating on the cure of bodily disease, do things that cause the patient as a person to suffer.

AN IMPENDING DESTRUCTION OF PERSON

Suffering is ultimately a personal matter. Patients sometimes report suffering when one does not expect it, or do not report suffering when one does expect it. Furthermore, a person can suffer enormously at the distress of another, especially a loved one.

In some theologies, suffering has been seen as bringing one closer to God. This "function" of suffering is at once its glorification and its relief. If, through great pain or deprivation, someone is brought closer to a cherished goal, that person may have no sense of having suffered but may instead feel enormous triumph. To an observer, however, only the deprivation may be apparent. This cautionary note is important because people are often said to have suffered greatly, in a religious context, when they are known only to have been injured, tortured, or in pain, not to have suffered.

Although pain and suffering are closely identified in the medical literature, they are phenomenologically distinct (Bakan, 1971). The difficulty of understanding pain and the problems of physicians in providing adequate relief of physical pain are well known (Marks and Sachar, 1973; Goodwin, Goodwin, and Vogel, 1979; Kanner and Foley, 1981; Zaner, 1981).

The greater the pain, the more it is believed to cause suffering. However, some pain, like that of childbirth, can be extremely severe and yet considered rewarding. The perceived meaning of pain influences the amount of medication that will be required to control it. For example, a patient reported that when she believed the pain in her leg was sciatica, she could control it with small doses of codeine, but when she discovered that it was due to the spread of malignant disease, much greater amounts of medication were required for relief. Patients can writhe in pain from kidney stones and by their own admission not be suffering, because they "know what it is"; they may also report considerable suffering from apparently minor discomfort when they do not know its source. Suffering in close relation to the intensity of pain is reported when the pain is virtually overwhelming, such as that associated with a dissecting aortic aneurysm. Suffering is also reported when the patient does not believe that pain can be controlled. The suffering of patients with terminal cancer can often be relieved by demonstrating that their pain truly can be controlled; they will then often tolerate the same pain without any medication, preferring the pain to the side effects of their analgesics. Another type of pain that can be a source of suffering is pain that is not overwhelming but continues for a very long time.

In summary, people in pain frequently report suffering from the pain when they feel out of control, when the pain is overwhelming, when the source of the pain is unknown, when the meaning of the pain is dire, or when the pain is chronic.

In all these situations, persons perceive pain as a threat to their continued existence—not merely to their lives, but to their integrity as persons. That this is the relation of pain to suffering is strongly suggested by the fact that suffering can be relieved, in the presence of continued pain, by making the source of the pain known, changing its meaning, and demonstrating that it can be controlled and that an end is in sight.

It follows, then, that suffering has a temporal element. In order for a situation to be a source of suffering, it must influence the person's perception of future events. ("If the pain continues like this, I *will be* overwhelmed"; "If the pain comes from cancer, I *will not* be able to take it.") At the moment when the patient is saying, "If the pain continues like this, I will be overwhelmed," he or she is not overwhelmed. Fear itself always involves the future. In the case with which I opened this paper, the patient could not give up her fears of her sense of future, despite the agony they caused her. As suffering is discussed in the other dimensions of personhood, note how it would not exist if the future were not a major concern.

Two other aspects of the relation between pain and suffering should be mentioned. Suffering can occur when physicians do not validate the patient's pain. In the absence of disease, physicians may suggest that the pain is "psychological" (in the sense of not being real) or that the patient is "faking." Similarly, patients with chronic pain may believe after a time that they can no longer talk to others about their distress. In the former case the person is caused to distrust his or her perceptions of reality, and in both instances social isolation adds to the person's suffering.

Another aspect essential to an understanding of the suffering of sick persons is the relation of meaning to the way in which illness is experienced. The word *meaning* is used here in two senses: in the first, to mean is to signify, to imply. Pain in the chest may imply heart disease. We also say that we know what something means when we know how important it is. The importance of things is always personal and individual, even though meaning in this sense may be shared by others or by society as a whole. What something signifies and how important it is relative to the whole array of a person's concerns contributes to its personal meaning. *Belief* is another word for that aspect of meaning concerned with implications, and *value* concerns the degree of importance to a particular person.

The personal meaning of things does not consist exclusively of values and beliefs that are held intellectually; it includes other dimensions. For the same word, a person may simultaneously have a cognitive meaning, an affective or emotional meaning, a bodily meaning, and a transcendent or spiritual meaning. And there may be contradictions in the different levels of meaning. The nuances of personal meaning are complex, and when I speak of personal meanings I am implying this complexity in all its depth—known and unknown. Personal meaning is a fundamental dimension of personhood, and there can be no understanding of human illness or suffering without taking it into account.

A SIMPLIFIED DESCRIPTION OF THE PERSON

A simple topology of a person may be useful in understanding the relation between suffering and the goals of medicine. The features discussed below point the way to further study and to the possibility of specific action by individual physicians.

Persons have personality and character. Personality traits appear within the first few weeks of life and are remarkably durable over time. Some personalities handle some illnesses better than others. Individual persons vary in character as well. During the heyday of psychoanalysis in the United States during the 1950s, all behavior was attributed to unconscious determinants: No one was bad or good; they were merely sick or well. Fortunately, that simplistic view of human character is now out of favor. Some people do in fact have stronger characters and bear adversity better than others. Some are good and kind under the stress of terminal illness, whereas others become mean and offensive when even mildly ill.

A person has a past. The experiences gathered during one's life are a part of today as well as yesterday. Memory exists in the nostrils and the hands, not only in the mind. A fragrance drifts by, and a memory is evoked. My feet have not forgotten how to roller-skate, and my hands remember skills that I was hardly aware I had learned. When these past experiences involve sickness and medical care, they can influence present illness and medical care. They stimulate fear, confidence, physical symptoms, and anguish. It damages people to rob them of their past and deny their memories, or to mock their fears and worries. A person without a past is incomplete.

Life experiences—previous illness, experiences with doctors, hospitals, and medications, deformities and disabilities, pleasures and successes, miseries and failures—all form the nexus for illness. The personal meaning of the disease and its treatment arises from the past as well as the present. If cancer occurs in a patient with self-confidence from past achievements it may give rise to optimism and a resurgence of strength. Even if it is fatal, the disease may not produce the destruction of the person but, rather, reaffirm his or her indomitability. The outcome would be different in a person for whom life had been a series of failures.

The intensity of ties to the family cannot be overemphasized; people frequently behave as though they were physical extensions of their parents. Events that might cause suffering in others may be borne without complaint by someone who believes that the disease is part of his or her family identity and hence inevitable. Even diseases for which no heritable basis is known may be borne easily by a person because others in the family have been similarly afflicted. Just as the person's past experiences give meaning to present events, so do the past experiences of his or her family. Those meanings are part of the person.

A person has a cultural background. Just as a person is part of a culture and a society, these elements are part of the person. Culture defines what is meant by masculinity or femininity, what attire is acceptable, attitudes toward the dying and sick, mating behavior, the height of chairs and steps, degrees of tolerance for odors and excreta, and how the aged and the disabled are treated. Cultural definitions have an enormous impact on the sick and can be a source of untold suffering. They influence the behavior of others toward the sick person and that of the sick toward themselves. Cultural norms and social rules regulate whether someone can be among others or will be isolated, whether the sick will be considered foul or acceptable, and whether they are to be pitied or censured.

Returning to the sculptor described earlier, we know why that young woman suffered. She was housebound and bed-bound, her face was changed by steroids, she was physically masculinized by her treatment, one breast was scarred, and she had almost no hair. The degree of importance attached to these losses—that aspect of their personal meaning—is determined to a great degree by cultural priorities.

With this in mind, we can also realize how much someone devoid of physical pain, even devoid of "symptoms," may suffer. People suffer from what they have lost of themselves in relation to the world of objects, events, and relationships. We realize, too, that although medical care can reduce the impact of sickness, inattentive care can increase the disruption caused by illness.

A person has roles: I am a husband, a father, a physician, a teacher, a brother, an orphaned son, and an uncle. People are their roles, and each role has rules. Together, the rules that guide the performance of roles make up a complex set of entitlements and limitations of responsibility and privilege. By middle age, the roles may be so firmly set that disease can lead to the virtual destruction of a person by making the perfor-mance of his or her roles impossible. Whether the patient is a doctor who cannot doctor or a mother who cannot mother, he or she is diminished by the loss of function.

No person exists without others; there is no consciousness without a consciousness of others, no speaker without a hearer, and no act, object, or thought that does not somehow encom-pass others. All behavior is or will be involved with others, even if only in memory or reverie. Take away others, remove sight or hearing, and the person is diminished. Everyone dreads be-coming blind or deaf, but these are only the most obvious injuries to human interaction. There are many ways in which human beings can be cut off from others and then suffer the loss.

It is in relationships with others that the full range of human emotions finds expression. It is this dimension of the person that may be injured when illness disrupts the ability to express emotion. Furthermore, the extent and nature of a sick person's relationships influence the degree of suffering from a disease. There is a vast difference between going home to an empty apartment and going home to a network of friends and family after a hospitalization. Illness may occur in one partner of a long and strongly bound marriage or in a union that is falling apart. Suffering from the loss of sexual function associated with some diseases will depend not only on the importance of sexual performance itself but also on its importance in the sick person's relationships.

A person is a political being. A person is in this sense equal to other persons, with rights and obligations and the ability to redress injury by others and the state. Sickness can interfere, producing the feeling of political powerlessness and lack of representation. Persons who are permanently handicapped may suffer from a feeling of exclusion from participation in the political realm.

Persons do things: They act, create, make, take apart, put together, wind, unwind, cause to be, and cause to vanish. They know themselves, and are known, by these acts. When illness restricts the range of activity of persons, they are not themselves.

Persons are often unaware of much that happens within them and why. Thus, there are things in the mind that cannot be brought to awareness by ordinary reflection. The structure of the unconscious is pictured quite differently by different scholars, but most students of human behavior accept the assertion that such an interior world exists. People can behave in ways that seem inexplicable and strange even to themselves, and the sense of powerlessness that the person may feel in the presence of such behavior can be a source of great distress.

Persons have regular behaviors. In health, we take for granted the details of our day-to-day behavior. Persons know themselves to be well as much by whether they behave as usual as by any other set of facts. Patients decide that they are ill because they cannot perform as usual, and they may suffer the loss of their routine. If they cannot do the things that they identify with the fact of their being, they are not whole.

Every person has a body. The relation with one's body may vary from identification with it to admiration, loathing, or constant fear. The body may even be perceived as a representation of a parent, so that when something happens to the person's body it is as though a parent were injured. Disease can so alter the relation that the body is no longer seen as a friend but, rather, as an untrustworthy enemy. This is intensified if the illness comes without warning, and as illness persists, the person may feel increasingly vulnerable. Just as many people have an expanded sense of self as a result of changes in their bodies from exercise, the potential exists for a contraction of this sense through injury to the body.

Everyone has a secret life. Sometimes it takes the form of fantasies and dreams of glory; sometimes it has a real existence known to only a few. Within the secret life are fears, desires, love affairs of the past and present, hopes, and fantasies. Disease may destroy not only the public or the private person but the secret person as well. A secret, beloved friend may be lost to a sick person because he or she has no legitimate place by the sickbed. When that happens, the patient may have lost the part of life that made tolerable an otherwise embittered existence. Or the loss may be only of a dream, but one that might have come true. Such loss can be a source of great distress and intensely private pain.

Everyone has a perceived future. Events that one expects to come to pass vary from expectations for one's children to a belief in one's creative ability. Intense unhappiness results from a loss of the future—the future of the individual person, of children, and of other loved ones. Hope dwells in this dimension of existence, and great suffering attends the loss of hope.

Everyone has a transcendent dimension, a life of the spirit. This is most directly expressed in religion and the mystic tradition but the frequency with which people have intense feelings of bonding with groups, ideals, or anything larger and more enduring than the person is evidence of the universality of the transcendent dimension. The quality of being greater and more lasting than an individual life gives this aspect of the person its timeless dimension. The profession of medicine appears to ignore the human spirit. When I see patients in nursing homes who have become only bodies, I wonder whether it is not their transcendent dimension that they have lost.

THE NATURE OF SUFFERING

For the purposes of explanation, I have outlined various parts that make up a person. However, persons cannot be reduced to their parts in order to be better understood. Reductionist scientific methods, so successful in human biology, do not help us to comprehend whole persons. My intent was rather to suggest the complexity of the person and the potential for injury and suffering that exists in everyone. With this in mind, any suggestion of mechanical simplicity should disappear from my definition of suffering. All the aspects of personhood—the lived past, the family's lived past, culture and society, roles, the instrumental dimension, associations and relationships, the body, the unconscious mind, the political being, the secret life, the perceived future, and the transcendent dimension—are susceptible to damage and loss.

Injuries to the integrity of the person may be expressed by sadness, anger, loneliness, depression, grief, unhappiness, melancholy, rage, withdrawal, or yearning. We acknowledge the person's right to have and express such feelings. But we often forget that the affect is merely the outward expression of the injury, not the injury itself. We know little about the nature of the injuries themselves, and what we know has been learned largely from literature, not medicine.

If the injury is sufficient, the person suffers. The only way to learn what damage is sufficient to cause suffering, or whether suffering is present, is to ask the sufferer. We all recognize certain injuries that almost invariably cause suffering: the death or distress of loved ones, powerlessness, helplessness, hopelessness, torture, the loss of a life's work, betrayal, physical agony, isolation, homelessness, memory failure, and fear. Each of these injuries is both universal and individual; each touches features common to all of us, yet each contains features that must be defined in terms of a specific person at a specific time. With the relief of suffering in mind, however, we should reflect on how remarkably little is known of these injuries.

THE AMELIORATION OF SUFFERING

One might inquire why everyone is not suffering all the time. In a busy life, almost no day passes in which one's intactness goes unchallenged. Obviously, not every challenge is a threat. Yet I suspect that there is more suffering than is generally recognized. Just as people with chronic pain learn to keep it to themselves because others lose interest, so may those with chronic suffering.

There is another reason why every injury may not cause suffering. Persons are able to enlarge themselves in response to damage, so that instead of being reduced, they may indeed grow. This response to suffering has encouraged the belief that suffering is good for people. To some degree, and in some persons, this may be so. If a leg is injured so that an athlete cannot run again, the athlete may compensate for the loss by learning another sport or mode of expression. So it is with the loss of relationships, loves, roles, physical strength, dreams, and power. The human body may lack the capacity to gain a new part when one is lost, but the person has it.

The ability to recover from loss without succumbing to suffering is sometimes called resilience, as though nothing but elastic rebound were involved, but it is more as though an inner force were withdrawn from one manifestation of a person and redirected to another. If a child dies and the parent makes a successful recovery, the person is said to have *rebuilt* his or her life. The term suggests that the parts of the person are structured in a new manner, allowing expression in different dimensions. If a previously active person is confined to a wheel chair, intellectual pursuits may occupy more time.

Recovery from suffering often involves help, as though people who have lost parts of themselves can be sustained by the personhood of others until their own recovers. This is one of the latent functions of physicians: to lend strength. A group, too may lend strength: Consider the success of groups of the similarly afflicted in easing the burden of illness (e.g., women with mastectomies, people with ostomies, and even the parents or family members of the diseased).

Meaning and transcendence offer two additional ways by which the suffering associated with destruction of a part of personhood is ameliorated. Assigning a meaning to the injurious condition often reduces or even resolves the suffering associated with it. Most often, a cause for the condition is sought within past behaviors or beliefs. Thus, the pain or threat that causes suffering is seen as not destroying a part of the person, because it is part of the person by virtue of its origin within the self. In our culture, taking the blame for harm that comes to oneself because of the unconscious mind serves the same purpose as the concept of karma in Eastern theologies; suffering is reduced when it can be located within a coherent set of meanings. Physicians are familiar with the question from the sick, "Did I do something that made this happen?" It is more tolerable for a terrible thing to happen because of something that one has done than it is to be at the mercy of chance.

Transcendence is probably the most powerful way in which one is restored to wholeness after an injury to personhood. When experienced, transcendence locates the person in a far larger landscape. The sufferer is not isolated by pain but is brought closer to a transpersonal source of meaning and to the human community that shares those meanings. Such an experience need not involve religion in any formal sense; however, in its transpersonal dimension, it is deeply spiritual. For example, patriotism can be a secular expression of transcendence.

WHEN SUFFERING CONTINUES

But what happens when suffering is not relieved? If suffering occurs when there is a threat to one's integrity or a loss of a part of a person, then suffering will continue if the person cannot be made whole again. Little is known about this aspect of suffering. Is much of what we call depression merely unrelieved suffering? Considering that depression commonly follows the loss of loved ones, business reversals, prolonged illness, profound injuries to self-esteem, and other damages to personhood, the possibility is real. In many chronic or serious diseases, persons who "recover" or who seem to be successfully treated do not return to normal function. They may never again be employed, recover sexual function, pursue career goals, reestablish family relationships, or reenter the social world, despite a physical cure. Such patients may not have recovered from the nonphysical changes occurring with serious illness. Consider the dimensions of personhood described above, and note that each is threatened or damaged in profound illness. It should come as no surprise, then, that chronic suffering frequently follows in the wake of disease.

The paradox with which this chapter began—that suffering is often caused by the treatment of the sick—no longer seems so puzzling. How could it be otherwise, when medicine has concerned itself so little with the nature and causes of suffering? This lack is not a failure of good intentions. None are more concerned about pain or loss of function than physicians. Instead, it is a failure of knowledge and understanding. We lack knowledge, because in working from a dichotomy contrived within a historical context far from our own, we have artificially circumscribed our task in caring for the sick.

Attempts to understand all the known dimensions of personhood and their relations to illness and suffering present problems of staggering complexity. The problems are no greater, however, than those initially posed by the question of how the body works—a question that we have managed to answer in extraordinary detail. If the ends of medicine are to be directed toward the relief of human suffering, the need is clear.

References

Bakan, D. (1971), *Disease, pain and sacrifice: Toward a psychology of suffering*. Chicago: Beacon Press.

Cassell, E. (1972), Being and becoming dead. *Soc. Res.*, 39:528–542.

Goodwin, J. S., Goodwin, J. M., & Vogel, A. V. (1979), Knowledge and use of placebos by house officers and nurses. *Ann. Intern. Med.*, 91:106–110.

Kanner, R. M., & Foley, K. M. (1981), Patterns of narcotic drug use in a cancer pain clinic. *Ann. NY Acad. Sci.*, 362:161–172.

Marks, R. M., & Sachar, E. J. (1973), Undertreatment of medical inpatients with narcotic and analgesics. *Ann. Intern. Med.*, 78:173–81.

Zaner, R. (1981), *The Context of Self: A Phenomenological Inquiry Using Medicine as a Clue*. Athens, Ohio: Ohio University Press.

Part I

THE NATURE OF PAIN

Dr. Eric Cassel, in his introduction, has addressed a most important issue in understanding the nature of suffering and its relationship to organic illness. Chronic pain patients are most noted by their long-term experience of suffering. The reduction and relief of suffering must be seen as a primary goal in the treatment of chronic pain patients. Health care professionals must clearly understand that the nature of suffering can be exacerbated by addressing the physical system without attention to its counterpart, the psychological system.

Drs. Willard Whitehead and Wolfgang Kuhn of the Department of Psychiatry and Behavioral Medicine, University of Louisville School of Medicine, review the elements of chronic pain, present the mechanisms of pain production, its modulation and treatment, as they are currently understood. In addition, pain classification and pain evaluation become core components in their treatment of the issues and aspects of chronic pain.

Dr. Erling Eng, clinical professor of the Department of Psychiatry, V.A. and University of Kentucky Medical Centers, addresses analytic issues of chronic pain by tracing the appearance of pain and the sequence of Freud's writings, elaborating on its significance in analytic thought, and focusing on the key operative idea of Freud—that cathexis becomes a core resource in the treatment of the chronic pain patient.

The economic, ethical, and psychosocial considerations of the chronic pain patient are addressed by Dr. Robert Marciani, an oral and maxillofacial surgeon. Addressed in his presentation are such issues as these: what does the treatment of pain do for the patient, what is the cost–benefit ratio to the patient and to the health care industry, and does the therapy reinforce secondary gain needs, thereby becoming a cofactor itself in the chronic pain syndrome? Any consideration of the theoretical bases of chronic pain must include issues related to ethnic factors influencing pain expression. Drs. Reid and Bush of Virginia Commonwealth University look at the implications for clinical assessment of ethnic factors in chronic pain expression. One of the most essential goals for medical professionals in the treatment of chronic pain is to appreciate the phenomenological reality of their pain expression, and by doing so, humanely and personally enhance the health and minimize the suffering of the chronic pain patient. These authors address the important issues of understanding pain expression as a crucial factor in the physician–patient relationship and the subsequent process of treatment that should occur in the treatment of chronic pain.

Finally, Dr. James C. Norton, associate professor of psychiatry and neurology, University of Kentucky College of Medicine, addresses compensation and litigation issues in disabled pain patients. Herein are addressed the ongoing problems and circumstances that the disabled pain patient experiences and its interface with the health care system. The variety of legal issues that patients with disabling pain and injury face, as well as the potential psychological effects of these procedures and of disability status, are addressed by the author. Health care providers in the treatment of chronic pain are encouraged to have a clear understanding of the legal realities that the patient faces. In addition to this, the professional is encouraged to understand that the disabled pain patient often has many difficulties in addition to the presenting complaint of pain, and these will often interact with the pain experience in complex ways.

1

Chronic Pain: An Overview

WILLARD WHITEHEAD, III, M.D. AND
WOLFGANG F. KUHN, M.D.

INTRODUCTION

Chronic pain is an intriguing phenomenon defying easy explanations and resisting generally accepted modes of treatment. It has drawn considerable interest over the past thirty years, yet the field awaits further advances before it can be called an exact science. The pathways and centers involved in pain transmission, evaluation, and modulation are not established with certainty, just as the chemical interactions involved in the pain process are not yet completely understood. There is debate as to the nature of chronic pain; we don't know if it is produced by a peripheral pathological process, or produced centrally, in a way similar to that in which visions are created in the brain of a dreaming person.

This chapter is designed to review elements of chronic pain regardless of controversy, and present mechanisms of pain production, modulation, and treatment as we currently understand them. Pain classification and patient evaluation will also be discussed; it is hoped that increased understanding of pain

Acknowledgment. The authors would like to thank Ms. Stacy S. Whitehead for her invaluable assistance in preparing and editing this manuscript.

5

mechanisms as well as of the patient and his problems will aid in selecting appropriate therapies, and will help patient and therapist alike gain greater control over this recalcitrant phenomenon.

The Taxonomy Committee of the International Association for the Study of Pain (IASP) defined pain as "an unpleasant sensory and emotional experience associated with actual or potential tissue damage, or described in terms of such damage." The Association added: "Pain is always subjective" (Wall, 1984, p. 1). Each individual learns about pain through experiences related to injury in early life. "It is unquestionably a sensation in a part of the body, but it is also always unpleasant and, therefore, an emotional experience" (Wall, 1984, p. 1).

> Many people report pain in the absence of tissue damage or any likely pathophysiological cause, usually this happens for psychological reasons. There is no way to distinguish their experience from that due to tissue damage, if we take the subjective report. If they regard their experience as pain and if they report it in the same ways as pain caused by tissue damage, it should be accepted as pain. This definition avoids tying pain to the stimulus. Activity induced in the nociceptor and nociceptive pathways by a noxious stimulus is not pain, which is always a psychological state, even though we may well appreciate that pain most often has a proximate physical cause [Wall, 1984, p. 1].

Chronic pain can be defined as pain lasting more than six months (Crue, 1985). The term may need further definition to exclude pain processes in which relief of pain beyond the six-month period is expected. An example of this would be headache pain secondary to trauma (personal communication, Grand Rounds). It is also important to consider whether the pain is secondary to a benign, progressive, or terminal process; these considerations have impact not only on definition, but also on treatment strategies.

Chronic pain is a health problem of major proportions, exacting a tremendous cost. It was estimated in 1981 that 700 million workdays are lost annually in industrialized countries because of it, at a, then, estimated cost of $60 billion per year (Bonica, 1981).

The clinician who treats chronic pain is dealing with a syndrome associated with a multitude of different problems, and must understand the patient's case intimately to be able to select the interventions most likely to be beneficial.

Chronic pain can be a syndrome with multiple etiologies operating simultaneously and changing over the course of illness. It has many elements: neurologic, physiologic, psychologic, sociocultural, motivational, cognitive, and behavioral (Kuhn, 1984). Any of these may offer a valid area of intervention. Usually, these elements interact, complicating diagnosis and treatment.

Patients tend to have difficulty comprehending why their problem is so difficult to treat, and see little sense in their suffering, not seeing any understandable function of their pain.

From the physician's point of view, there may be difficulties in diagnosing the sources of chronic pain and in accepting the fact that the treatment may involve more support and "care" rather than "cure." The chronicity of pain seems to fly in the face of patient and physician expectations that some sort of cure should be provided by the medical establishment. Lack of a cure is often seen as treatment failure, and frequently patient as well as doctor can become discouraged. Given these expectations and resultant feelings of disappointment and failure, it is no surprise that patients with chronic pain often follow a downhill course.

The clinician's best tools in aiding the patient rest in understanding the contribution of the diverse elements of chronic pain, understanding pain modulation, the evaluation and classification of pain, and treatment with appropriate medications and adjunctive therapies.

COURSE OF CHRONIC PAIN

As pain becomes chronic, patients tend to become dissatisfied and angry that no effective treatment of their condition seems to be forthcoming. Their anger tends to alienate physicians, who then often avoid contact with those complaining, dissatisfied people. Patients will often insist on further treatment in their quest for a "cure," and are likely to develop a state of hostile dependency on their physicians. In many cases the physician begins to doubt the veracity of the pain, labeling continued complaints as "functional" at best (Hackett, 1978). Patients often end up in a state of chronic disability. They are likely to lose self-esteem, as well as the esteem of friends and family, and find themselves in a state of bitter, disillusioned isolation (Hendler, 1982).

Chronic pain, once established, tends to perpetuate and accentuate itself as the patient changes physicians repeatedly as a result of frustration and disappointment (Violon, 1982). Patients often undergo repeated surgeries which can worsen the problem, become dependent upon narcotics and tranquilizers, or even become physiologically addicted, and frequently experience early withdrawl from pain medications as additional pain (Aronoff and Evans, 1982; Halpern, 1982).

Beyond patient and clinician, chronic pain has effects on others. The adoption of the "patient identity" leads to a role shift in the family and other social systems. An energetic, productive individual may become a social and economic liability (Hendler, 1982; Violon, 1982; Gallagher and Wrobel, 1982). Family and workmates have to make up for the loss of working capacity which tends to weaken support for the pained individual and leads to anger toward the pain patient.

Eventually pain can become the central issue in a patient's life. It may begin to function as a major coping mechanism, allowing the patient to avoid stressful issues because he is "in pain." This leads to further incapacitation, which aggravates the problem, and a morbid fascination on the part of patients with their own decline (Kuhn, 1984).

Other factors, such as litigation and compensation, compound the picture, leading to increased suffering, and adversely affecting prognosis (Gallagher and Wrobel, 1982). Pursuing claims, no matter how legitimate, may shift the patients' focus of attention to having been wronged and seeking to have their pride restored, rather than adjusting to a difficult situation while leading as normal a life as possible.

Patients with chronic pain are also likely to experience depression. The literature reports an incidence of depression ranging from 10 percent to eighty percent among persons who experience chronic pain. It is often not clear whether this depression preceded the pain or is secondary to it (Kramlinger, Swanson, and Maruta, 1983). While there is some question of how the depression evolves, it is important to remember that this indeed is likely to be a depressed group of patients. Beyond chronic pain related to injury or associated with depression, there is evidence supporting the hypothesis that chronic pain syndromes evolve as part of a larger process. The pain experienced by pain-prone individuals (Engel, 1959), or the development of painful processes such as rheumatoid arthritis, may in fact reflect other problems in life-style that predispose to the acquisition of chronic pain.

THE FUNCTION OF PAIN

It is noteworthy that one of the body's first responses to a stimulus evoking acute pain is an attempt at reversing the pain caused by the incident. Beyond withdrawing the injured part of the body or beyond receiving a signal that the injured part of the body needs attention or needs rest, the body takes steps to reverse pain input, to reduce perception of the pain signal. As commonly viewed, pain serves a protective purpose. That acute pain is a sense that adds to an organism's survival and state of well-being is seen in studies of people who lack the ability to sense pain (Beecher, 1959). People who cannot feel pain may experience mutilation and early death as they may not protect themselves when initially injured, and may not know that injuries are present (Beecher, 1959).

After some time, pain can lose its protective purpose, being present and continuous even when the noxious stimulus is removed. Thus, a valid warning against pain-provoking and damaging activities can turn into a useless burden inflicting needless suffering. When dealing with "referred pain," the patient may even be forced into a situation of protecting an uninjured body part, experiencing pain in an area of the body different from the injured one.

The meaning assigned to pain can further reduce its adaptive effects as patients worry about implications such as neoplasia and physical damage. Chronic pain even has implications extending into spiritual life. Many patients feel punished, angry with God, fate, or with themselves, for being forced to experience such a problem, and tend to feel helpless, out of control, and bitter.

Accurate diagnosis of the source of pain is essential so that the physician can clarify the function of chronic pain to the patient. When activity would be physically harmful, the patient needs to know that his decreased activity is beneficial and may need help in accepting a more sedentary life-style. When pain is less useful, when it has become physically meaningless, the patient may need help in learning to actively focus on living life regardless of the pain in order not to become incapacitated by it.

When chronic pain is worsened by an excessive degree of stress the patient can be taught to see the pain as a sign that he or she should reduce stressful activities in life. Regardless of this, changes in the nature of pain should not be dismissed; they may represent changes in the patient's condition that would reflect a different function of the pain. Having a chronic pain syndrome secondary to one process does not preclude a patient from developing pain secondary to another.

THE NEUROLOGY OF PAIN

Historically, physiologists believed that there were no specific nerves for mediating pain. Instead pain was viewed as resulting from overstimulation of nonspecific nerve endings. It is now understood that small unmyelinated C-fibers and A-delta fibers carry pain impulses from specialized nerve endings that serve as pain sensors in the skin, muscle, blood vessels, and organs; the A-delta fibers are class I and the C-fibers are class IV nerves (Hendler, 1982). Accompanying these two transmission systems are two types of sensory experience that lead to pain (Bowsher, 1983): pinprick sensations are carried by small myelinated fibers and deep pain is carried by unmyelinated axons.

In both cases, pain receptors and fibers are specific, and pain is never due to overstimulation of other types of receptors. Pinprick pain or pain resulting from thermal or mechanical insult causes reflex withdrawal from a potentially damaging stimulus. Deep pain is caused by tissue damage and causes tonic muscle contraction and immobility that splints a damaged area (Bowsher, 1983).

Central pain recognition circuits differ for each type of pain. When the pinprick sensation becomes pathologic, as in neuralgias, the patient experiences chronic shooting or lancinating pain. Such pain is presumed to be caused by paroxysmal discharge of central neurons, probably in the spinal or brain stem gray (Bowsher, 1983).

Unmyelinated nociceptive fibers from the skin, joints, and viscera enter the spinal cord and brain stem, where their cell bodies are located in the dorsal root. Similar neurons are in the Gasserian ganglion. All these neurons contain a biochemically active agent called substance P. Substance P appears to have a neurotransmitterlike action in these axons. Visceral fibers often travel via autonomic rather than systemic nerves, passing straight through the sympathetic or parasympathetic ganglia without relay. Many of the unmyelinated axons double back along the distal portion of the root to enter the cord or brain stem via the ventral root.

Both the thin myelinated fibers and the unmyelinated pain fibers end in the dorsal horn of the spinal cord and the medulla oblongata. Marginal cells receive pain input from the fine myelinated fibers. These marginal cells have long axons that cross to the other side of the spinal cord and ascend into the anterolateral funiculus on their way to reaching the thalamus. Information used to localize pinprick and hot–cold sensations is projected to the postcentral gyrus (Bowsher, 1983).

The unmyelinated substance P-containing fibers are associated with branches of large myelinated fibers whose main axons go without synapse to the dorsal columns to convey messages from low threshold mechanoreceptors regarding touch, pressure, vibration, and joint movement. These large axon collaterals exert presynaptic inhibition on small unmyeli-nated terminals and can reduce the amount of substance P produced in response to afferent impulses (Bowsher, 1983).

A temporary painful syndrome can result when, in a peripheral nervous cut, the small fibers regenerate before the larger fibers. Without the inhibition provided by the large axons, reinnervating skin can be extremely painful until the larger fibers regenerate. Similarly, herpes zoster, which selec-tively destroys ganglion cells of large fibers, leaves a patient with an imbalance of more small peripheral fibers than large ones so that any stimulation can cause great pain. The effect of the large axon mechanism is also exploited in "rubbing to make it better"—a stimulation of large low-threshold fibers reducing the effects of small fiber input. This mechanism is incorporated into the so-called Gate Control Theory (to be discussed later) and can be simulated through the use of a Transcutaneous Electrical Nerve Stimulator (TENS) (Bowsher, 1983).

It seems likely that the pathway for organic pain involves a polysynaptic projection from the spinal cord to the brain stem reticular formation, which then leads through the intralaminar (midline) thalamus to prefontal regions of the nonprimary cortex (Bowsher, 1983).

Pain information from the dorsal horn is transmitted in the dorsal column via the medial lemniscus to the thalamus and then to the cortex. This tract is useful in localizing the pain stimulus in the body. The neospinothalamic tract begins at the synapse in the dorsal horn, where it crosses and ascends to the lateral portion of the spinal cord. Fibers of this pathway extend into the ventroposterolateral and posterior thalamus, and syn-apse. This lateral pathway, the neospinothalamic tract, trans-mits sharp, localized pain via the mesencephalon to the thalamus and is somatotopically organized. This system is thought to carry acute pain. The paleospinothalamic tract carries less localized burning pain and dull pain. It arises from cells in lamina-regions I and V of the spinal cord and is not somatotopically arranged. It sends branches to the reticular formation of the brain stem and the hypothalamus, which is part of the limbic system, and then to the medial and intralaminar thalamic nuclei, with final transmission to the limbic forebrain structures. The limbic system is part of the archeocortex, or old brain, which is the seat of the emotions and other basic functions such as sexual activity. Chronic pain transmission is also thought to occur in this paleospinothalamic tract (Hendler, 1982). It is interesting that prefontal lobotomy can abolish the affective component of pain, presumably by interrupting the majority of diffuse thalamocortical projections (Bowsher, 1983).

THE NEUROPHYSIOLOGY OF PAIN

Recently, research has revealed intriguing facts about opiate receptors in the pain system. Exogenous opiates and endogenous opiates such as endrophins and enkephalins act on dorsal horn synapses of the "true" pain pathway, initially involving the articulation between unmyelinated primary afferents and gelatinosa cells. Other synapses at higher levels in the "true" pain system are also morphine sensitive and so are other synapses that are not in the pain pathways, including synapses in the corpus striatum and in some hypothalamic and limbic areas as well as those of the pneumotaxic center. It is because of opiate binding in the pneumotaxic center that morphine and related drugs have a depressant effect on respiratory function. Opiate binding in all of these synaptic sites is displaced by naloxone (Bowsher, 1983).

Enkephalins are pentapeptides secreted by terminals of certain short axon neurons, which are located at the majority of regions where there are opiate receptors. It has not yet been decided whether enkephalin should be classified as a neurotransmitter or neuromodulator since some of these neurons have been shown to secrete other transmitter substances. The most important question to be answered, however, is how enkephalinergic interneurons within the pathway can be activated. Those in the substantia gelatinosa have been subjected to intense study (Bowsher, 1983).

Fibers descending from the medulla oblongata control

enkephalinergic interneurons in the dorsal horn. The neurons from which these fibers descend are driven by cells in the gray matter surrounding the cerebral aqueduct in the midbrain called periaqueductal gray (PAG). Neurons in the PAG are highly sensitive to opiates, and microinjection of morphine into this region has a potent analgesic effect. When electrodes are implanted, PAG stimulation via neurons in the midline of the reticular formation of the medulla oblongata can activate enkephalinergic interneurons in the dorsal horn and suppress upward transmission of impulses generated by noxious peripheral stimuli. Axons of PAG cells excite neurons in the midline raphe of the medullary reticular formation, and raphe–spinal neurons, whose axons descend in the dorsolateral funiculus of the spinal cord, excite interneurons in the dorsal horn. The raphe–spinal neurons are called serotoninergic because their neurotransmitter is serotonin (5-hydroxytryptophane, 5-HT), and the interneurons of the dorsal horn are enkephalinergic. Thus the last and most important stage in the suppression of the upward transmission of pain-generated information is enkephalinergic, and analgesia brought about by stimulation of PAG with implanted electrodes can be reversed by naloxone (Bowsher, 1983). This system of pain modulation is part of the Endorphin-Mediated Analgesic System (EMAS) (Fields, 1981).

It appears as though there is yet another neurosynaptic transmitter mechanism involved in the neurophysiology of pain perception. It is located in the hypothalamus and appears to be mediated by catecholamines, especially norepinephrine. It has been shown that a decrease in the concentration of norepinephrine in the ventricular system leads to an increase in the effect of analgesia induced by various methods, such as electrical neurostimulation or morphine administration, with subsequent rise in pain threshold. Conversely, postsynaptic blockade of dopamine with an antagonist diminishes analgesia. It thus appears as though decreased norepinephrine action or increased dopaminergic activity will also decrease the amount of pain experienced (Hendler, 1982).

It is obvious that descending pathways are involved in controlling pain transmission from the intact cortex. They must be operative in stress-induced analgesia, the phenomenon whereby an injured soldier or athlete may be unaware of pain from an injury. Stress-induced analgesia may be biologically useful, aiding survival, and is naloxone-reversible. It is thought to be due to neurosecretion of beta endorphin by the hypothalamus in response to cortical command. The second type of cortically induced analgesia is hypnosis, which can be used to relieve pain and may not be naloxone reversible. Its mechanism of action is unknown (Bowsher, 1983).

Aside from these descending control systems, there are two more peripheral neurocircuits involved in pain modulation. These two circuits may explain the successful application of acupuncture and other pain interventions. A segmental neuronal circuit which, when stimulated by myelinated pinprick afferents, activates enkephalinergic interneurons in the dorsal horn of the spinal segment. These, in turn, block upward transmission of impulses arriving in unmyelinated (acute pain) primary afferents. A nonsegmental effect is less well understood but may work through ascending spinoreticular fibers transmitting pinprick type stimulation and acting at the level of the descending reticulospinal fibers in the medullary raphe or through spinothalamic collaterals which synapse with PAG cells (Bowsher, 1983).

Pain Modulation

In earlier years of pain study, pain was seen as a simple response to nociceptive stimulation. Later, sensory and affective components of pain were identified, and clinical experience led clinicians to believe that attitude and emotion had an impact on the pain experience. Melzack and Wall were the first to propose a system of pain modulation that could clarify these interrelations. Their theory holds that mechanisms operating in the dorsal horn of the spinal cord open or close "gates" which allow or prevent impulses generated by peripheral noxious stimuli to have access to higher centers (Bowsher, 1983). This system recognizes three factors concerned with pain transmission from the first central cells in the spinal cord: (1) The arrival of nociceptive messages; (2) the convergent effect of other peripheral afferents which may exaggerate or diminish the effect of the nociceptive message; and (3) the presence of central nervous system (CNS) control systems which influence the first central cells (Wall, 1984). These factors operate in a system built of four components: the afferent nerves, segmental interneurons in the dorsal horn, descending controls, and transmission cells (Wall, 1984). This modulating system affects conscious pain perception and can be influenced by awareness at three levels: affective–motivational, sensory–discriminatory, and cognitive–evaluative (Craig, 1984). Once activated, these central control systems can inhibit or facilitate pain input. Messages reflecting cognitive, attentional, and emotional factors descend from the brain through the spinal cord and influence message transmission from the periphery. Neurologically, components of the nervous system have been found to function in ways consistent with the gate control theory. The effects of large myelinated afferents on small fiber input has been discussed earlier in this chapter. In addition to this system, three other modulating systems are seen as components of gate control. These include a system of descending control, the endorphin-mediated analgesic system (EMAS), and a segmental as well as a nonsegmental neurocircuit (Bowsher, 1983), which have been discussed in a previous section of this chapter.

MECHANISMS INVOLVED IN THE CHRONICITY OF PAIN

The gate control theory offers an intriguing explanation of ways in which pain can be conceptualized and managed, but it does not explain how pain becomes chronic. Other factors must be considered if the mechanism by which acute pain becomes chronic is to be understood. Chronic pain is not seen as a prolongation of an acute process, but is assumed to involve changes in the peripheral nervous system (PNS) and CNS (Wall, 1984). It is proposed, and supported by some observations, that changes occur in injured nerve terminals, afferent fibers, and in the CNS following an injury, and that some of these changes contribute to the chronicity of pain. Some of these changes impact on gate control, while others involve the pathways on which pain is transmitted and modulated. These particular changes are referred to as changes in connectivity control. Changes occurring at levels of the tissue, nerve terminals, peripheral axons, central axons, and central cells will be discussed.

First, stimulation at the level of nerve terminals can produce changes in the tissue, in impulse conduction patterns, and nerve sensitivity. The effects of injury on C-fiber terminals may play a role in the periphery by way of the axon reflex which produces three local reactions to injury: vasodilation, neurogenic edema, and sensitization of nerve endings (Wall, 1984).

Such injury can also lead to a sequence of long-term changes in the CNS, possibly in response to transport of certain substances through action of C-fibers. It is proposed that C-fibers monitor the metabolic state of the tissue in which they terminate and release substances which produce central alterations over time. These alterations change connections by which nerve impulses are routed through the nervous system's connectivity control. Other changes can occur when nerve terminals are stimulated. Some high threshold afferents become more sensitive after stimulation and may fire without additional stimuli. This phenomenon can contribute to prolongation of pain even after mild injury. These changes in sensitivity might be mediated by direct changes in the structure of the terminal after a large stimulus, the presence of tissue breakdown products, or substances released from stimulated nerves (Wall, 1984).

Other changes may occur at the level of peripheral axons. When such an axon is cut and begins to regenerate, sprouts growing toward the periphery generate chronic afferent barrages. These barrages can act as false signals which can be interpreted in the CNS as if injury were in progress. When growing sprouts successfully reconnect, these spontaneous impulses decrease; however, if reconnection is not established, they can be produced indefinitely. Ways in which nerve sprouts differ from connected nerves also contribute to chronic pain. Nerve sprouts are sensitive to mechanical stimulation and alpha receptor binding of adrenaline. Thus, mechanical distortion as well as the release of noradrenaline caused by sympathetic arousal can generate barrages of nerve impulses in sensory afferents and generate pain (Wall, 1984).

Experimentally, nerve sprouts have also been observed to establish contact with other sprouts, thus allowing impulses to "jump" from one axon to another. This observation opens the possibility that an afferent barrage from a region of damage could be formed by direct transfer of efferent impulses into an afferent nerve (Wall, 1984).

Beyond changes in the tissue and peripheral nerves themselves, peripheral nerve damage may induce changes central to the lesion which are not reversed by treatment directed at the area of original injury (Wall, 1984). There seem to be at least three types of central change involving the dorsal root ganglia that may contribute to chronicity of pain. First, after peripheral nerve transection, nerve impulse generation begins in the region of the dorsal root ganglia. The ganglia also becomes sensitive to mechanical distortion and circulating adrenaline. Thus, there are two sources of abnormal peripheral afferent nerve impulses in chronic pain, one from the region of injury, and one from the dorsal root ganglion.

The second central change involves proteins and peptides produced by the dorsal root ganglion cells which are reported to be neurotransmitters. Some of these substances were previously discussed. They are transported to peripheral terminals and spinal cord terminals. When a peripheral nerve is cut, the concentration of these chemicals in the spinal cord afferent terminals in the substantia gelatinosa decreases. While some experiments do not support the idea that these substances are neurotransmitters, it is still possible that they are involved in producing slow changes of postsynaptic function which alter connectivity control (Wall, 1984). Third, in addition to changes in function induced by peripheral damage, cell death and degeneration of central axons can occur following an injury. Cells of dorsal root ganglia and the trigeminal nuclei can be lethally affected by insults such as amputation and tooth extraction, respectively. Death of these cells leads to anatomical deafferentiation, and it is possible that chronic peripheral nerve lesions produce pain in part through such irreversible degeneration of spinal cord afferents (Wall, 1984). Fourth, decrease in inhibition has also been observed as an effect of peripheral injury to central terminals in the spinal cord, especially involving the C-fibers. Interactive inhibitions of nerve fiber types, that is A on A, A on C, and C on C, may decline after nerve section. In such cases the injured fiber shows decreased ability to evoke primary afferent depolarization. The cells maintain ability to stimulate spinal cord cells, but lose ability to feedback on themselves and produce prolonged depolarization of their terminals which is associated with presynaptic inhibition (Wall, 1984).

Chronic pain may also involve the transport of chemicals from the periphery. C-fibers may continually relay messages from the periphery about the state of tissue in which the fibers terminate. When tissue is damaged, or the nerve is cut, a new chemical message could be transmitted since the fiber endings would be in a new chemical environment. It is proposed that these C-fibers have terminal arbors that anatomically innervate some cell regions they do not normally excite. Arriving chemical messages might release these ineffective synapses and make them operational so that receptive fields are enlarged (Wall, 1984).

Finally, some associated functions of the CNS may contribute to the development of chronic pain. When a noxious stimulus is applied with a warning event, some cells may "learn" to respond not only to the pain stimulus but also to the signals associated with the noxious stimulus which might warn of impending injury. Signaling of injury by even the first cells is dependent upon the arrival of nociceptive afferent impulses, other peripheral events, and upon the setting of excitability by CNS mechanisms. These CNS mechanisms may help explain varied response to injury, and the presence of such controls suggests that they can become locked into pathological conditions and exaggerate or create pain (Wall, 1984).

THE PSYCHOLOGY OF PAIN

Psychologically, pain is a multifaceted and multifactorial phenomenon. Attitudes and thoughts have significant impact on the perception and expression of pain. For instance, there are many known incidents of athletes who have finished important plays unaware of bone fractures received during the play (Beecher, 1959). Studies on the Beach of Anzio reveal that soldiers with horrible injuries requiring evacuation home suffered very little pain, but winced instead when receiving injections (Beecher, 1956). Patients with lesser, minor injuries that would eventually necessitate a return to the front, suffered much greater discomfort. Thus, even in situations where pain is acute, psychological factors play an important part in modulating pain perception and experience.

Pain perception changes during the course of psychological development, and psychological factors may come to play an important role in the experience of pain. Psychogenic parts of the pain experience are as unpleasant as somatic pain, and somatic and psychogenic pain may exist simultaneously.

An interesting finding is that dogs raised in isolation as puppies would later stick their muzzles into flame without showing any signs of pain reaction (Melzack and Scott, 1957). This finding points to the close relations between the functioning of the "pain apparatus" and individual psychological development.

It is assumed that newborns and very young infants are incapable of discriminating between pain and other unpleasant stimuli, and are also incapable of telling whether those stimuli arise from within or outside themselves (Freud, 1905; Mahler, 1952; Spitz, 1965). As maturation continues in the continuous presence of a nurturing and affectively connected caretaker, the infant learns to discriminate between "inside" and "outside" as well as to differentiate different feelings of displeasure, learning that those will subside once their source is dealt with (Mahler, 1952; Klein, 1957; Spitz, 1965). Theories hold that affective energy initially is diffusely invested throughout the body, and, only as development progresses, attaches itself selectively more and more to the superficial body structures and organs of perception. A certain amount of stimulation of those structures is necessary to initiate and maintain this process; in other words, pain is a necessary prerequisite for the development and differentiation of the pain-perceiving apparatus. The degree of sensitivity to pain, and the acuity of perception, are thus in part determined by the nature and intensity of painful stimulation (Petrie, 1967; Adler and Lomazzi 1973; Adler, Gervasi, and Holzer, 1973). Since identical lesions lead to different pain behavior in indolent as opposed to more sensitive individuals (Libman, 1934), it may be assumed that the degree of infantile investment of emotional energy in the pain-perceiving apparatus determines the clinical picture and therefore is relevant to the differential diagnosis of pain (Breuer and Freud, 1895). As the child learns to discriminate between the nature and extent of different sensory stimuli, increasing differentiation between self and others also takes place. It was observed that autistic children, who poorly perceived their separateness from external objects, tend to be much more insensitive to pain than other children (Mahler, 1952). Thus, our awareness of pain seems to be related to how we see ourselves related to our outside world, and not only to neurophysiologic events. Conditioned reflex learning based on synchronous occurrence of painful physiologic events and events within relationships takes place. Interaction between those factors occurs throughout development. Not only does the origination of pain become linked to the actions of other people, the child also learns that suffering and exhibiting pain behavior will lead to attention and an affective response from a caretaker. The awareness alone that a nurturing person has perceived the distress and is about to take some comforting action seems to alleviate distress and appears to be an important part of the placebo response (Beecher, 1962). Such awareness probably leads to a release of endorphins in the CNS (Levine, Gordon, and Fields, 1978). Eventually, by means of a conditioned reflex, the need for attention and affection can also lead to pain behavior and the experience of pain.

Also in childhood, aggression and pain become linked as children learn that through aggressive behavior pain can be produced in others, and others can react by inflicting pain on them. Since young children cannot differentiate between impulses to commit an aggressive act and the actual carrying out of those impulses, a mere aggressive impulse may suffice to induce guilt and a need for punishment. This psychological phenomenon can persist into adulthood and lead to the anticipatory experience of pain as punishment for feelings of aggression. This is an important part of the explanations of psychogenic pain in the form of so-called conversion symptoms, and the life-style of pain-proneness (Engel, 1958, 1959). Even the English language attests to this connection: the words *pain, punishment,* and *penalty* possess the same etymologic root. Not only aggressive impulses may elicit this emotional response; persons conflicted over their sexuality, who consciously or unconsciously perceive sexual impulses as undesirable and forbidden, will react with a similar need for punishment when sexually stimulated, and may also develop pain. Lastly, sexual and aggressive impulses may become linked in a sadomasochistic way, which can also lead to the experience of pain when erotic impulses occur.

The discussion of the psychology of pain is necessarily complex. The question may be asked whether chronic pain is a pathological emotion related to acute pain, as fear is to anxiety and as sadness is to grief (Swanson, 1984). Pain was considered an emotion by Aristotle, and this view persisted until delineation of the nervous system and the advent of neurophysiology (Craig, 1984). Yet the fact that a pain receptive system exists does not remove the emotional significance involved in the pain experience. Learning to respond to painful stimuli seems to be part of the process of socialization, and this process involves factors that associate pain experiences with emotions. As a human develops, this interplay grows so that a spectrum of pain situations exists involving variable ratios of organic and psychological components.

Pain experience may be viewed as a continuum with a purely organic form of pain on one end and a purely psychogenic form of pain on the other (Cooper and Braceland, 1950). The first part of the spectrum represents the "normal" person and reaction to pain. Psychological factors may alter the pain threshold, and distraction and autosuggestion can produce significant elevation in the pain threshold in normal persons. Even this normal perception contains a psychological component describable as "fight or flight" when the pain is sharp, and "withdrawal" when the pain is dull. The next range in the pain spectrum involves an abnormally heightened reaction to pain and is characterized by patients who overreact to painful experiences. These patients may suffer prolonged recovery following an injury and may complain unduly of stimuli which usually produce less psychic reactions. This hyperreaction to pain may be shaped by interpretation of the meanings of pain, attitude, cultural background, and life events.

Next on the spectrum there is an area in which "psychic perpetuation of organically induced pain" exists. Here the pain started on an organic basis but is perpetuated for psychological reasons. This may occur in cases of drug addiction, situations in which compensation is sought at some level in the psyche, and in instances where a person is unable to recover from the trauma involved in the injury. This perpetuation can also occur when a patient experiences relief and gratification through the patient role, becomes overly dependent on the health care system, and fearful of recovery.

Listed next is "gestalt" pain which is described as pain in which a primary role cannot be easily ascribed to either organic or psychic cause. Phantom limb pain might epitomize this type of pain, a pain in which neither physical nor psychological factors can be used to fully explain the existence of the pain.

In the next part of the pain spectrum, there appear for the first time problems which may be psychogenically determined, including such "psychosomatic" problems as migraine, cardiospasm, and certain kinds of low back pain. People who suffer these problems may maintain anxiety that results in a prolonged state of readiness for action which can be satisfied only by discharging in terms of somatic function. As a result, unresolved tension produces physiologic expressions which are perpetuated by emotional problems. When the psychic or emotional component of these disorders is not appreciated, the organic lesions may become persistent. In disorders such as Raynaud's disease and peptic ulcer there may, thus, be organically determined perpetuation of pain which is originally psychogenically induced. Surgical therapy may be required for a lesion that might have been healed with the proper medical and psychotherapeutic regimen.

At the extreme end of the spectrum exists "psychogenic pain." This is pain in which psychic conflicts are in some way experienced in a somatic fashion, without demonstrable organic pathology.

Up to this point, the discussion has taken into account psychological experiences that flavor the development of a person's ability to recognize and act on pain. It has been assumed that this pain was in response to end organ stimulation. Yet, there seems to be a set of patients who experience pain when no evidence of end organ stimulation is found (Engel, 1959). The term *psychogenic pain* has come to be used to describe pain in which no other cause has been demonstrated. Often physicians assume such pain to be "imaginary." This is somewhat puzzling, given the fact that we have no trouble in accepting the existence of dreams and hallucinations, knowing that these involve no peripheral nerve stimulation (Engel, 1959). By analogy, it is argued that a sensory pain experience could come about without peripheral stimulation as well (Engel, 1959). Pain can be provoked by peripheral stimulation, but this does not justify a belief that pain results only from peripheral stimulation. Pain is known to have an affective component bringing it into a central position in psychological development. It may also have several meanings for an individual which may play an important role in the development of psychogenic pain. First, pain warns of damage to the body and helps a person learn about dangers in the environment. Second, pain is part of relationships, and from infancy on, crying can lead to a positive emotional response. Third, in childhood pain becomes linked with punishment and its presence can signal to a person that he is "bad." In this way, pain can also become a way to expiate guilt and gain forgiveness as a person suffers pain to inflict punishment on himself, thus gaining relative comfort. Fourth, pain is associated with aggression and power. Fifth, pain is associated with threatened loss of a loved one; often people can experience pain in the body as a way of substituting for the lost person. And finally, pain can be associated with sexual feelings. At the height of sexual arousal pain may be mutually inflicted. However, when sexual behavior becomes threatening, persons may tend to experience pain rather than sex.

In the development of psychogenic pain, there are instances (Engel, 1959) in which certain patients gain pleasure through experiencing pain, the key being that the pleasure is a relative pleasure because the pain is experienced in place of something more distressing.

There seems to be a population of pain-prone patients who repeatedly or chronically experience chronic disability, sometimes without recognizable peripheral change (Engel, 1959). These patients have many features in common. They may feel guilt associated with a recent or ongoing event. The patients may appear chronically gloomy or depressed. Often, they enter situations and relationships in which they are defeated and seem not to learn from their experiences. Some of these patients may fear success and others may need to see themselves as martyrs who tolerate suffering, or as suffering persons to be pitied and cared for. These pain-prone patients are most likely to have come from families in which aggression, suffering, and pain played an important part in early relationships.

Psychogenic pain can be precipitated by three sorts of events. The first event is that of external circumstances failing to satisfy a patient's unconscious need to suffer. Psychogenic pain may occur as a response to a real or threatened loss. Following a death, permanent loss, or anticipation of loss of a loved one, the suffering person may symbolically equate a part of his body with the lost love object and utilize this part of the body for unconscious expression of feelings toward the lost person. Persons may also experience psychogenic pain when guilt is evoked by intense aggressive or forbidden sexual feelings.

Location and type of pain may be determined by two processes. First, a peripherally provoked pain experience from the past can be relived or reexperienced when pain is "needed." Second, a pain experienced by someone else or pain the patient imagined or wished another person would experience can be assumed. The second operates almost universally at an unconscious level (Engel, 1959).

When psychiatric diagnoses are applied, it appears that

conversion phenomena tend to occur in the majority of patients with the pain-prone personality. Another group suffers predominantly from depression, in which cases the experience of pain may serve to attenuate the guilt and shame involved with the depression. A patient may experience hypochondriasis, as is common in depression (Engel, 1959).

Psychological events that influence the pain experience can be elucidated by asking about fluctuations in the course of pain and association of life events with remissions and exacerbations. When an understanding of the influences of life on pain is reached, constructive changes in life-style can sometimes reduce suffering.

A mental status exam will help determine whether a psychiatric condition associated with chronic pain is present; for example, depression, conversion, psychosis, compensation neurosis, malingering, and pain-proneness (Hackett, 1978). Some authors note that chronic pain sufferers often mask depression well, and recommend the use of psychological testing such as the MMPI (Aronoff and Evans, 1982).

Some more subtle observations can be used to determine whether emotional problems may be contributing to the pain. The use of the MADISON scale has been suggested, MADISON being an acronym for words that characterize psychological aspects of chronic pain (Hackett, 1978). The first is M—multiplicity; pain may exist in varying forms and locations or may recur when one pain is successfully treated. A is for authenticity; the patient wants his pain to be accepted as authentic and real. D is denial of emotional problems; a patient with psychological overlay of pain is liable to paint a rosy picture in the face of horrible reality. I stands for interpersonal relationships; observation of the patient may yield grimaces or other negative reactions when difficult interpersonal relationships are discussed. S stands for singularity; pain presented as singular and unusual is likely to be psychologically influenced. O stands for only you; the patient seems to say that only you can help. Again this is an indicator that the pain may have some psychological component. Finally N stands for nothing helps or no change; physical pain generally fluctuates during the course of a day according to activity, concentration, and mood, and the observation that "nothing changes the pain" increases the likelihood that it has a psychological overlay. Patients who possess many of these characteristics are likely to have a significant psychological component in their pain syndrome.

SOCIOCULTURAL AND MOTIVATIONAL ASPECTS OF PAIN

The description of the model of "sick role" (Parsons, 1951) has proved to be a major contributor to the understanding of illness in our culture. According to this model, the sick person is not considered to be responsible for his illness, and is also considered exempt from the normal day-to-day obligations. However, the patient also is expected to see the sick role as something undesirable; in other words, the patient is expected to show a desire to get well. Furthermore, sick persons are expected to seek competent medical help and cooperate with the provider of such help.

This model seems to fit acute better than chronic illness (Gallagher and Wrobel, 1982). It has been suggested (Gallagher, 1976) that it be modified in the sense of patients expecting adaptation to their condition rather than a cure. It appears as though patients with a chronic condition, such as chronic pain, carry greater personal autonomy and more responsibility for maintenance of their health status than people with an acute condition. In chronic illness, the sick role does not necessarily seem to take precedence over other social roles. However, patients do not have all the resources of the healthy person to engage in the endeavors of normal life. Exemptions are necessary both on the part of expectations of the patient and expectations of society to accommodate the chronic impairment or limitation.

Szasz and Hollander (1956) described three possible kinds of physician–patient relationships: (1) active/passive; (2) guidance/cooperation; and (3) mutual partnership. In the first kind of relationship (active/passive), the physician makes all the decisions, and the patient passively accepts those. An example of this kind of relationship would be the relationship between surgeon and patient as intraoperative decisions are made. In the second model (guidance/cooperation), the physician does not make all the decisions but suggests to the patient a course of action which the patient is supposed to carry out. In the third conceptual model, mutual partnership, decisions concerning treatment are made jointly. Either party carries about an equal amount of responsibility for the treatment plan followed and the eventual outcome. In the treatment of chronic pain, aspects of the second as well as the third model prevail. The treatment of chronic pain is very much a cooperative venture, but the treatment team retains somewhat greater responsibility in terms of providing medical oversight.

While having an illness generally does not imply loss of social status, there are exceptions to this; some illnesses, such as venereal disease or mental illness, are socially stigmatized and are seen as very undesirable. Being in pain which is not responding to standard medical treatment, the chronic pain patient often finds himself in a similar position, having a condition so frustrating that, after some time, physicians are generally loath to treat it. This angers the patient, who may approach the next physician with some defensiveness, often alienating physicians right from the start. This leads to increased hostility in a relationship which the patient seems to need more and more desperately as his condition continues to plague him. Thus, patients are usually very frustrated, mistrustful, and suspicious by the time they are referred to a pain treatment facility. There, often somewhat to their surprise, they are taken seriously, and for the first time may have the experience that somebody "knows that they are hurting." While this may lead to a considerable feeling of relief, it also has potentially negative aspects to it in that it reinforces patients' notions that they are sick and disabled and must assume the sick role to the fullest extent. By the time patients reach pain centers and pain treatment specialists, they have often reached a point where pain is needed in their life-style because of the profound alterations forced upon the patient's life (Sternbach, 1974). An important part of treatment occurs when patients gradually but systematically recognize, with the help of their therapist, how many "benefits" the pain gives them: while causing suffering, it also provides a self-sustaining continuity, an identity, a means of dealing with stress by avoiding it, and a means of manipulating relationships.

It is well known that there are large cultural variations in the expression of pain and other emotional discomfort (Zborowski, 1969). For instance, while traditional American culture supports stoicism and discourages the liberal expression of discomfort, Italian and Jewish culture is much more tolerant of emotional expressions of every form. Culturally determined attitudes toward expression of pain are certainly learned behavior. While a person's ethnicity cannot be changed, the biographical particulars of pain-related learning experiences can be examined, thus adding to the understanding of pain and its meaning to the individual.

Our current medical culture can certainly also affect the expression of pain. As physicians and patients become more and more dissatisfied with the results of standard medical treatment, and as patients become angrier and angrier, they start being defined in terms of what they are not, such as "good patients" who promptly get better when expected, thus pleasing physicians as well as themselves. They are also given new, negative identities, as terms are used such as *compensation neurosis,* which, to patients, carries the meaning that they are parasites on the system; or *hysteria,* which means they are cowards or weaklings; *malingering,* which seems to denote that they are liars; and *psychogenic pain,* which at best implies that they are imagining the pain, at worst that they are "crazy" (Tunks and Roy, 1982). Being denied the reinforcers of a positive identity in a sociocultural system and acquiring a new, negative identity, complaints of pain now acquire a new meaning, namely as expression of defiance and hostility.

Each individual in society carries, at any given point, multiple roles. Thus, a person may be, at the same time, his children's father, his wife's husband, his parent's child, his family's provider, a member of his church, a worker in the workplace, and a participant in the activities of his social organizations. This role behavior is culturally determined and described. As persons enter maturity, it becomes important to attain mastery in all of these roles. They then serve as sources of positive self-concept, sense of achievement, and feelings of satisfaction. Disability, such as chronic pain, greatly diminishes feelings of mastery and achievement, thus reducing a person's self-esteem. However, assuming the sick role does not necessarily eliminate functioning in all other roles (Tunks and Roy, 1982); an abrogation of the role of breadwinner, for instance, does not necessarily mean an interruption in functioning in interpersonal roles. However, it appears as though disruptions of social or interpersonal life, rather than occupational life, carry the better prognosis.

Once a person's occupational functioning is affected, the very organizations and programs designed to assist his recovery and occupational rehabilitation, such as disability insurance or workers' compensation programs, can start working to his detriment. They seem to provide an incentive to remain sick, especially when a person's occupation is difficult, boring, or otherwise undesirable, such as changing shift work. There is often anger at the amount of benefits received, since they may appear to be a pittance compared to what the person expected. There is fear that benefits might be discontinued as rehabilitation progresses and people are judged to be no longer disabled due to participation in rehabilitation activities several hours a day. A sudden termination of such benefits leads to panic and disorganization on the part of the disabled worker, and thus to a failure of the rehabilitation program. This being the case, chronic pain may lead to an adversarial relationship between patient, employer, and employment-related assistance programs. To this may be added hostility from other employees, who are envious of the chronic pain patient's seemingly easier status and doubting of the veracity of his symptoms. In addition to this, problems with repeated absences from work because of chronic intermittent disability often lead to a termination of employment on medical grounds. Thus, the patient exits from the system.

Once the occupational role is gone, the role as provider for the family is gone with it. The resulting phenomenon usually is a role shift in the family; patients may now become dependent upon the spouse, who often will have to function as the sole breadwinner. Thus, the previous head of the household is delegated to a secondary role. Also, the relationships with other family members change since disabled persons are often sidelined from customary family functions because of their limitations.

Of course, the previously held sense of mastery and degree of control over one's destiny no longer exists. This loss can diminish a person's expectations of earning his own leisure and security, and result in guilt feelings over being dependent upon the rest of the family and not contributing economically. Under this pressure, patients often regress to levels of adjustment held earlier in personal development, leading to additional dependency, a needy and clamoring posture, and a defeated and passive attitude which creates much pessimism about the potential of future rehabilitation.

COGNITIVE AND BEHAVIORAL ELEMENTS OF CHRONIC PAIN

Behavioral psychology uses operant learning as an explanation of the process of chronic pain development. Respondent pain is defined as a response to antecedent stimulation within the organism, a signal of disease or dysfunction. Operant pain is pain expression shaped by reinforcement. Prolonged respondent pain can lead to operant pain. This may come about because of the effect of pain on its observer, and the observer's altered behavior to accommodate the pain. These accommodations can be rewarding to the pain sufferer and increase the possibility of pain behavior. When pain behavior receives direct positive reinforcement, it is likely to persist. For instance, it is reinforced when pain enables the patient to avoid unpleasant activities or when health behavior is discouraged. Such reinforcement can lead to continued pain behavior, even after successful surgical and medical intervention have been accomplished. In such cases, altering contingencies so that health behavior is rewarded while pain behavior is not, is expected to have positive results (Grezsiak, 1982).

Those who propose operant treatment of chronic pain syndromes do not suggest that responses to reinforcing environmental events is conscious or deliberately manipulative, but that pain patients do indeed experience significant subjective distress even when behavior is being reinforced by environmental consequences. Reports exist of patients believed to have significant operant components to their pain who are initially suspected of being malingerers. On observation, these patients continue to show evidence of disability even when unaware of being observed (Cameron, 1982).

Studies have been described in which chronic pain patients were asked to immerse their hands in ice water in a laboratory situation. In one set of observations, the patient–subject was led to perceive the experimenter as a sympathetic person prepared to reinforce pain behavior. In a second set of observations it was suggested that pain tolerance and coping would be rewarded. Subjects in the first group exhibited pain behavior after only 74 seconds, while most of the second group could endure pain exposure for a full 360-second trial (Cameron, 1982).

Operant analysis of chronic pain behavior suggests two intervention strategies. One model predicts that environmentally controlled pain behaviors will decrease in frequency if reinforcing consequences are withheld. The second model predicts that a patient's functional status will improve if "well behaviors" which are incompatible with pain behaviors are rewarded (Cameron, 1982). These considerations have therapeutic implications.

Social attention and analgesic medications are common reinforcers of pain behavior. Medication serves as a negative reinforcer by reducing pain, and behavioral approaches diminish this problem by providing medications at fixed intervals rather than contingent on pain. Social attention can be withheld in order to extinguish pain behaviors and may be important in reinforcing healthy behaviors. Care must be taken, however, to avoid appearing callous and to provide a reasonable level of attention so that patients do not feel poorly treated (Cameron, 1982).

While most operant programs described in the literature involve inpatients, it also seems important to alter a patient's social environment in order to increase the possibility that pain behaviors not be reinforced and that healthy behaviors will continue to be reinforced. It might be possible to increase the effectiveness of operant programs by training family members in the uses of operant conditioning. Patients can also be taught adaptive behaviors not already in their repertoire (Cameron, 1982).

Cognitive theory holds that when one of a class of responses to distress is elicited, such as anxiety, depression, or pain, other members of the class may also be experienced. Cognitive mediation is needed before characteristics of the specific affect (i.e., pain, anxiety, or depression) are developed. Cognitive approaches train patients in strategies to enhance self-control over the pain situation.

Cognitive approaches may include relaxation, imagery, cognitive relabeling, and reinterpretation of pain related to experiences, day-to-day problem solving, assertiveness training, and systematic desensitization. One cognitive treatment rationale is that disturbing moods and behaviors associated with the pain result from certain thought processes. Many cognitive approaches are designed to substitute rational coping skills and self-statements for catastrophic thoughts. Others reduce the psychological reaction to pain by training the patient to mentally create and focus on pleasant physical sensations.

Chronic headaches of vascular and tension types have responded to cognitive treatment approaches, and cognitive approaches can be effective in treating groups as well as individuals (Cameron, 1982).

Cognitive approaches can be applied to the sensory–discriminatory, affective–motivational, and cognitive–evaluative components of treatment approaches based on Melzack and Wall's gate control theory. The sensory–discriminatory aspect can be modified by training a patient to alter sensory input through relaxation and biofeedback. The cognitive–evaluative component and affective–motivational components can be modified by strategies designed to counteract thoughts of helplessness and reinforce thoughts of self-control (Grez-siak, 1982).

CLASSIFICATION OF CHRONIC PAIN

Given the broad spectrum of functions that influence the development and experience of the chronic pain symptoms, it is obvious that evaluation and classification are difficult. Because of the difficulty in correlating much complex information, formal chronic pain classification systems have been devised to simplify research and aid in selecting treatment strategies. No one single system seems to answer all the requirements of an evaluation system, but some are useful in establishing clinical or experimental information.

Some authors support the use of the McGill Pain Questionnaire (Melzack, 1980), which uses words found to correlate with the sensory, affective, and evaluative aspects of the pain experience.

When applied to patients suffering postherpetic neuralgia, phantom limb pain, metastatic carcinoma, toothache, degenerative disc disease, rheumatic or osteoarthritis, labor pain, and menstrual pain, it was found that each of these eight syndromes produced a different constellation of verbal responses. It was concluded that each type of pain is characterized by a unique cluster of verbal descriptors, and that patients with similar disease use similar words to describe their experience. While this evaluative method might be useful in screening, it is easy to see that the clinician needs a more exact method of determining the origin of a chronic pain syndrome. Unidimensional approaches of using symptoms to produce a diagnosis seem inadequate when applied to cases of chronic pain (Brena, Crue, and Stieg, 1984). Many multidimensional approaches to classification of chronic pain have been proposed to solve this problem. One system proposes a three-factor index for assessment of pain states using estimates of the patient's somatic inputs, anxiety, and depression. This construct is called the SAD Index, but it is said that this model fails to incorporate relevant social and environmental factors and is of limited diagnostic value (Brena, et al., 1984). There exists a computerized "pain profile" for classification of each patient with pain. The model is based on comparison of indices representing pathological, psychosocial, and behavioral dimensions of pain.

While this model is an excellent tool for teaching and research it is said to be time consuming and limited in clinical value.

In 1975 a two-axis model for quantification and classification of chronic pain states was proposed which was based on the Emory Pain Estimate Model (EPEM) (Brena, et al., 1984). In this system an operational definition of chronic pain is achieved by the analysis of three quantifiable sets of information: medical findings, behavioral data, and the relationship between medical–behavioral correlates. These correlates exist in four different classes of chronic pain patients. Assessment of the medical findings includes evaluation of pathological and physiological–functional assessments which are depicted on a zero to ten horizontal scale, while measurements of pain behavior are graphically depicted on zero to ten vertical scale, crossing the horizontal scale at midpoint. Medical scores are based on a physician's assessment of all available medical data, and behavioral scores are based on information generated by the patients through paper and pencil testing (Brena, et al., 1984).

It has been found that the four classes describe significantly different groups of chronic pain patients:

1. Class I patients score above 5 on the behavior vertical scale and low on the medical scale. These patients display conditioned behavior which exceeds demonstrable medical findings. These patients best fit the description of patients with "psychogenic pain disorders" described in the *Diagnostic and Statistical Manual of Mental Disorders,* Third Edition (DSM-III) (1980).
2. Class II patients score low in both sets of variables. These patients are functional despite sometimes dramatized pain complaints with poorly defined anatomical patterns. Many headache patients fall into this class of chronic pain.
3. Class III pain patients score high in both pathological and behavioral scales. They are disabled by documented pathological conditions as well as by conditioned factors similar to those in Class I patients.
4. Class IV patients score high on the medical scale and low on the behavior scale. These patients have well-

documented pathological lesions, but remain functional. Class IV patients might be referred to as underreactors to pain and in general display effective coping skills and adjustments to their pain situation.

The use of this scale has clinical benefit as patients who fall into the different categories are likely to share similar characteristics. Class I patients exhibit primarily learned behavior which is characterized by the following sets of symptoms referred to as the 5-D syndrome of chronic pain: *d*ramatization of complaints; *d*isuse (i.e., the consequences of inactivity on various body systems); *d*rug misuse; *d*ependency; and *d*isability.

Class II patients show normal levels of activity during daily living. Many of the patients in Class II are incapable of physically pacing themselves. Pain complaints are often responses to periods of sustained activity without appropriate rest, which result in discomfort and decreased activity. Simple counseling can help these patients accept their limitations while training in relaxation and proper time management skills may allow adjustment in life-style and a return to wellness.

Class III patients display learned behavior associated with a documented pathological condition. These patients may display many of the symptoms of Class I patients. When the pathological disorder cannot be corrected and/or when the condition is stabilized, these patients are good candidates for programs of appropriate rehabilitation.

Class IV patients demonstrate competent coping in the presence of pathological conditions. Management of their illness should be careful and restrained so as not to interfere with their ability to cope. Overtreatment of Class IV patients may convert this functional person into a Class III patient through iatrogenic complications.

A totally different classification system for chronic pain has been proposed partly in response to controversy over the EPEM-based classification system, especially taking issue with the notion of ongoing end organ pathology in chronic pain. This system is based on the premise that "true" chronic pain is never produced by incoming stimuli but is always a centrally produced phenonemon (Brena, Crue, and Steig, 1984).

The system recommends the use of a temporal classification to correlate the underlying etiology of pain with mechanism of ongoing pathophysiology. In this system the first four categories, acute, subacute, recurrent acute (with underlying chronic pathophysiology), an ongoing pain (due to underlying malignant disease), were conceived as pain largely due to peripheral nociceptive input. The term *chronic pain* is reserved to describe continued subjective pain in the absence of any demonstrable peripheral nociceptive input (Brena et al., 1984). This system points out the significance of the central mechanisms in the genesis of chronic pain, rejecting the notion that psychogenic or chronic pain results from continued nociceptive input. It heavily supports the theory that there is a centrally produced form of chronic pain, and it is critical of the EPEM-based model because of the fear that, by failing to recognize central production of pain we might endanger patients and expose them to unnecessary surgery as well as use of drugs, thus further contributing to their problems (Brena et al., 1984).

A five-axis classification system has been recommended for clinical use by the IASP (Buckoms, 1985). The IASP recommended this be combined with a standard set of definitions as a nontheoretical and comprehensive system of classifying pain patients. The axes include: (1) region of pain; (2) system of pain; (3) temporal characteristics of pain; (4) patient's statement of intensity and time lapsed since onset of pain; and (5) etiology of pain.

While the system offers categories suitable for both central and peripheral genesis of pain, it may lack the flexibility needed to denote a change from a purely physical to a more psychogenic problem.

GENERAL ASPECTS OF CHRONIC PAIN MANAGEMENT

Evaluation and treatment of a chronic pain syndrome can be a complex task owing to the number of factors that can contribute to chronic pain. Management of a chronic pain syndrome requires application of the best diagnostic and evaluative procedures available in order to form an understanding of the cultural, social, motivational, emotional, somatic, and psychic components operative in the chronic pain syndrome. Evaluation and management are often done in specialized, multiple-discipline pain management centers (Kuhn, 1984), but might also involve appropriate, well-coordinated referrals to inpatient detoxification units, orthopedists, neurologists, surgeons, anesthesiologists, internal medicine specialists, rheumatologists, physiatrists, psychologists, and psychiatrists.

When referrals are made, it is important that the patient and consultants be aware of the role each is expected to play in the coordinated approach to management. This can be a major role of the therapist who is primarily interested in pain management.

Because of the many factors and mechanisms involved with chronic pain, treatment is difficult and complex, and no one single method is likely to be successful as treatment. A variety of therapeutic approaches used in combination seems to produce the best results (Melzack, 1980; Halpern, 1982; Roy and Tunks, 1982). Each set of treatment approaches must be individualized. Often, treatment is being provided by a multidisciplinary team.

In designing and implementing a management program, it is important to remember that patient motivation is crucial and often determines whether or not treatment is likely to be successful. Owing to the importance of motivation, it is often difficult, but important, for both patient and physician to hold in the forefront the possibility that the chronic pain syndrome may never be "cured," and that often the best that can be done is to reduce the impact of the pain on life-style. Neither the patient nor clinician stands to lose when this realistic and accepting attitude is maintained. However, several frank and honest discussions are often necessary before patients are ready to accept this. It is often necessary that patients be brought to the realization that conventional measures, such as additional pain medications and surgeries, offer no further hope. On the other hand, care has to be taken that patients don't perceive this as a message that "the pain is all in your head." They have to learn that theirs is a chronic and complex condition which can be expected to improve considerably with the right treatment, even though they may have to learn to "live with" some pain.

In the treatment of all pain, acute as well as chronic, appropriate surgical and medical procedures should be applied only if the source of pain is known to be organic and such treatment is likely to improve it. Selected patients with ongoing nociceptive input may require nerve blockage or neurosurgical measures, such as tractotomy (Aronoff and Evans, 1982). In most chronic pain conditions which started with organic damage, there is considerable psychological overlay, and if the original pain-producing organic condition is stable and non-progressive, a rehabilitation approach to restore coping skills and manage life with a minimum of discomfort may be attempted first with good chance of a successful outcome. When traditional medical intervention is necessary due to a life- or function-threatening condition, such intervention should be matched with structured pain rehabilitation (Brena, 1984). When end organ damage is suspected as a source of nociceptive input and the source of input is beyond surgical or medical intervention, several approaches can be chosen to diminish suffering.

PHARMACOLOGICAL MANAGEMENT OF CHRONIC PAIN

Analgesic drugs can be considered the first line of approach in all pain treatment (Bowsher, 1983). Aspirin, acetominophen, and other nonsteroidal anti-inflammatories can serve as a basis for most pain relief programs. When these fail to offer adequate relief, use of narcotic analgesia can be considered, but these are generally recommended only in acute cases in which rapid recovery is expected or when the condition is felt to be terminal. When a narcotic analgesic is to be used over a long period of time, choice of medication should be made with extreme care. Propoxyphene napsylate has been successfully used as an opioid substitute. Codeine is commonly utilized for extended periods. When a maintenance dose of analgesic is used, the potential for abuse and tolerance must be considered. It is necessary to obtain informed consent from the patient and use of medication must be closely supervised. A regular physical exam should be performed to minimize the possibility that physical problems have been hidden by the use of medication (Schooff, Buck, and West, 1984).

While narcotics may thus be used temporarily in conditions with ongoing nociceptive input, they definitely are contraindicated and sedative-hypnotics are vigorously discouraged in chronic "nonmalignant" pain patients, where such peripheral input is no longer thought to exist (Halpern, 1982).

Neurogenic pain suffered in cases of trigeminal and postherpetic neuralgia, causalgia, Sudeck's atrophy, lightning pains of tabes dorsalis, and thalamic syndrome may never yield to analgesics, and it is wise to avoid the use of analgesics in such patients (Bowsher, 1983).

Prolonged, continuous treatment with sedative-hypnotics and minor tranquilizers, alone or in combination with strong narcotic analgesics, can also create drug dependency (Halpern, 1982). In chronic nonmalignant pain, drug dependency may complicate the patient's condition and can eventually become a patient's primary problem. Significant increases in the number of pain-related hospitalizations, surgeries, time spent resting, and significant decreases in physical activity have been reported in chronic pain patients on narcotics. When patients were removed from sedative-hypnotics and narcotics, they became more ambulatory, more able to engage in activity, and utilized fewer health care resources. There may be tremendous improvement in mood, pain, behavior, anxiety, and sleep following detoxification of chronic pain patients (Halpern, 1982).

It has been our clinical experience that patients with low levels of psychic dependence who lack physical addiction to narcotic analgesics, spontaneously decrease use of medication as pain management regimens are implemented. However, this patient group may not be large and more addicted patients fare poorly with this regimen.

Inpatient withdrawal from addicting agents is generally recommended as a first step in treating chronic pain patients who are addicted to narcotics, sedative-hypnotics, and/or alcohol (Halpern, 1982; Schooff, et al., 1984).

Detoxification programs for patients with chronic pain who are addicted to medications have repeatedly been proposed (Schooff et al., 1984; Halpern, 1982). While the details of these programs will not be discussed here, it is important to bear in mind that chronic pain patients are indeed likely to have addictions to both narcotics and sedative-hypnotics. Patients must first be stabilized on appropriate doses of sedative-hypnotics and/or narcotics before dosage reduction begins, and it is recommended (Schooff et al., 1984) that patients be withdrawn from the sedative-hypnotic prior to withdrawal from the narcotic analgesic. Tricyclic antidepressants can be used as adjunctive measures during withdrawal and may be especially helpful in allaying anxiety and helping the patient to sleep. Hydroxyzine can be used in conjunction with the use of antidepressants to aid in sleep as well, at doses of 100 mg per night. When further anxiolytic medication is needed, hydroxyzine may be given in 50 mg doses three times a day (Halpern, 1982).

Beyond use in controlling anxiety, aiding in sleep, and use in patient detoxification, tricyclics also have been found useful in treating chronic pain syndromes.

Doxepin and amitriptyline, tricyclic antidepressants with a high potential for serotonin reuptake inhibition, are most recommended for use in treating chronic pain. Serotonin-containing neurons exist in EMAS. Serotonin agonists interfere with opiate and stimulation-produced analgesia; therefore, serotoninergic tricyclics may produce analgesia in animals directly or by enhancing the action of opiates (Fields, 1981). However, antidepressants with a different mode of action are also mentioned (Kuhn, 1984; Moore, 1980). Some authors recommend doses that would be considered subtherapeutic for treatment of depression, others suggest the usual antidepression dosage range.

Low-dose, high-potency neuroleptics are also occasionally suggested for treatment of general chronic pain states in conjunction with antidepressants (Merskey and Hester, 1972; Taub, 1973). The underlying assumption is that adrenergic arousal causes an increase in the acuity of pain perception, whereas central adrenergic blockade such as the effect of neuroleptics has the opposite effect, thus reducing pain perception.

Some authors recommend the use of tricyclic antidepressants in combination with the neuroleptic perphenazine as one of the principal pharmacologic methods of treating central pain states (Halpern, 1982), while others recommend the use of tricyclic antidepressants with high serotoninergic reuptake inhibition as the treatment of choice in treating neurogenic pain with a burning quality (Bowsher, 1983). Also, the use of anticonvulsant medication to treat the lancing, stabbing pain of neurogenic origin has been suggested (Bowsher, 1983). Carbamazepine is recommended as the drug of first choice for lesions above the face, whereas sodium valproate 200 mg three times a day, is described as the drug of choice for shooting pains below the face. Whichever of these two drugs in not used first should be used as a second choice. The drug of third choice is phenytoin. Combined use of anticonvulsants and tricyclics can be undertaken in cases of neurogenic pain (Bowsher, 1983).

An additional approach can involve the use of a phenothiazine derivative, methotrimeprazine, which may be an analgesic as potent as morphine and has been used in treatment of postoperative pain, cancer pain, and chronic pain of various causes (Fields, 1981). The use of the drug has not been associated with addiction potential; however, it is sedating and produces hypotension and extrapyramidal side effects.

Many patients who suffer chronic pain also experience depression, either as a result of the pain experience or perhaps as a precipitant. In either case, treatment of the depression may improve the patient's ability to tolerate pain. When pain is thought to be secondary to a psychiatric disorder, specific treatment for that disorder is indicated.

Concomitant with the institution of an appropriate pharmacologic approach, nonpharmacological measures should be considered and used as indicated as part of a comprehensive treatment program. These include activities such as psychotherapy, biofeedback, relaxation, stress management, and time management as well as physical therapy. Procedures such as acupuncture and stimulation therapies might also be considered.

NONPHARMACOLOGICAL ASPECTS OF CHRONIC PAIN TREATMENT

The gate control theory, as well as other theories, emphasizes the role of psychological variables and the way they affect reactions to pain. As discussed previously, psychological factors and attitudes affect the pain experience in a very complex way. It is therefore not surprising that psychotherapy, both on an individual and a group basis, plays a large role in the treatment of chronic pain. Its value has been recognized for some time (Pilowsky and Bassett, 1982). Psychotherapeutic approaches allow patients to assess the role of pain in their lives, develop alternative coping mechanisms, deal with secondary gain, grieve for the loss of pain as a coping mechanism and life-style, and learn ways of accepting a degree of disability without becoming incapacitated by it ("learning how to live with pain").

Patients are often not very psychologically minded, which often makes it difficult to engage them in psychotherapy. This task becomes easier if all attempts at psychotherapy convey unambiguous concern (where attitude and nonverbal messages often carry more weight than verbal statements). Much tolerance of negative countertransference is necessary, since patients tend to be frustrated, hostile, and suspicious. For large stretches of time, a cognitive approach may have to be used before emotions can be addressed in a productive way. It seems important that physical measures (paying attention to new physical complaints when appropriate; touching) not be neglected.

Group psychotherapy programs have certainly proven their worth in chronic pain states. Transactional, educational, and cognitive therapeutic models have been suggested; it seems that the most promising approaches strongly endorse cognitive-behavioral aspects, education, and relaxation techniques. Patients who manage to change their conceptualization of their pain problem as they participate in group therapy are likely to benefit the most. Therefore, a group approach should provide opportunities for positive expectations, change in cognition, and an eventual sense of mastery (Baptiste and Herman, 1982).

Among the behavioral techniques used for treatment of chronic pain are operant conditioning with reinforcement of wellness behavior, and cognitive therapy, which is based on the premise that thoughts are behavior ("thinking behavior"). Patients usually carry many faulty assumptions regarding the significance of pain and life events, engage in "catastrophizing" of trivial events, and tend to establish attributions which seem to make problems insoluble and render the "victims" helpless. A cognitive-behavioral approach can correct many such maladaptive patterns of cognition as part of an overall treatment plan.

Additional behavioral techniques are biofeedback, autogenic training, and deep muscle relaxation. The therapeutic principle common to them seems to be relaxation. Biofeedback has been shown effective in controlling pain of tension headache, and is considered very useful in other pain syndromes also, by means of increasing relaxation. It was concluded that its effect is mediated mostly through distraction of attention, suggestion, relaxation, and sense of control over pain. Biofeedback was used in conjunction with hypnosis and a positive response was seen in 58 percent of the cases (Melzack, 1980). Few studies have supported the use of hypnosis by itself in treating chronic pain, but it appears as though it had been effective in the treatment of selected individuals (Melzack, 1980). It has been suggested that hypnosis operates through a mechanism of CNS analgesia not reversible with nalaxone (Bowsher, 1983).

In conditions with some ongoing nociceptive input, some techniques addressing this can be utilized. Transcutaneous electrical nerve stimulation (TENS) operates by selective stimulation of large-diameter myelinated axons. This technique can provide dramatic relief, especially when used postoperatively, and in cases of chronic pain associated with peripheral nerve damage. It is most effective when stimulation is applied proximal to the site of injury (Fields, 1981). Dorsal column stimulation with implanted electrophysiological devices is also effective in pain associated with nerve damage, but effectiveness has been noted to diminish in many patients with chronic pain. Infection, CSF leakage, pain, and cord trauma at the site of implantation have limited the clinical usefulness of dorsal column stimulating devices (Fields, 1981).

The families of patients should always be involved in the treatment process, since they are main providers of support, and also will have to adjust the family system to reaccept a more functional individual into it. Sometimes when it seems that a particularly strong need for homeostasis of the family system keeps the patient locked into the sick role, formal therapy is necessary. It has been noted that there seems to be a peculiar way of handling fantasy, affect, and cognition in families of chronic pain patients, most visibly affecting the "significant other" (Mohamed, Weisz, and Waring, 1978). In such families, it may be impossible for patients to regain a higher functional status without causing major disruption of family functioning. These families need therapeutic assistance, for which behavioral, cognitive, and structured family therapy approaches have been suggested.

No matter what the combination of treatment modalities used, an invaluable adjunct to treatment is attendance at self-help groups, which have sprung up all over the country, often following the model of Alcoholics Anonymous. Peer support and encouragement helps to motivate patients who might have given up hope that they, or anybody else, might be able to do anything to improve their lot. Chronic pain sufferers also seem to be much more capable of accepting confrontation and direction from someone "who's been there," than from one of the very ambivalently viewed authority figures, such as physicians. Also, the opportunity to help somebody else reduces their focusing on themselves and their self-pity, which can reach enormous proportions. These groups have been of help in enabling large numbers of pain sufferers to change their attitude and regain some control of their lives. Many have been motivated to seek appropriate treatment for the first time.

One additional recommendation is vocational retraining. Opportunities for this exist in many states, even in situations of chronic disability of long standing, and the main reason why patients have not utilized them are insufficient motivation, psychological incapacitation, discouragement, and hopelessness. Vocational assistance and retraining in a motivated and medically as well as psychologically improving patient can greatly facilitate the return to a productive life-style with concomitant increase in self-esteem.

Finally, it is important to hold in mind the possibility that even the most meticulous evaluation can miss subtle abnormalities and early lesions. New pathological processes can have an onset after initial work up. Vigilance must be maintained that progressive, correctable processes are identified as they occur over the course of chronic pain management. New complaints, or problems which do not respond as expected may indicate a need for further evaluation.

REFERENCES

Adler, R., Gervasi, A., & Holzer B. (1973), Perceptual style and pain tolerance; II. The influence of an anxiolytic agent. *J. Psychosom. Res.*, 17:381–387.
——Lomazzi, F. (1973), Perceptual style and pain tolerance; I. The influence of certain psychological factors. *J. Psychosom. Res.*, 17:369–379.
American Psychiatric Association (1980), *Diagnostic and Statistical Manual of Mental Disorders*, 3rd ed. Washington, DC: American Psychiatric Press.
Aronoff, G. M., & Evans, W. O. (1982), Evaluation and treatment of chronic pain at the Boston Pain Center, *J. Clin. Psychiat.*, 43 (Sec. 2):4–7.
Baptiste, S., & Herman, E. (1982), Group therapy: A specific model. In: *Chronic Pain: Psychosocial Factors in Rehabilitation*, eds. R. Roy & E. Tunks. Baltimore: Williams & Wilkins, pp. 166–178.
Beecher, H. K. (1956), Relationship of significance of wound to pain experienced. *J. Amer. Med. Assn.*, 161:1609–1613.
——(1959), *Measurement of Subjective Responses*. New York: Oxford University Press.
——(1962), Pain, placebos and physicians. *Practitioner*, 189:141–155.
Bonica, J. (1981), Editorial. *Triangle*, 20:1–6.
Bowsher, D. (1983), Pain mechanisms in man. *Resident & Staff Physician*, 29:26–34.
Brena, S. F. (1984), Chronic pain states: A model for classification. *Psychiat. Ann.*, 14:778–782.
——Crue, B. L., & Steig, R. L. (1984), Comments on the classification of chronic pain: Its clinical significance. *Bull. Clin. Neurosci.*, 49:67–81.
Breuer, J., & Freud, S. (1895), Studies on Hysteria. *Standard Ed.*, 9:132–141 London: Hogarth Press, 1957.
Buckoms, A. J. (1985), Recent developments in the classification of pain. *Psychosomat.*, 26:637–645.
Cameron, R. (1982), Behavior and cognitive therapies. In: *Chronic Pain: Psychosocial Factors in Rehabilitation*, eds. R. Roy & E. Tunks. Baltimore: Williams & Wilkins, pp. 79–103.
Cooper, I. S., & Braceland, F. J. (1950), Psychosomatic aspects of pain. *Med. Clinics N. Amer.*, 34:981–993.

Craig, C. D. (1984), Emotional aspects of pain. In: *Textbook of Pain*, eds. P. D. Wall & R. Melzack. New York: Churchill Livingstone, 1985, pp. 153–161.

Crue, B. L. (1985), Multidisciplinary pain treatment programs: Current status. *Clin. J. Pain*, 1:31–38.

Engel, G. L. (1958), "Psychogenic" pain. *Med. Clin. N. Amer.*, 42:1481–1496.

———(1959), Psychogenic pain and the pain-prone patient. *Amer. J. Med.*, 26:899–918.

Fields, H. L. (1981), Pain II: New approaches to management. *Ann. Neurol.*, 9:101–127.

Freud, S. (1905), On narcissism: An introduction. *Standard Edition*, 14:183–194 London: Hogarth Press, 1957.

Gallagher, E. B. (1976), Lines of extension and reconstruction in the Parsonian sociology of illness. *Soc. Sci. Med.*, 10:207–218.

———Wrobel, S. (1982), The sick-role and chronic pain. In: *Chronic Pain: Psychosocial Factors in Rehabilitation*, eds. R. Roy & E. Tunks. Baltimore: Williams & Wilkins, pp. 36–52.

Grezsiak, R. C. (1982), Cognitive and behavioral approaches to management of chronic pain. *NY State J. Med.*, 82:30–38.

Hackett, T. P. (1978), The pain patient: Evaluation and treatment. In: *MGH Handbook of General Hospital Psychiatry*, ed. N. Cassem. St. Louis: C. V. Mosby, pp. 41–63.

Halpern, L. (1982), Substitution–detoxification and its role in the management of chronic benign pain. *J. Clin. Psychiat.*, 43 (Sec 2):10–13.

Hendler, N. (1982), The anatomy and psychopharmacology of chronic pain. *J. Clin. Psychia.*, 43 (Sec. 2):15–20.

Klein, M. (1957), *Envy and Gratitude: A Study of Unconscious Sources*. New York: Basic Books.

Kramlinger, K. G., Swanson, D. W., & Maruta, T. (1983), Are patients with chronic pain depressed? *Amer. J. Psychiat.*, 140:747–749.

Kuhn, W. (1984), Chronic pain. *S. Med. J.*, 77:1103–1106.

Levine, J. D., Gordon, N. C., & Fields, H. L. (1978), The mechanism of placebo analgesia. *Lancet*, 2:654–657.

Libman, E. (1934), Observations of individual sensitiveness to pain. *J. Amer. Med. Assn.*, 102:335–341.

Mahler, S. (1952), On child psychosis and schizophrenia: Autism and symbiotic infantile psychosis. *The Psychoanalytic Study of the Child*, 7:286–305. New York: International Universities Press.

Melzack, R. (1980), Psychologic aspects of pain. In: *Pain*, ed. J. Bonica. New York: Raven Press, pp. 143–154.

———Scott, T. T. (1957), The effects of early experience on the response of pain. *J. Comp. Physical Psychol.*, 50:155–163.

Merskey, H., & Hester R. A., (1972), The treatment of chronic pain with psychotropic drugs. *Postgrad. Med. J.*, 48:596–598.

Mohamed, S. N., Weisz, G. M., & Waring, E. M. (1978), The relationship of chronic pain to depression, marital adjustment, and family dynamics. *Pain*, 5:285–292.

Moore, D. P. (1980), Treatment of chronic pain with tricyclic antidepressants, *S. Med. J.*, 73:1585–1586.

Parsons, T. (1951), *The Social System*. Glencoe, IL: Free Press.

Petrie, A. (1967), *Individuality in Pain and Suffering*. Chicago: University of Chicago Press, 2nd ed., 1978.

Pilowsky, I., & Bassett, D. (1982), Individual dynamic psychotherapy for chronic pain. In: *Chronic Pain: Psychosocial Factors in Rehabilitation*, eds. R. Roy & E. Tunks. Baltimore: Williams & Wilkins, pp. 107–125.

Roy, R., & Tunks, E., eds (1982), *Chronic Pain: Psychosocial Factors in Rehabilitation.* Baltimore: Williams & Wilkins.

Schooff, K. G., Buck, R., & West, P. (1984), Psychiatric consultation for the chronic pain patient who abuses drugs. *Psychiat. Ann.*, 14:801–807.

Spitz, R. A. (1965), *The First Year of Life: A Psychoanalytical Study of Normal and Deviant Development of Object Relations.* New York: International Universities Press.

Sternbach, R. (1974), *Pain Patients: Traits and Treatment.* New York: Academic Press.

Swanson, D. W., (1984), Chronic pain as a third pathologic emotion. *Amer. J. Psychiat.*, 141:210–214.

Szasz, T., & Hollander, M. A. (1956), The basic models of the doctor-patient relationship. *Arch. Intern. Med.*, 97:585–592.

Taub, A. (1973), Relief of Postherpetic neuralgia with psychotropic drugs. *J. Neurosurg.*, 39:235–239.

Tunks, E., & Roy, R. (1982), Chronic pain and the occupational role. In: *Chronic Pain: Psychosocial Factors in Rehabilitation*, eds. R. Roy & E. Tunks. Baltimore: Williams & Wilkins, pp. 53–67.

Violon, A. (1982), The process involved in becoming a chronic pain patient. In: *Chronic Pain: Psychosocial Factors in Rehabilitation*, eds. R. Roy & E. Tunks. Baltimore: Williams & Wilkins, pp. 20–35.

Wall, P. D. (1984), Introduction. In: *Textbook of Pain*, eds. P.D. Wall & R. Melzack. New York: Churchill Livingstone, 1985, pp. 1–16.

Zborowski, M. (1969), *People in Pain.* San Francisco: Jossey-Bass.

2

The Neurosis of Pain: Analytic Issues in Chronic Pain

ERLING ENG, PH.D.

I

There are some things to be mindful of if we wish to speak of pain in the context of psychoanalysis. To begin with, psychoanalysis starts with the notion of trauma, literally a wound, with its connotation of "pain." Efforts to determine a primary trauma move historically in the direction of understanding man as a suffering animal. The late Freud extends the classic topos of man's lack of specialization, using Bolk's observations on human birth as premature (1926), compared with other animals. Freud makes vulnerability the starting point for understanding human consciousness and self-experience.

All discussions of pain use words. Although we may "see" that another person is in pain, we will not advance very far in determining its precise character without the other's words, or putting words to the other.

Words that carry the meaning of pain are many and various. For example: *ache, misery, pain, stitch, throe, twinge,* or *discomfort, distress, hurt, suffering, agony, torment, torture* (Webster). If we were to explore the etymology of these pain words, our realization of the varieties of passive experience would be still further deepened.

Any discussion of pain must consider the situation in which it is reported. This is usually the medical one. Almost always, mention of pain is a virtual appeal to another, above all to a doctor to "do something about it," namely, "to take it away." The doctor is further presumed to be able to tell "what it really is," a belief which conflates the sufferer's experience with the etiological account. With this, the patient's discomfort has been transformed into an opportunity for the doctor to demonstrate his competence in removing the pain. Its meaning for the patient is generally ignored.

Freud kept listening to the patient. As he listened, he also paid attention to what the patient's words evoked within his own sensibility. Now, "pain" was taken as a kind of obscure knowledge, meaningful but enigmatic to begin with for both patient and doctor. The pain became the condition for a relationship of understanding between them, one whose experienced modifications in the course of a joint inquiry might furnish clues through which both the pain and their relationship could become more meaningful.

Any discussion of pain in psychoanalysis necessarily starts and finishes with language; concordantly, it begins and ends with pain, not as symptom but as a condition of a relationship, a relationship no less one of discovery than of "treatment."

In what follows, I intend to show how the preoccupation with pain, together with trauma, anxiety, repression, and inhibition, guide the enterprise of Freud throughout. In the first part, I shall take a chronological course; in the second part his metapsychology of pain will be spelled out.

The earliest reference to "pain" (Schmerz) in Freud's writings occurs in Draft G, "Melancholia," composed early in 1895. Seeking to account for the components of melancholy, Freud gave it this formula: "Psychic inhibition with instinctual impoverishment and pain concerning it"(1895, p. 205). Inhibition of the psychic-sexual sphere was a "contraction" which prevented a discharge of nervous excitation which produces pain. "The dissolution of associations is *always painful* (Freud's emphasis). Through *inward bleeding* (Freud's emphasis), as it were, there occurs an impoverishment of unbound, stored-up excitation, manifested in the other instincts and performances. As inhibition, this contraction acts like a *wound* [my emphasis] (cf. the theory of physical pain), analogous to pain" (1895, pp. 205–206). Although Freud wishes to formulate a purely neurophysiological explanation, his language remains ambiguously psychological, even interpersonal. For example, he refers to "pain about," the "instinctual impoverishment," and that "the dissolution of association is always painful." Moreover, even though he makes a distinction between psychic pain and physical pain, he moves freely between the two emphases, one of psychic contraction, the other of "inward bleeding." Their difference is not significant within Freud's broadly conceived biological standpoint.

Later in 1895, Freud sketched his *Project for a Scientific Psychology*. After introductory sections on his quantitative viewpoint, neuron theory, contact gates, biological standpoint, and the problem of quantification, he begins with a section on pain.

Freud initially views pain as arising from an overwhelming of the "psychic neurons" by external excitation. *"Pain is thus characterized as an eruption of excessively large Q's into phy and psy: that is of Q's, which are of a still higher order than the phy stimuli"* (1895, p. 307). Q stands for quantity of excitation, and *phy* refers to a neuron system mediating stimuli from outside the body. The *psy* is a neuron system transmitting intrabodily stimuli, those of hunger, thirst, sexual need. The latter system is linked with the external world through the *phy* system. Now pain is to be understood as the breakthrough of excessive excitation from without, so that both systems are penetrated, conflating them, and leaving a trace "as if lightning had struck" (Freud) in the *psy* system mediating inner stimuli. Although Freud does not make the inference explicit, it stands to reason that this latter trace would now be experienced much as a bodily need in its organic tendency to repetition.

In a subsequent part of his sketch, Freud refers to the "lived experience (Erlebnis) of pain" (p. 320). He has since introduced another kind of neuron, a perception neuron, into his theory, one accounting for conscious experience. The breakthrough of excitation into the system dealing with inner stimuli results in a heightened level of tension, one reacted to by the perception neuron as "unpleasure," with a tendency to a

modifiable discharge in certain directions, and a linkage between this tendency and a memory image of the pain-arousing
object. Whenever the memory image of the unpleasure-
evoking object occurs, a condition of unpleasure (Unlust) is
produced, with the same tendency to discharge as that of a lived
experience (Erlebnis) of pain. The source of the unpleasure
with which the memory image has been invested is assigned to
"secretory" neurons responsible for raising the level of internal
tension. These "key neurons" are activated when a certain level
of excitation is reached in the *psy*-system. Freud observes finally
that "since the release of unpleasure can be extraordinary with
only a slight investment of the hostile memory, we may conclude that pain in particular leaves behind an abundance of
facilitations" (1895, p. 321).

With Freud's recourse to "secretory" or "key" neurons, the
contrived explanatory apparatus begins to wobble. To be sure,
Freud is attempting to account for his observations, using the
current scientific language of his profession, but his observations are also personal. Thus it is that Freud, in straining his
language to the very limit, not only seeks to make his theory
more adequate, but also to clarify an understanding of pain for
his own life as well (1894, p. 64). Several years later, as if in
acknowledgement of this less apparent function of his neuron
theory, he was to write: "Ganglion cells can be fantastic too"
(1900, p. 87).

Following his initial formulation, his next treatment of
pain appears in the *Three Essays on the Theory of Sexuality* (1905).
After having abandoned his earlier scientific project, he has
since published his book on dreams, and has begun to focus on
sexual phenomena. He first of all observes that there are both
passive and active forms of pleasure in pain. Freud wonders
whether sadism, which appears to be an intensification of the
aggression implicit in all sexual activity, is not primary, and
masochism simply its modification through being redirected
toward the own self. He observes: "A sadist is always at the same
time a masochist . . ." (1905, p. 159). He concludes that such
active and passive tendencies are linked with the opposition of
masculine and feminine tendencies within human bisexuality.
Here pain is understood as an experience in which sadist and

masochist are not merely partners, but as an experience relating to the conjunction of masculine and feminine components in bisexuality. Now pain for Freud, to quote Alice, is "becoming curiouser and curiouser."

For his earlier neurons as the basic elements of his combinatorial formulations, Freud has now substituted the urges or "instincts" (Triebe), which he defines as organismic tendencies stemming from inner stimuli, in contrast to externally induced excitations. At this point he seems more interested in how pain-inflicting behavior can enhance sexual activity than relating sexual feeling and cruelty to one another in a psychological fashion. Once again, we may suspect that he is engaged not merely in explaining the facts but in attempting to clarify at the same time the structure of his own experience, experience instantiating the issues under discussion. This modus operandi had been elaborated in *The Interpretation of Dreams* (1900), where the linkage of scientific observation with interrogatory self-awareness is central.

Before leaving *Three Essays*, an incidental note: in this monograph Freud refers to "the fact that symptoms involve *suffering* (Freud's emphasis), and it almost invariably dominates a part of the patient's social behavior." With this observation, Freud has crossed over into the interpersonal realm, so that he can now add: "It is also through the medium of this connection between libido and cruelty that the transformation of love into hate takes place . . ." (1905, p. 166). This reference to suffering marks a shift from the theater of neurons in his scientific psychology to the world of theater, and its involvement of display with pain. With this we have entered the dramatic sphere, as in Freud's essay from the same period on "Psychopathic Stage Characters" (1905–1906), where he considers the possibility of the human display of one's pain as an assertion of autonomy, "A rising rebellion against the divine regulation of the universe, which is responsible for the existence of suffering," so that "pleasure is derived, as it seems, from the affliction of a weaker being in the face of divine might" (p. 306). With this reference to a tie between suffering and self-assertion, Freud has abandoned the ground where neuronal explanations with their connotation of passively suffered pain rather than active suffering of the ego mirror the medical preoccupation with a pain reified in the concern for instant relief. "Suffering of every kind is thus the subject matter of drama and from this suffering it promises to give the audience pleasure," (p. 307). Freud dwells on the difference between the dramatist and physician: "If we are sick, we have one wish only: to be well again and to be quit of our present state. We call for the doctor and medicine, and for the removal of the inhibition on the play of fantasy which has pampered us into deriving enjoyment even from our own sufferings" (1905–1906, p. 307). Psychoanalysis occupies the twilight zone between theater and medicine in its concern with the latent drama of the medicinal complaint in the treatment relationship.

It deepens our understanding of Freud's allusions to the Oedipus plays when, in his treatment of cruelty and theater, he refers in the same essay to Sophocles' *Ajax* and *Philoctetes*. Sophocles, of all the Greek dramatists, spoke most movingly of the pain and suffering in human existence. For Freud, the gratification for the audience of such dramas derives from the spectacle of pain as evidence of human assertion in the face of adversity, adversity which changes historically. "It must be an event involving conflict and it must include an effort of will together with resistance. This precondition found its first and grandest fulfillment in the struggle against divinity" (1905, p. 307). Freud continues: "The hero's next struggle is against human society" and still later "the struggle that causes the suffering is fought out in the hero's mind itself . . ." Freud depicts self-assertion as value, in the face of the gods, society, and the instincts. Ultimately, as Freud writes in his book on Leonardo (1910), we can see the possibility of conflict within the ego itself, between the ego ideal and representations of the instincts.

Because pain, suffering, and human autonomy are all involved with the struggle against the divine and/or nature, it is necessary to consider the idea of the ego more closely. First of all, the ego refers to an organization serving self-preservation and enhancement of identity. What is experienced as inimical to such living identity in its various changing phases is ascribed to the not-self from the very beginning. The not-self is initially the repository of all "unpleasure" (Unlust). Complementarily, the nascent ego is a pleasure-ego (Lust-Ich).

Pain (Schmerz) is a form of unpleasure deriving from the membership of our body in the world, the latter with its core of not-self. To the degree, however, that as body-I-am, in contrast to the body-I-have, I still connect with the alienated "unpleasure," a world-pain (Weltschmerz) is returned to the original pleasure-ego, tempering it with a sense of the reality principle and necessity (Freud's Ananke).

In explicating the origins of love and hate, Freud furnishes another example of creative embeddedness. He does so by showing that love and hate are not the simple opposites they appear to be, but that they are inextricably intertwined in the emergence of the ego; love as it were representing a moment of pull, hate a moment of push or repulsion. Along with the progressive unfolding of sexual instincts, there is a concomitant development of the ego as a synthesis of representations. The emergence of a constituted ego represents an enhanced embeddedness of the early pleasure-ego both in the body and the world. The idea of "regression in the service of the ego" is a way of referring to just this approximation of the self-identity toward a unity of self and world out of one's own experience in time. Now, recalling the overwhelming of the *psy* or inner stimuli system by the *phy* or outer stimuli system in the experience of pain (in Freud's initial account) so that the two become fused, we can see how a scission of the love and hate moments of the ego, together with formation of complementary and opposing identities, becomes possible.

Although Freud, to my knowledge, is silent on this, let us recall that experiences of divided ego (i.e., out-of-body experiences), supervening on conditions of extreme pain are not uncommon. When pain has persisted for an extended period or has become unusually intense, a partial or complete switch into a condition of reduced pain or utter peacefulness may occur. One might characterize such an altered consciousness as a "lucid faint." A part of the ego, as it were, now floats as if disembodied above the scene of strife where the person's own body can be seen in the midst of the action. A remarkable serenity and sense of control may accompany such a detachment from the immediacy of pain. Soldiers tell of having experienced such states in combat when they had given themselves up for lost. Such splitting of the ego in a situation of extreme pain and suffering obviously has a self-preservative value. Its activation in combat is ego syntonic, given the extreme polarization of the situation in terms of life and death. But the experience of such a detached serenity, with its accompanying sense of being removed from harm can, if persevered in as phantasy, render one hors de combat in the ordinary affairs of postwar civilian life—as indeed is the case for those combat veterans unable to return from that extremely polarized world, where love and hate were not experienced as synergic, but as virtual ontological opposites.

Freud's meditation on pain and suffering, with its strange modicum of pleasure, is continued in *Beyond the Pleasure Principle* (1920). With this work, Freud reaches back to draw on the findings of his scientific psychology of 1894 to 1895. From wondering about the way in which pain inflicted by another can enhance pleasure, Freud now inquires how the self-inflicted suffering of the nightmare might entail a bit of ego gratification. The example he begins with is that of the nightmare of the war veteran. He asks how it is possible for such a dream to be understood as the fulfillment of a wish, in view of the self-inflicted character of its distress.

Freud shows us how the nightmare of the soldier represents a resistance of the ego against the acknowledgment of its fundamental helplessness. In combat, conditions of survival entail a focus on action, openness to a full sense of one's condition. An extreme focus on the outer world, the world of Freud's *phy*-system, is ego syntonic. But a memory of the inner stimuli remains, a memory now ascribed to a subaltern ego, whose dominance is dreaded. Should this vulnerable self emerge, it would be endowed with all the fear-magnified violence of the seemingly dispassionate combat veteran by whom it was excluded.

When Freud undertakes to give a biological account of the nightmare, he begins from the evocation of an image of life in a situation of defensive battle: "This little fragment of living substance is suspended in the middle of an external world charged with the most powerful energies; and it would be killed by the stimulation emanating from there if it were not provided with a protective shield against stimuli" (1920, p. 27). We may suspect, once again, that the situation of combat has *already* been understood as the condition of organismic life. This accords with Freud's express debt to the Darwinian view. The protective shield to which Freud refers is formed by a partial death, as it were, of the vital surface, while "in highly developed organisms, the receptive cortical layer of the former vesicle has long been withdrawn into the depths of the interior of the body" (p. 27–28). This interior layer is now also receptive to "excitations from *within*" (Freud's emphasis) (p. 28). But while there is a barrier toward the external stimuli, there is no barrier toward stimuli from within. When these give rise to excessive unpleasure, they are attributed to the world without. Now the perceptual barrier may be brought into play against this illusion-charged antagonist. This is the basis for "projection."

It is now that the possibility of trauma may supervene: "We describe as 'traumatic' any excitations from outside which are powerful enough to break through the protective shield. When such excitation breaks through the protective shield, it also puts the pleasure principle, which requires intactness of the inner cortical layer, out of action. Now there is flooding by unbound stimulus excitation" (p. 30). Freud distinguishes "the specific unpleasure of physical pain" as "probably the result of the protective shield having been broken through in a limited area" (p. 30). When external stimulation has broken through the inner cortical layer, it is experienced as much from within as from without, accompanied by a quasi-psychotic rending pain. Although it would appear that this explanation of trauma corresponds to the older shock theory of trauma, Freud is careful to note a difference: "What *we* [Freud's emphasis] seek to understand are the effects produced on the organ of the mind by the breach in the shield against stimuli and by the problems that follow in its train. And we still attribute importance to the element of fright" (p. 31). The fright, Freud tells us, is caused by the "lack of any preparedness for anxiety, including lack of hypercathexis of the systems that would be the first to receive the stimulus" (p. 31). It appears that Freud is once again pursuing his analysis in terms of an apparatus to such a degree that something overlooked in his starting point will become visible when the accumulated refinements begin to challenge the credibility of the model itself.

Freud hypothesizes that the anxiety dream, the nightmare, and traumatic neurosis all stand for an effort to belatedly secure the preparedness ("hypercathexis") that would have effectively formed a barrier against the stimuli that became traumatic. With this, Freud has acknowledged a principle in addition to that of wish gratification in dream formation, namely, a compulsion to repeat in an effort to retroflectively secure protection against what, in the absence of an adequate defensive hypercathexis, resulted in trauma, with its accompanying pain. Since it is the hypercathexis which is preventive of trauma, hypercathexis of an injured organ in the case of physical injury can likewise account for the relative absence of anxiety often observed in such cases (p. 33). In a sense, the physical injury with its hypercathexis can be considered as helping to bind the excitation, thus diminishing the anxiety.

What is new here is just the emphasis on the need for the hypercathexis or the preparedness. But when we speak of preparedness, we necessarily invoke a world for which one seeks preparation. With this, the closed framework of Freud's cathectic analysis is violated, because of the necessity for admitting the world as phenomenologically given. Now we may ask, does the world as given, as primordial, stand for what can be utterly overwhelming in every case for the infantile ego? At the same time, does this original, open, undeveloped ego represent a minimal involvement with the world, preserved as a nostalgia of freedom, of which even pain is a partial memory, but now in terms of bodily experience? If so we would expect to find in pain both the wish for bodily dissolution, and a resistance to the wish.

Freud's most focused inquiry into the nature of pain is to be found at the end of his 1926 work, *Inhibitions, Symptoms, and Anxiety*. In his late work, Freud starts from where he had left off in his earlier discussion of the war neuroses. There he alluded to the likelihood that trauma results from the cooperation of inner need and external stimulation. If the inner need is not present, the situation is merely one of danger. The possibility, however, of *anxiety* arises with the ego, and is occasioned by loss of perception of the object. An experience of actual loss of the object is the source now of *pain*, this time of excessive stimulation from within rather than from without: "It cannot be for nothing that the common usage of speech should have created the notion of internal, mental pain" (1926, p. 171). Freud locates the "point of analogy" between physical and mental pain in the fact that both in the case of loss of a love object and in that of a bodily injury, there is an intense preoccupation with the missing or injured object or part, "an object-presentation which is highly cathected by instinctual need plays the same role as a part of the body which is cathected by an increase of stimulus" (p. 171–172). Now, Freud discovers pain to result from a state of mental helplessness accompanying the high level of cathexis. Such a high level of cathexis of the representation of the lost object results in a sense of separation within the ego subject, like the pain experienced with the death of a loved one, and which it is the task of mourning to transform. What is new in this reading of pain is the way in which physical and mental pain are linked by the common factor of intense cathexis. That such pain represents a rift in the ego is borne out by Freud's closing comment, in which he characterizes mourning as the dissolution of a painful cathexis of a lost love object.

Finally, in his posthumously published *Outline of Psychoanalysis* (1940), the topic of pain merges with that of the separation of the sexes and of the apparently insatiable fantasy of psychic integration in terms of possessing the genital complement of the opposite sex, the male with his castration anxiety, the female with her wish for a penis. Freud's work closes on the theme of sexual separation, already invoked in *Beyond the Pleasure Principle*, and more than three decades earlier, in his letter of August 28, 1883, to Martha Bernays, his betrothed: "I'm only half a human being in the sense of the old platonic fable which you surely know, and my cut surface gives me pain when I don't keep occupied" (Freud, 1960, p. 49).

II

In the first part I have taken up Freud's effort to understand pain by discussing his writings on the subject in chronological sequence. Now I wish to take up the problem in a
broader context afforded by the introduction of new relevant
material. Above all, I wish to show how the elusiveness of the
meaning of pain in psychoanalysis derives from its root in the
idea of biological evolution with its necessary blending of
personal history and phyletic endowment.

Pain, in the context of psychoanalysis, means, above all, *in
the situation of psychoanalysis*. The psychoanalytic situation is one
in which any particular thematic pain is considered to be ideally
resolvable in terms of the constitutive stress of the psychoanalytic situation itself: namely, as constituted in the communicative differences between analyst and analysand. In this
situation, pain is ultimately not extraneous, but a source of
certain disclosures into which the pain is considered to be
ideally capable of being resolved. A principle difficulty is that
the psychoanalytic situation is conventionally viewed only in the
light of its affective disturbances, without regard for those of its
properties which afford the possibility of a *certain kind of healing*.

In talking about pain in psychoanalytic perspective, it is
necessary to note that psychoanalysis represents an effort to
understand human experience in terms of the idea of evolution
generally, and specifically in terms of natural selection.

Basic for Darwin's psychology, as for that of Freud, is the
triad of pain, wound, and ego, the last understood as brain, or
neural organization, as in Freud. In the notebooks of Darwin's
annus mirabilis, 1838, we find the following observations:
"When one is simply habituated in life time to any line of action,
or thought, one feels pain at not performing it (either if
prevented or over-tempted)" (October 8, 1838). And: "Think,
whether there is any analogy between grief and pain—certain
ideas hurting brain, like a wound hurts body" (November 28,
1838). *Pain, brain,* and *wound* are also the key terms of Freud's
thought in the inception of what he came to call psychoanalysis.
In Freud's (like Darwin's) unpublished writings, where he
sought to define his starting point, we find definitions of pain,

trauma (wound), and ego (as neuronal organization) treated in that order in his *Project for a Scientific Psychology* (Freud, 1895). Considering the implicit tension between any kind of ego identity, neuronal or otherwise, and the constant change implicit in evolutionary natural selection, the possibility of *trauma* for the ego must be granted at the outset. The ego as inclusive of a barrier function grounds afresh the possibility of a new trauma. Freud first of all defines trauma: "A trauma would have to be defined as an *accretion of excitation* in the nervous system, *which the latter has been unable to dispose of adequately by motor reaction*" [Freud's emphasis] (1895, p. 137). In the "Project," it is pain which is treated after trauma: "The nervous system is contrived in such a way that the major external Qs (quantities of excitation) are kept off from the phy-(sical system) and still more from the psy-(chic system): by the nerve-ending screens, and by the merely indirect connection between psy-(chic system) and external world. Is there a phenomenon which can be brought to coincide with the failure of these contrivances? Such, I think, is *pain*" (1895, pp. 306–307). Only after taking up trauma and pain does Freud come to the issue of the neuronal organization corresponding to Darwin's "brain," and which Freud terms *the ego*:

> With the hypotheses of *"wishful attraction"* [Freud's emphasis] and of the inclination to *repression* [Freud's emphasis], we have already touched on a state of *psy*- which has not yet been discussed. For these two processes indicate that an organization has been formed in *psy*- whose presence interferes with passages of [quantity] which on the first occasion occurred in a particular way [i.e. accompanied by satisfaction or pain]. This organization is called the "ego" . . . the ego is to be defined as the totality of the *psy*-cathexes at the time, in which a permanent component is distinguished from a changing one. [1895, pp. 322–323].

This triad of pain, trauma, and ego in the *"Project for a Scientific Psychology"* (1895) recurs in *Beyond the Pleasure Principle* (1920) and in "Inhibitions, Symptoms, and Anxiety" (1925). Their tie derives from the fundamental presupposition of evolution, namely, the mutual dependency between the resources of the phylum or species, and those of individuals within such a phylum or species. The classical nineteenth century statement of this relationship was Haeckel's (1866) "fundamental biogenetic law." Darwin's "natural selection" represents the coping stone of this structure of thought by introducing the world as controlling instance, one regulating the commerce between the species or phylum and individuals. In the perspective of evolutionary thought the psychic sphere is ambiguously ontogenetic *and* phylogenetic. Given the reciprocity between individual contributions to the species and the species endowment of individuals, every element of human experience may have either positive or negative survival significance depending on the circumstances, while "circumstances" vary, depending on the amplitude of the context considered. In this perspective, pain and trauma can be discovered to have developmental value in a world which requires changes of individuals, if not their death. Indeed pain and trauma are inseparable from the ego identity of a human being and/or human collective. By the same token, the ego as an organization, in resistance to necessary change, can have a destructive consequence. Thus at one point Freud glimpsed the possibility of the ego principle as having the value of an impulsion to death, given its fixated character with its potential for maladaptation.

In the late thought of Freud the dual of phylum and individuum continues to hold sway, when the three instances of his tripartite personality model are distinguished only as moments of process in which the I supersedes the It. The It, the I, and the Higher-I are each partly conscious, partly unconscious, repeating the complementarity of ontogenetic and phylogenetic contributions. This is something like an uncertainty principle for psychoanalysis, at once biological and psychological.

Given this state of affairs, the senses of life and death, pain, trauma, and ego are all ambiguous apart from specific lived situations. Existence involves both registers, that of the biological collective and that of the individual. What is of positive value in one register may be of negative value in the other.

What enhances the life of the individual may prove destructive for the species, what is destructive for the individual may prove of benefit for the species. Psychoanalysis is rooted in the exploration of the ties between the history of one's biological development and that of one's individual experience in the interest of attaining their greatest mutual enhancement. Such enhancement for Freud is represented by his use of I to refer to an organization in which a higher kind of I (superego) emerges out of that ego which is set over against an id. It would be more to the point to refer to this more comprehensive I as the self, understanding by self an organization of experience at once biological, social, and psychological, in the course of becoming.

The rigor with which Freud applies the idea of evolution to human experience accounts for his unswerving adherence to a Lamarckian (also ancient Greek) postulate of the inheritance of acquired characters, no less collective than individual. In fact the Lamarckian postulate, also accepted by the aged Darwin, stands for the recognition that the idea of evolution has radical consequences for man's understanding of himself. So too, the experience of pain has extreme consequences for human self-understanding, as the book of Job attests. We may see this in the way the issue of pain poses a central problem for religious faith. All such concern with theodicy resurfaces in the evolutionary idea, now as a *biodicy*, one which receives scientific sanction in the achievement of Darwin. This also provides the basis for a new science, that of psychoanalysis, indifferently biological and psychological.

If the ego is inseparable from pain and trauma, then pain is of indeterminate value, always to be understood in terms of ego situated in the world, and thus involved with the issue of self-identity. "Tell me your relationship to pain, and I will tell you who you are" (Juenger, p. 145, 1934). Or, as is always acknowledged in pain research, pain is what the person in pain interprets as pain. This, incidentally, removes pain into that sensibility from which all speech takes its rise and to which it returns.

In his essay, "Creative Writers and Day-dreaming", Freud makes reference to the famous passage in Goethe's *Torquato*

Tasso: "When man in pain turns mute—A god gave me the gift—To say what I suffer" (1908, p. 146n). It would not be too much to say that Freud's entire opus, from his dream book on, is an effort to learn, from his patient, the language he needs to say what he too has suffered. The result of all his efforts was to discover the "chronic pain" of that which cannot *yet* be said. But as the word *chronic* indicates, there is always a temporal horizon with its promise of meaning. This is the sense of Freud's lifelong preoccupation with pain of every sort, pain which remains inseparable from the impossibility of exhausting it. He sought to learn how to understand it out of the difficulties of his patients in saying their pain. The continuing evolution of his terminology through the years, retentive of earlier meanings while productive of new ones, attests to his unremitting effort to say what he and we suffer. This effort made him the writer he was. When asked by Abraham how he was able to write so much after long days of seeing patients, he answered: "I have to recuperate from psychoanalysis, otherwise I can't stand it" (1965, p. 122). "Pain" and "suffering" are to be understood together. It is in the saying of *what* I suffer that speech is discovered to have been the gift of a god. In saying what I suffer, I realize who I am, my responsibility. Such healing speech is the gift of "our [psychoanalysts'] god Logos." It is not surprising that Freud had such an affinity for Sophocles, whose language it has been said speaks of dreadful things with healing words. Like the dramatist, Freud grasped the tie between the pathology of the psyche and the meaning or logos latent in pathos, in the forms of suffered logos, the logopathies of "nervous disorders" and "sexual perversions," as in Charcot's theater of pain he attended in Paris as a young man, or as in the *Ajax* and *Philoctetes* of Sophocles, whose suffering protagonists he mentions in his 1906 essay "Psychopathic Characters on the Stage."

It is necessary to keep in mind the inseparability of Freud's search for a language adequate to his own suffering from the attentive hearing he gave to that of his patients. He never ceased using their words as clues in the discovery of his language, to realize as he said, "the I where It was."

On the saying by sufferers of chronic pain there follows a

second silence, one which replaces their initial muteness. This silence, one may say, is that of logopathic presence, as it is conveyed in classic theater, music, portraits, and self-portraits like those by Rembrandt. By "logopathic" I refer to passively suffered experiences charged with meaning and value. All of this is known, but rarely acknowledged by those who write about pain.

Pain is a matter of verbal report. If a patient does not report pain, there is, strictly speaking, no "problem" of pain. But what of pain which is not directly experienced, is masked, as say, in some depressions? Here too psychoanalysis understands loss as lying at the heart of pain, of all pain, even if this cannot be empirically demonstrated. Pain in psychoanalysis stands for objectless need, desire without an object, objectless desire. If the patient complains of pain in the absence of any conventionally credible evidence for its possibility, the pain remains a problem for the caregiver, unless, as is often the case, he wishes to dismiss the patient's complaints. It is a well-known fact that under certain conditions pain is present only when one's attention is drawn to it, as when questioned. In my own work with pain patients, only a few questions are asked about the pain, and those in the beginning.

In my experience with war veterans who suffer pain from having been wounded as well as from posttraumatic stress disorder, the blending of pain complaints from bodily wounds with pain from the loss of comrades is particularly striking. But this is a topic for a different time and place.

What of chronic or intractable pain? Here too it is necessary to ask: chronic or intractable under what conditions? I have known a war casualty who has suffered for thirty years with phantom pain following amputation of both legs. But his report of severe and virtually unremitting pain is accompanied by a smiling expression that seems to give the lie to its reported severity. How can such a strange combination of pain and humor be understood?

Let us consider what we can learn from those who in the midst of extreme pain or suffering have experienced out-of-body or near-death states. At such times there is a sudden shift from extreme stress to detached calm, sometimes with a survey of one's body and the situation in which it remains trapped. In near-death experience there may also be an over-view, now temporal, as when one's entire life seems to flash before one's eyes. The possibilities of spatial and temporal modes of out-of-body experience show that we can inhabit the world in two different ways, proximally as body ego or distally as motile in the world. Body and world are to be understood as reciprocally involving, neither one for itself alone, with ab-sence, imaginary or otherwise, of the other. Because of this amphibolous structure of our experience we are capable of experiencing pain proximally or distally. It is the proximal mode of experience we speak of as "physical," while experience in the distal mode increasingly assumes a "mental" character. Needless to say, practical limits are set to the conversions of one into the other by the difference between the ontogenetic and phylogenetic contributions. The two kinds of contribution are always related in terms of relative dominance or recession.

For Freud, who took for granted the "fundamental bioge-netic law," which in one form or another ruled biological thought from the birth of the modern evolutionary idea at the beginning of the nineteenth century, it was above all the twofold character of human experiencing at once phylogenetic and ontogenetic, which enabled him to comprehend the possi-bility of pain, with its compassion, in a more deeply integrated manner. Pain is the hallmark of a survivor, conscious of its mortality. Given the twofold root of human experience, onto-genetic and phylogenetic, it is possible for an individual to emphasize one or the other position. The importance of the position occupied is shown by the word Freud employed in his treatment of pain, and of the ego's origin, in his "Project for a Scientific Psychology" (1895): "Besetzung," (occupancy) strangely rendered into English as "cathexis." We shall have more to say about this in the third section of this chapter.

In the healing of pain, the psychoanalyst, as far as possible, becomes the container or place in which pain of the trauma can be located, and from where it can be relived, this time with greater clarity. In the psychoanalytic, evolutionary perspective, all pain is *ideally* understood as evidence of an earlier trauma. Indeed, all origins in evolution are necessarily catastrophic (i.e., traumatic). Although Freud does not go any farther back than the emergence of animate from inanimate life, there is nothing in principle to prevent one finding in Freud's position that of Fechner (1873), whose importance Freud acknowledges, and who understood both the animate and the inanimate as descended from an undifferentiated "cosmorganic" matter. Moreover, even though not so intended by Freud, the primal trauma could even be viewed as implicit in the separation of a divine creation from its divine maker, as understood in terms of human separation, one repeated in the Garden through the Fall incurred by disobedience. In the analytic situation, pain, like a hieroglyphic tablet, needs to be deciphered, to be rendered transparent to an earlier interior text. In the analytic situation it is through the place of the analyst that a fragment of the scene of the earlier trauma, a primal scene, is in part beheld, in part constructed by the partners. The scene, here and now of the analytic situation, guides the disclosures of meaning, so that the analysand is able to become aware of what he or she suffers, at once more immediately and yet with a certain distance. The pain comes to be experienced in a new key, through which it becomes transparent to a mythic suffering of things, persons, and times to one another.

It is the caregiver's containment of the mute pain of the complainant which enables her or him to say what he or she suffers. The caregiver has provided an out-of-body locus for the careseeker to occupy in developing the scene of which he has in part become the mute witness. The careseeker is thus enabled to say what he sees *now*. Intractable pain, as an event of consciousness, is taken to imply an antecedent primal scene. A violent origin of the world is presupposed in any evolutionary attempt to understand pain which starts from consciousness, thus the quasi-historical, quasi-mythic references in Darwin, followed by Freud, to the murder of a primal father out of sexual jealousy, entailing subsequent guilt and remorse, which inspired morality in revulsion against the crime. Crime and punishment are the mythic phylogenetic roots of pain. The metapsychology of archaic events *assumed as inscribed* in human biology provides the frame within which the paradoxes of posterior traumata may be clarified, pain finally becoming tolerable through being rendered meaningful.

However strange such an understanding, even intractable pain may be seen to follow from a rigorous evolutionary understanding of pain which starts with consciousness itself as evolutionarily significant. Beginning with consciousness within an evolutionary perspective, the fundamental biogenetic law accepted by Freud and Jung, and implicit in all depth psychology, becomes heuristic in human efforts for self-knowledge and self-control. Given the fundamental biogenetic law, it should also be pointed out that an understanding of consciousness in the light of evolutionary idea also allows for the possibility that "phylogeny *pre*-capitulates ontogeny"; that is, unconsciously prestructures its course. This would be one way of understanding Freud's "Unconscious" within the evolutionary frame of reference. In an evolutionary perspective the course of phylogeny, however mythically imagined, from which individuals emerge, must have produced a kind of template through which their present existence is realized. Individuals realize such existence through their efforts to transliterate the language of that template (read "genetic code") into language formed from their experience. "Where It was, there shall 'I' become" (1933, p. 80).

For understanding pain in a psychoanalytic context, it is necessary to start from consciousness as evolutionarily significant. In an evolutionary understanding both pain and consciousness are directly or indirectly of survival value. And it is in working out the way in which the individual and phyletic registers of experience are interwoven that psychoanalysis has evolved. In such a task Freud's "metapsychology" refers to the language which enables mediation between the two registers.

For Freud, as for Schopenhauer and Nietzsche, consciousness and thus world, relieves the pain implicit in the phyletic historical organism, just as the phylogenetic resource of sexuality may be sought as relief from the pain of consciousness. This is the taproot of a psychology which starts from consciousness, one in which the experience of pain is rigorously unwrapped within the idea of evolution. Within such an evolutionary perspective any distinction between mental and physical is no longer feasible. All pain is in a sense compassion: the "com" here understood as the bond within each of the basic dualities, mind and body, male and female, active and passive. Thus too, all passion, insofar as it is evolutionary, is compassion, since the species or phylum is collective, the outcome of a selection of individuals, the species diverging in turn into a variety of individuals from which fresh selection follows.

In this way the otherwise strange Lamarckism of the late Darwin and of Freud becomes comprehensible, an adherence to the idea of a collective inheritance of the memory traces of individuals. We need only to understand this in a more fundamental way than its abstract language suggests or a positivistic biology allows. When we do so, we can see that in evolutionary perspective the past is somehow included in the present, albeit only as a mythic potential. At the same time memories of individuals must be distinguished from what is genetically transmitted. This has been true since Weismann. If the past is present, but not in a way that can be directly inferred from the experiences of individuals, then it must be mythically accessible. A possibility of its imaginary reality is given by the necessarily deep continuity between species identity and that of any individual within such a species. For Freud it was the "mythic impulsions" (Triebe) which mediate between the ontogenetic and the phylogenetic. This mediation is one which occurs in both directions, however indirectly, through the world in which both are present and contained.

A word about "pleasure" and "pain" in Freud's usage: it is characteristic for him that to "pleasure" he opposes not "pain," but "unpleasure" (Unlust). This word Freud found ready-made in German. Freud understood the infant ego as one which attributed all negative experience to the nonego, retaining pleasure as a property of the ego, thus constituting a primitive "pleasure-ego."

The implicit relegation of unpleasure to the nonego is consistent with Christian, Orphic, and Buddhist traditions. What makes Freud's understanding different is the evolutionary biological distinction between phylum and individuum. Now the unpleasure of the world, which is also unpleasure of the individuum, insofar as its body is of the world, can be alleviated by an alteration in the economy of the impulsions, insofar as the stress itself in part holds a knowledge of the difference necessary for its reduction. The implication of Freud's view of pain as a mode of unpleasure is that of the possibility of healing, already implied in the invocation of trauma. We shall see that in theory there is no limit that can be put on the possibility of healing from pain in psychoanalysis, given the interplay, however mediated, between structure and function in an evolutionary understanding of organismic consciousness. For the difference between the individual order of action and that of phyletic instinctuality means that there is an ever-present possibility for the ego to be traumatized, that is, to become incapable of discharging its excitation. Now the healing in psychoanalysis occurs through quantic discharge of the excessive excitation through speech, speech with another who has realized his own trauma and pain of the ego, and who has found the language necessary for evoking such knowledge on behalf of another in and through his own speech.

Out-of-body and near-death experience both attest to our capacity to occupy a position in the world, even to the extent of becoming free of any bodily distress. There seems to be no limit to the kinds of pain from which relief may be realized in this way, as the evidence from hypnosis already shows. Both the ability of steadfast believers to resist torture, and the selfless death of martyrs, attest to this power to rise above the downward pull of pain into concreteness and psychic constriction.

The hidden root of all evolutionary theory is that of a capacity for self-division, and with this a repression of the suffering part. In human experience this takes the form of liberation through experience of the world from the unpleasure of irritability, a basic feature of animal life. Relief from stimuli (Latin "goads") is afforded by the world as a kind of lived vision, representing the position of the other, as in out-of-body or near-death experience. In his dream book, Freud understood dreams as a shift toward an out-of-body position, one which affords distance to nocturnal excitations. In the same way, objects of libido may be seen as positions through which one secures a limited kind of out-of-body freedom. The affordance of this out-of-body position in the analytic situation replaces the historically earlier intrusive out-of-body position adopted by the hypnotist. In the analytic situation representations of historically occupied out-of-body positions enter into play, and may be detected in the field of the analyst's free-floating attentiveness. Such occupancies (Besetzungen), are souvenirs of historically dated unpleasures, including traumata, the outdated measures of defensive attachment which limit current possibilities of occupying relevant out-of-body positions. Needless to say, all creative activity occurs through the utilization of such out-of-body movement, the sense of "being with it," even though primordially it may also be seen as a defensive move to secure distance from the elementary unpleasure of being alive in a world apparently largely inanimate. The extent to which occupancy of an out-of-body position can afford relief from pain is, as mentioned, also apparent in the use of hypnosis to reduce pain. It can be seen in the treatment of war neurosis in which the reliving of past experience in the form of fantasy, however nightmarish, is invoked in the service of eventual relief from pain. No matter how disturbing a nightmare may be, the fact that it is experienced as coming from without (i.e., as in the world), enables it to serve as a shield against a more deeply intimate pain.

Ideally, pain can always be surmounted, since the movement of occupancy is inseparable from consciousness. The exaltations or literal ecstasies of out-of-body and near-death experiences are evidence. In such experience—like that of the lucid dream as well—the character of consciousness as occupancy is immediately experienced, that is, lived. This may be seen as the purposiveness (telos) of psychoanalysis. Darwin's own acknowledgment of such purposiveness took the form of his late acknowledgment of Larmarck.

To have introduced the evolutionary idea as I have in a volume devoted to the management of chronic pain will seem to some as philosophical idealism. After all, what could be more immediate and more concrete than pain, or rather, not concrete, but singular and individual. Your pain can never be my pain, and my pain is never unaffected by my attitude toward it, and my understanding of it.

That I have the capability for occupying different positions, within the body as well as various positions out of the body, points up the motility of the ego, a movement recognized by Freud in his idea of occupancy by the ego, or even by the libido.

The implicit ideal of psychoanalysis is a perfect motility of the ego, both cross-generational (phyletic), as well as throughout individual life. In this understanding, unpleasure (Unlust) is a constitutive quality of individual existence, given the unattainability of such perfect motility. And within the gamut of unpleasures, pain can now be seen to stand for the infrangible bounds of the individual human being, standing for the ruptured continuity between the ego and the phylum. Within the presupposition of the evolutionary standpoint, pain attests, when consciousness is recognized as the indispensable starting and ending position, to an ego torn between generational and transgenerational modes of existence. "Where It was, there shall 'I' be" (1933, p. 80). Such an I would be one of a paradoxically sheer motility. The ideal of the motile ego is recognized in the part attributed to empathy in psychoanalysis. The primordial trauma which is the hallmark of the ego in psychoanalysis stands for the mythic separation of the individual from the phylum in birth and throughout life, only to be suspended in death. The phyletic–individual horizon lies at the heart of psychoanalysis as an evolutionary doctrine of a protean motile ego.

For Freud the dream is a minimal out-of-body experience. Freud's own earliest out-of-body experiences were induced with cocaine in the 1880s and 1890s, even as his own death was eased with an administration of morphine he requested in the pain of terminal cancer. It may also be recalled that once, many years earlier, he was heard to murmur, while coming to after a faint, another out-of-body state, "How sweet it must be to die" (Jones, 1953, vol. 1. p. 317).

The motility of the ego within the body and within the world is still rooted in the body. The possibility of such motility is given, however, only by the potential of the ego to leave the body, also connoting the possibility of my own death. If pain announces the latency of my own death, it also conveys the promise of a complete freedom. When this tie of freedom and death is understood it enables a more positive approach to the fantasies of suicide that often accompany chronic pain.

Ultimately, pain stands for our simultaneous attachment and opposition to this attachment to the body, and may serve or disserve the emergence of the ego. As long as we are attached to the body in a submissive way—and to a degree this is necessary throughout life—ego motility is hindered. We remain backward looking, confined to constricting occupancies. Our resistance, our incapacity for an absolute birth of the ego, is measurable in terms of pain. Absolute birth of the ego can only be imagined in our present condition as a *fulfilling trauma*. Short of this, trauma is experienced as loss, even though its deepest and necessarily unconscious promise is that of an absolute birth. The latent sense of any "birth trauma" is the promise of a completion of the birth of the ego. Failing this, only that unpleasure which accompanies pleasure like its shadow offers a clue to this possibility of a further birth of the ego. Needless to say such sense of the ego can only be realized within this very life.

One place where Freud hints at this hidden potential of ego identity in pain is in the following passage from "Mourning and Melancholia":

> Each single one of the memories and expectations in which the libido is bound to the object is brought up and hypercathected, and detachment of the libido is accomplished in respect of it. Why this compromise by which the command of reality is carried out piecemeal should be so extraordinarily painful is not at all easy to explain in terms of economics. It is remarkable that this painful unpleasure is taken as a matter of course by us. The fact is, however, that when the work of mourning is completed, the ego becomes free and uninhibited again. [Freud, 1917, p. 245].

The deeper sense of life is given in the realization of the higher sense of mourning, i.e., deoccupancy enabling freedom of reoccupancy. The intuitive understanding of this possibility serves to account for the "remarkable" fact "that this painful unpleasure is taken as a matter of course by us."

III

In the first section of this chapter, we have shown how an ensemble of root notions, such as *trauma, pain, anxiety,* and *ego* form an organic whole for Freud's "Scientific Psychology." In the second section, we have shown how these root notions are to be understood within the context of the evolutionary idea, for which consciousness has survival value. In this section, we intend to develop an original element of Freud's thought, one which makes it possible to understand pain in terms of psychoanalysis. Freud's innovation is the concept of "Besetzung," translated in the *Standard Edition* as "cathexis." While *Besetzung* is a graphic word in German, referring to not merely a neuronic "charge" as in Freud's "Scientific Project," but more usually to the casting of a play, military occupation, or to a "busy" telephone line, the neologism "cathexis" remains opaque in meaning. While this enhances its value as a technical term, it prevents that expansion of meaning which Freud came to realize in the way he employed Besetzung. Its value for Freud was that it is an action noun, one which may be used subjectively or objectively as the occasion requires, without being capable of exhaustive definition in either the subjective or objective direction.

A more appropriate translation of Besetzung would be "occupancy." Occupancy implies something which enters into something else, without specifying either the entrant or that into which it enters. Freud variously shifts his emphasis in one direction or the other, emphasizing either the object or subject of occupancy. The space of the movement of occupancy itself represents the space of the ego, understood as intentional motility, always embodied. As embodied, one may speak of the ego in an objective way, as Freud does in his early "Project," where he speaks of the ego as "the sum of its occupancies." But if that which it occupies serves to define the ego, it also needs to be remembered that it is also the ego which defines that which it occupies. Thus we are returned to the amphibolous character of *occupancy* as a primordial term, inclusive of both subject and object meaning. We may conceive of any particular occupancy as proceeding either from the subject or object pole of a relation, or more precisely, as their synergy. This of course relates ego and world to one another as wholes, each one implicitly comprising the possibility of the other. While Freud does not develop the implications of his use of occupancy to this extent it should be understood that these possibilities remain in the idea itself, and can be shown to play a part in the subsequent evolution of Freud's thought. It is necessary to stress these implications if we are to understand pain and trauma in a perspective which accords with Freud's evolutionary standpoint as well as with his elemental understanding of the problem of pain.

How is pain to be understood in terms of the indeterminancy of occupancy? The necessary condition for pain according to Freud is a threat of loss, whether of body, person, place, time, value, and so on, any one of which represents an occupancy by and of *the ego*. We may speak of "the ego," despite the indeterminacy of occupancy, because of the inseparability of ego from body in our experience. Even if our experience of ego is not concrete, inasmuch as occupancy is intrinsic in all experience, it always nevertheless involves an element of materiality, one deriving from the primordial mythic occupancy implicit in the idea of psyche or soul.

The inseparability of occupancy and motility of the body ego makes possible its response to loss or threat of loss to the body ego, by an intensification of occupancy of what is threatened. Pain presupposes prior occupancy by the psyche of the body, threat to which is countered by heightened occupancy on the part of the libido. Insofar as we are concerned with libido, it is that aspect of it which relates to loss, or the genesis of pain. We return to the theme of threatened loss to the body ego. It is the continuation of a threat to the body ego, already constituted through a primary occupancy, that now results in stress between the possible loss and the heightened occupancy by the body ego of the threatened part, value, or person.

Chronic pain in this context can be represented as a clonic process whose tension between the threatened loss and the enhanced body ego occupancy is mutually binding and splitting.

Modification of such chronic pain might in theory be

effected through (1) reducing threat, as through medical intervention; (2) reducing the heightened body ego occupancy of the threatened part, value, or person, as through disciplines involving control of the self; (3) investing as much of the ego which is not primarily body-involved in persons, values, or activities of contrasting meaning, such as realizing identification with figures who have mastered similar threats or losses. A fourth possibility is opened up by Freud's distinction between representation and affect attached to that representation, both of which are involved in an occupancy with adequate discharge. To the extent that the affect and representation have become separated, adequate discharge of vital tension is hindered. Insofar as threat of body ego loss has continued in the splitting off of affect from representations of life history losses, a reunion of representation and affect, enabling an adequate discharge of repressed pulsions, would also effect a reduction of unconscious pain. This, it seems to me, is the original contribution of psychoanalysis to the healing of pain, insofar as it is accessible to psychotherapeutic intervention.

There is, however, another kind of pain which, while not itself curable, represents the possibility for treatment of the pain which we have just discussed. For Freud, this pain is subsumed under that of sexual desire, understood as the longing for a lost integrity. In his *Beyond the Pleasure Principle*, Freud, somewhat like Fechner, conceives of life itself as an outcome of the disintegration of a primordial cosmorganic matter. We bear intrinsically its souvenir in our constitution and strive throughout our life to recover its lost condition. But the effort to do so, starting from our monadic state, involves an infringement of others' autonomy. The different world religions all implicitly recognize a distinction between such meta-cosmic pain and the secondary metapsychological pain we start from. In Freud's work it is his idea of a "mortality urge" (Todestrieb) which ties such metacosmic trauma and pain to his metapsychological exposition of pain and trauma.

In short there are two kinds of pain: one metacosmic and one metapsychological. The former makes possible the latter, the latter instantiates the former as experience.

The inseparability of sensitivity to pain and consciousness

entitles us to speak of human psychalgesia. Such psychalgesia enables us to better understand human susceptibility to prejudice, crime, addiction, and war. Insofar as such painful susceptibility of the psyche is linked with the experience of time, we may speak of chronalgesia as standing for the tie of pain with time in human experience. The collective modes of representation of such chronalgesia lie at the basis of religious observances, carnival and sacrificial, including those of war (Girard, Caillois). In psychoanalysis the recognition of an inherent trend of life to return, however vainly, to its origins, is based on the presence of such chronalgesia.

Psychoanalysis understands pain finally as that moment of experience which corresponds to the expanding movement of the cosmos in the "big bang" theory of the origin of the universe. Inseparable from this still continuing movement of creation is the differentiation of the fragments resulting from the primordial dispersion. Pain now stands for the necessary tension between the expansive moment of this cosmorganic movement and the contractive moment of each monadic fragment on itself, a "primary narcissism." The openness and indeterminancy of the fragment derives both from the forgotten memory of an integral whole from which it derives, no less than from a fantasy of a whole yet to be realized. This is the condition within which the sense of Freud's dictum that the ego is the actual locus of anxiety is to be understood. The motility of the ego is to be understood as an expression of never-ending occupancies in the service of relieving the pain resulting from the trauma of continuing creation. It was in his *Beyond the Pleasure Principle* (1920) that Freud gave expression to this cosmalgic vision implicit in his erotomorphic metapsychology. Parallel works contemporary with those of Freud, and of similar thrust, were the *Thalassa* of Ferenczi, (1938) his close associate, and *The Book of the It* (1923) by Groddeck, his acquaintance. Such "cosmalgology" stands in a tradition of thought which reaches back through the doctrines of the Kabbala, gnostic Christianity, Plato, to the cosmopsychology of the presocratic physiologoi, the earliest philosphers of a science of nature.

REFERENCES

Bolk, L. (1926), *Das Problem der Menschwerdung*. (The Problem of Hominization.) Jena: Gustav Fischer.

Caillois, R. (1980), *Man and the Sacred*. New York: Greenwood.

Fechner, G. T. (1873), *Einige Ideen zur Schoepfungsgeschichte und Entwickelungsgeschichte der Organismen, Tuebingen: Archiv diskord*, 1985. (Some Ideas on the History of the Creation and Development of Organisms).

Ferenczi, S. (1924), *Thalassa: A Theory of Genitality*. New York: Psychoanalytic Quarterly, 1938.

Freud, E. L. (ed.) (1960), *Letters of Sigmund Freud*. New York: Basic Books.

Freud, S. (1892–1894), Extracts from Freud's footnotes to his translation of Charcot's *Tuesday Lectures. Standard Edition*, 1:137–143.

———(1894), The neuropsychoses of defence. *Standard Edition* 3:25–68. London: Hogarth Press, 1962.

———(1895), Project for a scientific psychology. *Standard Edition*, 1:295–343. London: Hogarth Press, 1966.

———(1900), The Interpretation of Dreams. *Standard Edition*, 4. London: Hogarth Press, 1953.

———(1905), Three essays on the theory of sexuality. *Standard Edition*, 7:123–243. London: Hogarth Press, 1953.

———(1905–1906), Psychopathic characters on the stage. *Standard Edition*, 7:303–310. London: Hogarth Press, 1953.

———(1908), Creative writers and day-dreaming. *Standard Edition*, 9:141–154. London: Hogarth Press, 1959.

———(1910), Leonardo and a memory of his childhood, *Standard Edition*, 11:59–138. London: Hogarth Press, 1957.

———(1917), Mourning and melancholia. *Standard Edition*, 14:237–258. London: Hogarth Press, 1955.

———(1920), Beyond the Pleasure Principle. *Standard Edition*, 18:1–64. London: Hogarth Press, 1955.

———(1926), Inhibitions, symptoms and anxiety. *Standard Edition*, 20:75–172. London: Hogarth Press, 1959.

———(1933), The dissection of the psychical personality. *Standard Edition*, 22:57–80. London: Hogarth Press, 1964.

———(1940), An outline of psychoanalysis. *Standard Edition*, 23:139–208. London: Hogarth Press, 1964.

———Abraham, K. (1965), *Briefe 1907–1926* (Letters 1907–1926). Frankfurt/Main: S. Fischer Verlag, 1965.

Girard, R. (1977), *Violence and the Sacred*. Baltimore: Johns Hopkins.

Groddeck, G. (1923), *The Book of the It*. New York: International Universities Press, 1976.

Gruber, H. (1974), *Darwin on Man*. New York: E. P. Dutton, 1974.

Haeckel, E. (1866), *Generelle Morphologie der Organismen. Allgemeine Grundzuege der organischen Formen-Wissenschaft, mechanisch begruendet durch die von Charles Darwin reformirte Descendenztheorie* (General Morphology of Organisms. Essentials of an Organic Science of Forms, Mechanically Grounded in the Theory of Descent Reformed by Charles Darwin). Bd. 2,300. Berlin: George Reimer.

Jones, E. (1953), *The Life and Work of Sigmund Freud*. Vol. 1. New York: Basic Books, 1953.

Juenger, E. (1934), Ueber den Schmerz (On Pain). *Saemtliche Werke*, 7:143–191. Stuttgart: Klett-Cotta, 1980.

Strachey, J. (1962), Appendix. The emergence of Freud's fundamental hypotheses. *Standard Edition*, 3:62–68. London: Hogarth Press, 1962.

3

Chronic Pain: Economic, Ethical, and Psychosocial Considerations

ROBERT D. MARCIANI, D.M.D.

The economic, ethical, and psychosocial aspects of chronic pain are important perspectives of a very complex health issue that are often neglected in the search for the cause and the relief of pain. Everyone involved in patient care must show an awareness of these fundamental questions: What does the treatment do for the patient? What is the cost: benefit ratio to the patient, the health care industry, and the service provider? Does the therapy reinforce secondary gain needs, thereby becoming a cofactor itself in the pain syndrome?

Pain is "an unpleasant sensory and emotional experience associated with actual or potential tissue damage or described in terms of such damage" (International Association for the Study of Pain [IASP]). Pain may be a consequence of some psychiatric disorders (Walters, 1961; Merskey and Spear, 1967; Sternbach, 1968) or produce psychological changes (Sternbach, 1974; Merskey, 1980a) by a prolonged experience of noxious stimulation that produces secondary emotional changes similar to those of patients with pain primarily due to psychological causes (Livingston, 1943; Mitchell, 1965; Woodforde and Merskey, 1972; Greenhoot and Sternbach, 1974; Merskey, 1980b). These secondary changes may improve; for example, following surgical intervention for pain relief (Sternbach and Timmermans, 1975). In contrast, abnormal illness behavior can occur when the pain syndrome is caused by a personality or a maladaptive response to psychological stress.

Economics and ethics are two fundamental issues of chronic pain patient care. Separately viewed, the cost of chronic pain treatment is staggering and impacts on many facets of the health care system. The ethics of chronic pain care are often interrelated with economic considerations.

ECONOMIC CONSIDERATION IN CHRONIC PAIN

Economic and psychosocial factors influencing the course of disability and recovery in chronic low back pain have been vigorously discussed. Spangfort (1972), in a prospective study of back pain patients in the State of Washington, found that 18 percent of 1135 people sampled had back pain and 4 percent had previously received back surgery. Three percent of all hospital admissions were for back pain, and 40 percent had had a previous back injury. Seventy-eight percent of complaints were not supported by physical evidence, and 25 percent of all industrial injuries in the State of Washington were related to the low back.

Bonica (1974) reported that 7 million Americans are disabled annually because of low back pain, 200,000 undergo back surgery, and more than 250 million work days are lost. Bonica (1982) also reported that the direct and indirect costs of back pain approached $24 billion per year in the United States. Beals and Hickman (1972) prospectively studied industrially injured patients operated on for back pain and found that only 36 percent returned to productive labor after surgery. Kelsey, White, Pastides, and Biske (1979) reviewed records from an Eastman Kodak plant as part of an industrial medicine study. Over a ten-year period, 35 percent of the sedentary workers and 45 percent of those doing heavy work visited the medical department for back pain.

Kelsey et al. (1979) also referred to a National Safety Council study that reported injuries to the back constituted 15 to 18 percent of all occupational injuries in the United States and that 2 percent of all United States employees had compensable back injuries each year. Carron, DeGood, and Tait (1985) studied 198 patients suffering from chronic low back pain treated at the University of Virginia Pain Center and 117 similar patients seen at the Auckland Hospital Pain Clinic, Auckland, New Zealand. Every patient at both institutions completed a self-report questionnaire prior to beginning comparable outpatient treatment programs. Approximately 55 percent of the sample from each country returned a follow-up questionnaire one year later. Analyses of the results indicated that despite nearly similar between-country reports of pain frequency and intensity, the United States patients, both at pre- and posttesting, reported greater emotional and behavioral disruption as a correlate of their pain. United States patients consistently used more medication, experienced more disphoric mood states, and were more hampered in social-sexual recreational, and vocational functioning. Patients from both countries demonstrated a nearly equal degree of pre- to postimprovement; however, the relative initial differences favoring the New Zealanders remained constant across both questionnaire administrations. At the onset of treatment, 49 percent of the United States sample and only seventeen percent of the New Zealand patients were receiving pain-related financial compensation. At follow-up, patients from both countries receiving pretreatment compensation were less likely to report a return to full activity, although the relationship appeared more pronounced in United States patients.

The differences in response to treatment as a function of country or origin were small. National differences in emotional and behavioral disruption existed both pre- and posttreatment. The authors concluded that several factors in the New Zealand compensation/disability/rehabilitation system distinguished it from the United States system and contributed to lesser life disruptions. Among these were: (1) the availability of worker's compensation unrelated to on-the-job injury; (2) the absence of adversarial relationships among employer, insurer, and claimant—no-fault compensation; (3) the rapidity of rehabilitation intervention; (4) substantial penalties for refusal of alternate employment; and possibly, (5) cultural differences related to functional capacity.

Carron et al. (1985) believed the key to understanding the differences between the two countries was related to the first two of the above-mentioned factors. They interpreted their findings and concluded that the fundamental difference was that the United States system was adversarial compared to the New Zealand entitlement system. In New Zealand it is not necessary to prove injury at work to receive income compensation. An employed wage earner in New Zealand is entitled to 80 percent of preaccident income up to a maximum of $600 a week to age sixty-five. Only at that age does the New Zealand equivalent of Social Security come into effect. An injury "off the job" simply defers the payment of compensation until after the first week of lost employment. By contrast, in the United States, claims are processed much more slowly and often require a claimant to "prove" both the actual presence of an injury or disability and that it was acquired on the job.

Marked differences in rehabilitation programs exist between the United States and New Zealand. In New Zealand there is a rehabilitation assessment team which evaluates patients for occupational therapy within thirty days of injury. Unemployment and disability benefit problems are immediately processed for settlement when disability persists over thirteen weeks or when an obvious totally disabling injury exists. A liaison representative may make the referral for occupational retraining based on a physician's report. The same process in the United States involves a substantially more elaborate rehabilitation apparatus which only occurs after all the physicians involved agree that rehabilitation is possible and that the disability has stabilized.

In the New Zealand system when the injured worker is found capable of performing a new job after rehabilitation, but cannot find a job, the Special Placement Division of the Department of Labor will find employment for him in the private sector or in a sheltered workshop with the government as the employer of last resort. If the worker will not accept a new job for which he is considered qualified, his weekly compensation payments are decreased by the amount he could earn for working. By contrast, in the United States, new employment opportunities may be limited and employment-seeking assistance so variable that the employer or insurer usually has little leverage to return the worker to productive employment. A more serious consequence of the United States system is that the patient is encouraged to maintain his disability status, especially when he has a limited education, low skill levels, and unemployment rates are high.

Singer (1978) found in the ten years between 1967 and 1976, only 2 percent of Social Security disability recipients were rehabilitated. The periodic medical review process so common in the United States has become a barrier to financial rewards one must periodically clear by failure to improve. Miller (1976) reviewed time-limited insurance data and the Social Security system and found (1) that open-ended compensation clearly prolonged disability, and (2) the return to employment was greater by as much as 25 percent if the period of benefits is time limited. These findings suggested that patients who receive worker's compensation or are awaiting litigation after an accident are neurotics or malingerers who are exaggerating their pain for financial gain. Melzack, Katz, and Jeans (1985) reported findings that patients who receive worker's compensation are no different from patients who do not. These findings were developed using a new method of analyzing the McGill Pain Questionnaire (MPQ). Since the MPQ is usually scored by using rank values rather than more complex scale values, the negative finding might be attributable to the loss of information by using rank values.

A study of 145 patients suffering low back and musculoskeletal pain revealed that compensation and noncompensation patients had virtually identical pain scores and pain descriptor patterns. The results showed that patients who receive compensation do not report higher levels of pain than patients who do not receive compensation, and are consistent with the conclusions of other studies. Taken together, the results indicate that the phrase "compensation neurosis" is an unwarranted, biased diagnosis and that disability and pain are not "cured by a verdict." Compensation patients do not exaggerate their pain or show evidence of neurosis or other psychopathological symptoms greater than those seen in pain patients without compensation.

Melzack et al. (1985) concluded that compensation often does not play a significant causative role in chronic pain and disagreed with the description of patients receiving compensation as sly, devious, neurotics and malingerers who are faking their pain to win or maintain comfortable financial compensation for the rest of their lives. They urged that each patient be judged individually, and that all cases not be lumped together under a single label. Using a method proposed by Brena and Chapman (1981), all pain patients were considered according to a defined set of physical and psychological criteria so that four distinct groups were distinguished from one another. Melzack et al. (1985) further conceived that a person who receives compensation is primarily the victim of an accident who tries to cope with the resulting disability, pain, loss of income, and disruption of patterns of day-to-day life. As a victim, he deserves the kind of psychological counseling that is now commonly advocated for victims of disaster such as floods and earthquakes. The sudden disruption in the person's normal working pattern, as well as his customary role in the family and community, would be expected to produce grief, sadness, and bereavement over genuine losses. Accidents, whether large or small, underscore our sense of vulnerability. Even such minor losses which occur after a mugging or a robbery in one's home may produce long-lasting psychological effects. An accident that results in prolonged disability and pain has no less an impact on a person's psychological and physical well-being.

WORK AND SOCIAL JUSTICE

Pope John Paul II has stated that:

> Human work is a key, probably the essential key, to the whole social question. It is in their daily work, however, that persons become the subjects and creators of the economic life of the nation and make the most important contributions to economic justice. All work has a threefold moral

significance. First, it is a principal way that people exercise the distinctive human capacity for self-expression and self-realization. Second, it is the ordinary way for human beings to fulfill their material needs. Finally, work enables people to contribute to the well-being of the larger community. Work is not only for oneself. It is for one's family, for the nation and for the benefit of the entire human family (quoted in Wintz, 1987).

The unemployed, irrespective of cause, do not share this basic fulfillment.

MORAL PRINCIPLES OF ECONOMIC LIFE

Drawing upon scripture and the social teachings of the Catholic church (Wintz, 1987), the U.S. bishops focused on six key principles as a basis for a just economy. The moral principles outlined in the bishops' pastoral message are a reaffirmation of the "golden rule" and can be used to generally outline the rights and obligations of all those individuals and institutions involved with chronic pain, including the patients.

1. Every economic decision and institution must be judged in light of whether it protects or undermines the dignity of the human person. The economy should serve people and not the other way around.
2. Human dignity can be realized and protected only in community. The obligation to "love our neighbor" has an individual dimension, but it also requires a broader social commitment to the common good.
3. All people have a right to participate in the economic life of society. It is wrong for a person or group to be unfairly excluded or unable to participate or contribute to the economy.
4. All members of society have a special obligation to the poor and vulnerable.
5. Human rights are the minimum for life in the community. In Catholic teaching, human rights include not only civil and political rights, but also economic rights.

All people have a right to life, food, clothing, shelter, rest, medical care, education, and employment.

6. Society as a whole, acting through public and private institutions, has the moral responsibility to enhance human dignity and protect human rights. In addition to the clear responsibility of private institutions, government has an essential responsibility in this area.

Chronic pain has a major impact on the economics of the health industry, the legal industry, the social services industry, and the family unit. As such, depending on one's perspective, pain can be viewed as a villainous disrupter of a family's well-being, a welcomed source of legal and medical "business," or a persistent, enigmatic clinical problem that consumes large amounts of a clinician's time, often without a resolution of the problem.

There are many moral and ethical health care issues that are vigorously debated, especially those involving acute or fatal diseases. The ethical questions that arise with chronic pain are much more subtle and less visible. A seriously ill child requiring a bone marrow transplant costing tens of thousands of dollars will receive media coverage and the public's attention, if not its sympathy and financial resources. In the case of the leukemic child, the illness is unequivocally diagnosable and the treatments clear and well accepted by traditional medicine. Substantial health care resources will be mobilized in an attempt to extend the patient's life, if not to cure the disease. Although there might be considerable debate as to the cost-benefit ratio and overburdening of the health care system, consensus would be more readily achieved concerning the attempt to salvage a life that has the potential to be useful and of high quality. Moral and ethical questions are raised when charlatans and misguided therapists offer unscientific treatments of little proven efficacy to extremely desperate, vulnerable, gravely ill patients.

RIGHTS AND RESPONSIBILITIES

Chronic pain conditions usually are not caused by life-threatening diseases, therefore, urgency of care and survival are not at issue. The moral and ethical dilemmas that develop can be examined from the perspectives of the patient, the therapist, and the financial support services. Each of these cohorts must be accountable to the standards of their individual groups and society in general. The responsibilities of each group represent a distillation of religious and societal values that are derived in the United States primarily from Judeo-Christian teachings and the philosophies of the founding fathers.

Rights and Responsibilities of the Patient

1. To have reasonable access to quality health care.
2. To be honest and forthright in recounting the nature of the painful state.
3. To resist overdramatization of the painful condition for secondary gains.
4. To use the health care system prudently.

Rights and Responsibilities of Health Care Providers

1. The freedom of entrepreneurship, business, and finance should be protected, but the accountability of this freedom to the common good must be assured.
2. To develop a strong doctor–patient relationship in which the professional spends considerable time with the pain patient.
3. To avoid excessive use of laboratory tests and paraprofessional personnel as a substitute for patient contact when such a relationship counteracts economics.
4. To avoid treating pain as a diagnosis and not as a symptom.
5. To avoid using therapy as a diagnostic tool.
6. To evaluate the "entire patient" with a thorough, com-

plete history and physical examination that precedes laboratory testing and is not limited to a specialty area of interest.

7. To be aware of the multifactorial nature of pain and practice a coordinated multidisciplinary approach to pain.

Rights and Responsibilities of Financial Institutions and Government Agencies

1. The financial resource institutions involved in health care are entitled to reasonable profits.
2. The desire to maximize profits and reduce costs must be fulfilled by good business practices; reducing or avoiding support for legitimate services for profit taking should be discouraged.

MEDICAL ETHICS

The phrase "medical ethics" has been described as "ambiguous" by A. W. Price (1985) in his paper describing Aristotle's ethics. The ambiguity exists between the application of moral concepts to medical practice, and the application of medical concepts to moral thinking. In Aristotle's ethics the end of action, and the starting point of deliberation, is eudaimonia, commonly translated as "happiness" or the "activity of soul exhibiting excellence, in a complete life" (Nicomachean Ethics, 1098a16ff, in Ackrill, 1974). No one deliberates whether to be "happy," just as no doctor deliberates whether to heal.

Medicine is often an art and less a science. When particular cases, such as chronic pain dilemmas, fall under the art percept, how far can the therapist deviate from accepted standards of care and still be ethically correct? Aristotle excluded grounding practical decisions upon a priori principles. He supported treating written laws like flexible rods used in making the Lesbian molding: the rod "adapts itself to the shape of the stone and is not rigid, and so too the decree it adapted to the facts" (Nichomachean Ethics, 1137b31f, in Ackrill, 1974). Aristotle expected a judge not to be bound by the letter of the law, but "to say what the legislator himself would have said had he been present" (Nichomachean Ethics, 1137b22f, in Ackrill, 1974). Price (1985) concluded further that Aristotle did not intend agents such as judges, to dispense with principles or ignore the laws. Moreover, the internalization of principles is implicit in Aristotle's general conception of moral development, which he adapted from truisms about physical training: just as bodily strength comes from habituation to food and exercise, and the strong man becomes stronger, so too, temperance comes from habitual abstention from pleasure, and the temperate man can do this best (Nicomachean Ethics 1104a30ff, in Ackrill, 1974).

Habituation or the adoption of practices of chronic pain care can be presented in general terms, and prescriptions for care can be outlined for those disease states that are diagnosed and are known to respond to specific treatments. However, principles need, like laws, to be modified in the light of experience. The therapist who knows what he or she is doing will act virtuously intending that such action will produce an acceptable result.

Plato's moral theory interpreted by Mary Margaret Mac-Kenzie (1985) can be applied to the pain therapist as he approaches "how best to live." She stated that individuals always pursue happiness is taken as obviously true. Equally obvious, however, is that we are often mistaken about where our happiness lies. Nonetheless, says Plato, what we really desire is happiness; anything that we appear to desire which turns out badly for us is not the object of our real desire. Thus, desire is for true happiness, and falling short of that goal may be explained in terms of having made a mistake about the objectives.

This view may be too simple when applied to the pain therapist. It ignores the possibility of psychological conflict, financial conflicts, and denies weakness of the will—knowing the better and doing the worse. Plato moved away from the Socratic influence and developed a more complex view of our psychological makeup (Plato 1945, *The Republic*). The soul (the person) has three parts: reason, spirit (the source of moral indignation), and appetite. The pain therapist may have the appetite for a form of treatment that reason tells us to avoid. Plato's tripartite analysis still requires that bad result cases caused by appetite overcoming the prudence of reason count as ignorance, the failure of reason. He who fails to get good results, therefore, is still ignorant, and so acting involuntarily. Reliable success, on the other hand, only occurs once the lower elements of the soul are subdued and reason is in control.

MacKenzie (1985) further interpreted Plato's analysis of the soul. In his early dialogues Plato claimed that the virtues— wisdom, temperance, justice, pity and courage—are a unity, held together by the central function of wisdom. The wise man knows what is right and what is wrong, and does what is right. In *The Republic*, the rule of reason is likewise the cohesive factor; true virtue only and always occurs in the person whose reason is in charge.

MacKenzie (1985) concluded that Plato's moral theory was incompatible with our notions of responsibility and culpability. We are inclined to assert responsibility even for failure, and we exculpate ourselves completely only at the risk of destroying our sense of self. She further repudiated Plato's moral theory on the grounds that it is reductionist dogma that does not fit the realities of moral life.

The Most Reverend J. S. Habgood (1985), Archbishop of York, presented medical ethics from a Christian view. He began with the assertion that all ethics, including medical ethics, has a theological dimension. Specific Christian insights concerning death, suffering, human nature, and human creatureliness can help to expose more fully the moral issues at stake in some of the dilemmas faced by doctors. The real resources of theology are not in some intellectual scheme, but in the awareness of a power greater than our power, a care for individuals greater than our own care, and a forgiveness greater than our own capacity for failure and error.

THE DEFINITION OF A PROFESSION

Originally the word *profession* meant "to profess" religious vows. Medicine was a profession along with the clergy, because its members shared a common "calling," and law was considered professional through a similar educational background in the medieval university.

Allen R. Dyer (1985) described the concept of a profession as it has been analyzed in sociological, legal, philosophical, and historical perspectives. He emphasized the importance of an ethic or service as well as technical expertise as defining characteristics of professions. Some level of skill or expertise is generally held to be requisite for professional status, and that self-conscious reflection on standards of conduct is one of the defining characteristics of a profession. According to Wilensky (1964), any occupation wishing to exercise professional authority must find a technical basis for it, assert an exclusive jurisdiction, link both skill and jurisdiction to standards of training, and convince the public that its services are uniquely trustworthy.

Dyer (1985) stressed the theme of trustworthiness as the pivotal criterion of professional status. The understanding of someone as a "professional" ultimately depends on the ability to trust that individual with personal matters. The various articulate codes of ethics of professional groups all stress the maintenance of the trustworthiness of members of the professional groups through control of entry into and exit from the professional group and disciplining or removing deviant members.

HEALTH FRAUD AND QUACKERY

Health fraud is becoming more widespread each year (Phillips, 1986). Despite efforts of many groups to combat health fraud, Americans spend more than $20 billion per year on products and treatments that are unproven, ineffective, and sometimes harmful. Bogus remedies and quackery are big business in the United States. A report issued by the health and long-term care subcommittee estimates that $4 to 5 billion a year is spent on cancer remedies of no proven value. Another $2 billion is wasted on worthless "cures" for arthritis, and $3 billion more for other questionable treatments. It is also estimated that at least $10 billion is spent on diet products and gimmicks.

The Food and Drug Administration (FDA) conducts many regulatory and educational activities against health fraud (Haffner, 1986). The FDA categorizes fraudulent products according to the risk they present. A direct health hazard is a product that presents an immediate potential harm to the user or patient when used as directed. Indirect health hazards are products that are safe and effective when used as intended but may become potentially harmful when fraudulently promoted for other uses. A third category includes no substantial health risks but major economic fraud or minor economic cheat.

Quackery and arthritis treatment have consistently been identified by government agencies through antifraud surveillance and enforcement activities. Unfortunately, many other pain sufferers are victims of questionable treatment practices that are devoid of reason, logic, and commonsense interpretation of the obvious. The public is decidedly more vulnerable to questionable medical care when the therapy does not necessarily involve a product and when a respected health profession gives, at the least, tacit consent to the practice.

Faith T. Fitzgerald (1983) described her experience with progenitors and adherents of naturalism, health foods, faddism, and "nontraditional" medicine. She readily acknowledged that despair and illness breed illogical and magical thinking; previously, however, she assumed that careful clarification and education in medical "reality" would overcome and replace erroneous thinking. Much to her chagrin, Dr. Fitzgerald discovered three different processes in her interactions with the proponents of "alternate" health care: the true believer, the mercantilist, the American public.

The True Believer

Practitioners in this group are characteristically proponents of "total healing." Judy the Holistic Health Lady ran an establishment for total healing that relied on deep massage, herbs, enemas, thinking the right thoughts, and an amorphous naturalism. She was unshakable in her convictions and would not respond to expostulations about the historical impotency of herbal remedies and massage in major illnesses. Her concepts of health were heavily interrelated with mysticism and religion. Many people attribute sickness to the direction of some divine agent, often as a penalty for bad behavior. Sin for them is "unnatural" action, and sickness the wrath of that offended deity. Holistic medicine, which contains a generous dose of naturalism has been described as "a pabulum of common sense and nonsense offered by cranks and quacks and failed pedants who share an attachment to magic and an animosity toward reason" (Glymour and Stalker, 1983). Fitzgerald (1983) equated holistic medicine with religion and offered an incisive insight into why holistic practice can be so convincing. As a religion, it stands on a different plane of thought than does science. Understanding the fervor of advocates of some alternative modes of therapy may be best accomplished by thinking of them as members of a fundamentalist religion. The arguments of science against their beliefs are doomed to fail. The true believer is not amenable to scientific reason.

The Mercantilist

Anna, the Body-Wrap Lady, owned a series of profitable studios across the country, where she reshaped people with her secret body-wrap solution (patent pending) and techniques. The wrapping purportedly cleansed the body of toxins, reduced body fat, restored youth and beauty, and might lead to weight loss. The mercantilist differs decidedly from the true believer. The former's basic motivating force is not complex neoreligion but greed. The mercantilist is a con artist who does not believe in the efficacy of the "treatment." He preys on the gullible and distorts science to his own commercial advantage. As in quackery through the ages, the true product being sold is hope. If the product does not sell or becomes too controversial, the mercantilist deftly switches to another "cure" without hesitation.

The American Public

The American public is both the audience and the ultimate consumer of the care and services of traditional and nontraditional healers. Dr. Fitzgerald (1983) believes that, for many consumers, magic is as acceptable as reason, if it accomplishes what was promised. Their allegiance is to efficacy rather than logic, and they are generally naive about the scientific process. Testimonials carried far more meaning for them than the fact that the process makes no sense. Many people express the belief that well-being is normal and that if one does not brim with vibrant health, therapy is required. If traditional health care does not maintain a state of complete physical, mental, and social well-being for a consumer, alternative therapies may be sought.

Dr. Fitzgerald (1983) further concluded that alternate health care providers are a reality that traditional therapists most recognize. Some are true believers who cannot be swayed by logic, reason, or demonstration. It is fruitless often to entertain debate. The ethical practitioner must continue to maintain a forceful presence and constantly interject logic, common sense, and the opportunity for patients to return to traditional care.

The mercantilist is the most dangerous because he is motivated by profit. He is more likely to do harm as a result, and often misuses traditional therapy for personal gain. He is more likely to advocate unnecessary surgery and apply therapy indiscriminately. He may be a traditional health care provider whose judgment is periodically skewed by economic considerations. The true mercantilist will always be present and must be vigorously prosecuted.

Patient's Ethical Obligation for Their Health

In contemporary medical ethics health is rarely acknowledged to be an ethical obligation (Sider and Clements, 1984). This oversight is due to the preoccupation of most bioethicists with a rationalist, contract model for ethics in which moral obligation is limited to truth telling and promise keeping. Such an ethics is poorly suited to medicine because it fails to appreciate that medicine's basis as a moral enterprise is oriented toward health values. In Western societies, ill persons are viewed as having a social obligation positively to value health and to cooperate with doctors in order to regain it. Health is a basic human good, the pursuit of which is an ethical obligation which we have toward ourselves and others. In coming under the care of doctors, patients enter a relationship defined and oriented by the importance of health values. Consequently, doctors are not only dispensers of health information or suppliers of contractual services, but they influence a patient's moral health decisions. Patients are free under any set of circumstances to refuse treatment. In doing so, they risk violating their moral obligations to maintain their own well-being. Failure to accept timely treatment may also prolong the cause of the illness, thereby, adding to the expense of the care. This expense will ultimately be borne by all the members of the health care system. The complexities of health care economics is such that we are all morally obligated to use the system prudently. Chronic pain patients who excessively use their health care privileges for secondary gain are behaving immorally.

BRIAN'S STORY

Many of the economic, psychosocial, and ethical elements of chronic pain are illuminated in the case report of a fourteen-year-old boy with severe facial pain (Marciani, Humphries, Maxwell, Costich, Weigert, and Engleberg, 1985). Brian was admitted to the hospital with chronic facial pain and psychosocial dysfunction. His facial pain complaints began one year before admission when, while eating breakfast, he screamed and began to cry because of jaw joint pain and difficulty opening his mouth. The boy was receiving active orthodontic treatment and a possible relationship between the pain and teeth movement was considered. A tentative diagnosis of a temporomandibular joint (TMJ) disorder was advanced and the braces were removed. The boy experienced several days of continued pain. He was referred to his pediatrician, who could find no cause for the symptoms, and referred the patient to an ear, nose, and throat specialist. The otolaryngologist thought the symptoms were a result of the prolonged orthodontic treatment. He then referred the patient to the orthodontist, who disagreed with the etiology of the pain and discomfort and referred the patient to a TMJ clinic for additional evaluation. At that point, the patient was having involuntary opening and closing movements of his mouth, ear noises, and dizziness. A bite guard did not alleviate his symptoms. After several weeks of further observation, the boy was seen by an oral surgeon who injected steroids into the jaw joints as symptomatic treatment in the absence of other clinical and radiographic findings. The procedure failed to relieve the boy's discomfort. A psychiatrist was consulted to evaluate the patient for evidence of an emotional basis for his severe pain and extreme social withdrawal.

For several months the persistent facial pain caused Brian to withdraw from school, peers, siblings, and outside activities. The psychiatrist described a chubby, pale, quiet boy, neatly dressed in jeans, T-shirt, and tennis shoes. His mother had to dress him. His hair was long and uncombed; he had refused to have a haircut because cutting it was too painful. He was pleasant and he tried to be cooperative, but he appeared to be in a great deal of pain. He slurred his speech and frequently clutched his jaw with a worried look on his face. He had a peculiar, unsteady gait, but he never fell as he walked. He said that at times he felt dizzy, which he attributed to the pain medication he was taking. He admitted to feelings of hopelessness, ineffectiveness, and desperation, but he denied suicidal ideation or intent, and he did not appear to have any disorder of thinking.

The family was then referred to a well-known midwestern clinic, where aspirin, a heat lamp, and psychiatric treatment were recommended. After his return from the clinic, the patient was referred to a child psychiatrist and was hospitalized in an adult psychiatric unit at a local hospital for two weeks. He improved, but upon returning home lapsed into the same symptom complex. School was missed often because of the pain, and a pediatric neurologist was again consulted for further examination. The neurologist treated the boy with medication, including methysergide maleate (Sansert), without apparent relief. He was hospitalized again in the adult psychiatric unit of the same local hospital for a week, without any improvement. The family was referred to a psychiatric center in another city, but did not believe the boy would benefit from this transfer. His mother then admitted him to an inpatient adolescent service at a local University Medical Center. A psychiatrist member of the adolescent service who met the patient when he was admitted was immediately struck with his defeated posture. His chin was tucked to his chest and he mumbled his words. The boy had milieu therapy, individual therapy, psychoanalytically oriented group therapy, and recreational therapy for the first eight weeks of hospitalization. At the end of eight weeks with no improvement in the patient, a dexamethasone suppression test and a urinary 3-methoxy-4 hydroxyphenly (MHPG) test were conducted and the results correlated well with depressive illness. Antidepressant therapy with imipramine, resulted in a dramatic improvement of the boy's psychosocial behavior. Tricyclic levels were measured to make sure that he was given a therapeutic dose of imipramine. Clinical response was seen about four weeks from the time medication was started and three months after the patient's hospitalization. He continued showing clinical improvement, and on discharge was able to resume school full time.

According to the mother, approximately $64,000 was spent on the patient's care. Ten thousand dollars in costs were incurred for outpatient visits and the first two hospitalizations, and $54,000 for a 158-day stay at the University Medical Center. The carrier for the boy's major medical insurance first contested the appropriateness of the length of stay but finally agreed to pay.

Brian's case illustrates dramatically that the etiology of chronic facial pain tends to be multifactorial and often obscure. This is clearly evident in Brian's history and underlies the diagnostic, therapeutic, economic, and sociologic dilemmas common to many patients with chronic pain. In essence, the obscure nature of the patient's complaints and the scarcity of clinical findings precipitated a cascade of health-care events that exhausted his family's resources and delayed effective treatment. Of particular importance in this case, and worthy of further review, are the absence of a definitive early diagnosis, the treatment of symptoms, the input from multiple doctors, the absence of a central coordinating doctor, the patient's need for secondary gain, and the peripetetic tendencies of the patient's family.

The patient was examined and in some cases treated by various specialists of medicine and dentistry for presumptive diagnoses of internal derangement of the TMJ, myofascial pain, arthritis, atypical facial pain, and trigeminal neuralgia, without substantial clinical, historical, or laboratory findings consistent with these diseases. Although there was some sharing of clinical findings among the practitioners involved in Brian's case, no integrated, multidisciplinary approach was established. As a result, each specialist, in his turn, had a limited view of Brian's pain complaints consistent with his area of interest, thereby minimizing a "whole patient" examination.

In the process of migrating from doctor to doctor, the patient was offered exploratory TMJ surgery, received a TMJ steroid injection, and consumed anti-inflammatory and muscle-relaxant drugs. With each diagnostic and treatment failure, the patient's family appeared less willing to accept a psychosocial diagnosis (a diagnosis that had been presented very early in the course of his care), and became more intent on finding a new doctor in their search for an "organic" cause of Brian's facial pain. After many months of unsuccessful symptomatic treatment, his severe chemical depressive disease became obvious.

What seems clear in retrospect is that if this patient had had a complete examination early in his care, the skillful diagnostician would have concluded that something more was amiss than pain caused by braces. Fortunately, with the exception of the injection in his jaw joint, he was not subjected to any irreversible treatment.

Fundamental questions of ethics must be considered when dealing with chronic pain patients: (1) Is the standard of practice too remote from the patient? (2) Are ill-advised laboratory tests being ordered as a substitute for doctor–patient contact? (3) Does a time-consuming doctor–patient interaction counteract the standard of care and impact negatively on the economics of practice?

The care of patients with chronic pain is enhanced when pain is treated as a symptom and not as a diagnosis; when practitioners avoid using therapy as a diagnostic tool; when history and physical examination are thorough as befits the multifactorial etiology of pain; when a coordinated multidisciplinary approach to patient care is practiced; and when a vigorous doctor–patient contact precedes laboratory testing. Patients whose history and clinical findings are inconsistent with symptoms and show obvious coexisting secondary needs should have psychosocial evaluation.

Health care is most effective and economical when the doctor treats patients, not symptoms or ailments. Hence, when one finds oneself treating symptoms irrespective of the presenting complaint, prudence demands that the appropriateness of treatment be immediately reviewed.

IDENTIFICATION OF PATIENTS AT RISK FOR UNNECESSARY MEDICAL CARE OR EXCESSIVE SURGERY

Chronic head and neck, generalized musculoskeletal, and abdominal pain may be associated with a variety of psychological and psychiatric conditions, particularly somatoform and anxiety disorders. Therefore, patients presenting with persistent pain complaints must also be evaluated for affective disorders. Unfortunately, a pattern of persistent pain and illness behavior may place a patient at high risk for excessive surgical and medical interventions, because formal psychological or psychiatric work-up and treatment is often overlooked. DeVaul and Faillace (1978) suggested that a particular pattern of persistent pain and illness insistence characterize those patients at high risk for excessive surgery and acute medical treatment. These patients presented with a childhood history of abuse or deprivation, a family history of multiple surgeries, and a history of pain-related surgeries, especially for similar pains; they reported multiple physician contacts and disappointment with therapeutic results. Their present complaints included persistent pain unrelieved by previous medical and surgical intervention, and associated with a conviction of organic cause and denial of any other problem. The complaint of unbearable pain, coupled with the insistence that it was an acute illness that the physician must cure, was followed by nonresponsive or deteriorating symptoms, irrespective of increased treatment.

The search for a method of detecting a similar group of patients presenting with facial pain and mandibular dysfunction has resulted in confusing and contradictory findings. The Minnesota Multiphasic Personality Inventory (MMPI) has been employed in a number of studies designed to identify the personality characteristics specifically related to facial pain patients. Schwartz (1974) and Shipman (1973) reported characteristic MMPI profiles for facial pain patients. However, other studies, which have included control groups, have failed to provide any support for such distinct profiles. Marbach and Lund (1981) were unable to distinguish between functional and organic TMJ and other facial pain syndromes using psychological variables. Similar studies by Moss and Adams (1984) assessing personality, anxiety, and depression in mandibular pain dysfunction subjects did not demonstrate any differences compared to control groups without facial pain. Another study (Marciani, Haley, Moody, and Roth, 1986) involving 130 patients evaluated for facial pain complaints who were also screened for psychosocial variables using anxiety and depression inventories, indicated that there were no significant differences in inventory scores between pain patients and the control group without facial pain complaints.

Taken together, these studies of patients presenting with facial pain suggest that abbreviated psychological inventories do not discriminate sufficiently to separate TMJ patients with pain or organic origin from those with persistent pain and illness insistence of psychogenic origin who are at risk for excessive and unnecessary surgery. These findings also suggest that clinicians who evaluate and treat chronic pain patients must rely on subjective observations and findings to establish a profile of proneness to surgery or other unnecessary care.

The conflicts that often exist between the chronic pain patient and the therapist attempting to treat the patient may be of a magnitude that precludes satisfactory care. The characteristics of patients who have a decreased likelihood of pain improvement must be recognized and considered in the treatment plan for the patient. Of equal importance, health care workers should recognize in themselves and their colleagues those characteristics that interfere with ideal care for the patient. Patient characteristics of illness persistence and surgical proneness which incorporates the recommendations of DeVaul and Faillace (1978) and Brena and Chapman (1981) have been found useful in identifying a complex pain problem (Marciani, Haley, Moody, and Roth, (1987).

PROFILE CHARACTERISTICS OF SURGICAL PRONENESS AND ILLNESS PERSISTENCE

Present Complaint

1. Persistent pain of several months duration that is unrelieved by previous medical, dental, and surgical therapy.
2. The patient is convinced that there is an organic cause for the pain and denies any other problem.
3. Dramatization of the pain state in a manner that is inconsistent with physical exam and test findings of known pain syndromes.
4. Pain is unbearable and immediate treatment is required, therefore, conveying a sense of emergency.

Past Medical History

1. Childhood history of abuse or deprivation.
2. Family history of multiple surgeries.
3. History of pain-related surgeries, especially for similar pains (polysurgery).
4. Multiple contacts with health professionals and disappointment with therapeutic results (polydoctor).
5. Lack of reported relief with large doses of narcotics and other medicines (polypharmacy).

Dependency

1. The patient seeks the implicit responsibilities and privileges associated with the sick role.
2. The patient controls his surroundings and attempts to orchestrate events to facilitate and further sanction the legitimacy of his pain state. Immediate treatment supplies the power of social sanction.

Drug Abuse

1. Patient suggests or demands narcotic and nonnarcotic analgesics.
2. Refused appropriate treatment because of "current circumstances" and requests analgesics.
3. Reports multiple drug allergies.

Disability

1. Seeking job or accident compensation for pain caused by an injury.
2. Seeking compensation for pain related to occupational diseases.

Dysfunction

1. Bodily impairments related to various physical and emotional factors.

Identification of Clinician Characteristics and Circumstances That Place Patients At Risk For Excessive Medical Care or Unnecessary Surgery

Ego

1. Easily frustrated by the failure to "make the patient better."
2. Unwillingness to involve other health care specialists in the care of the pain patient.

3. Misrepresenting the appropriateness of care in the absence of scientifically proven results.
4. Continuing therapy without evidence of foreseeable substantial results.

Competence

1. Does not have sufficient training and experience to understand and diagnose the common pain maladies manifesting in a specific anatomical area.
2. Applies one form of therapy to a variety of pain states, thereby imparting a "silver bullet" mystique to the treatment.
3. Routinely practices symptomatic management of pain.
4. Uses a "shotgun" therapy approach to the pain problem in an attempt to establish a diagnosis.
5. Supports relatively obscure and unsupported simple explanations of complex pain states.

Affect

1. Impatient
2. Not a good listener
3. Intolerant
4. Cynical
5. Dislikes people

Economics

1. Overriding personal circumstances, such as multiple marriages, mega-mortgages, Mercedes, and nonhealth related business distractions that foster a sense of financial urgency.
2. The revenue generated from the care of the patient is more important than the care of the patient.

The dilemma that the chronic pain patient often presents to well-trained and ethical practitioners is not easily resolvable. Patients with persistent illness traits generally should be evaluated for the severity of their disease and the extent of their illness behavior. The case of Brian, the young man with persistent jaw pain and loss of function, illustrates many of the key issues previously discussed.

Brian's dramatization of the pain state (slamming his fists on the table and screaming in pain) was inconsistent with the usual findings of patients with TMJ disease or associated muscle of mastication abnormalities. The pain persisted for several months and was unrelieved by dental, medical, or initial psychiatric treatment. His family was convinced that there was an organic cause for the pain and repeatedly refused to accept a diagnosis of primary psychiatric illness. The pain was so unbearable that it required several emergency visits to doctors. Brian's father was a large, burly man with an athletic background who felt he had little in common with his son. He could not understand the boy through most of his childhood because Brian was so uninterested in the activities his father found enjoyable. He believed that Brian's succumbing to his pain made him something of a "wimp," and he clearly stated that he was at odds with the boy's mother because of her overprotectiveness.

Brian's mother was an intense, hard-working person who was desperate to find a solution to her son's problems. She was thoroughly disgusted with Brian's caregivers and their failure to localize and effectively treat his difficulty. His first psychiatrist reported that the mother read extensively about the problem and, after consulting with her neighbors routinely, had a new suggestion for Brian's treatment with every visit. Over the initial eight months of therapy, she continued to hover around him closely, helping him dress, and making few demands upon him. He relished the sick role and the privileges it gave him in his family unit. His older sister resented the extreme involvement of her mother in his care, as did his younger sister, with whom the boy had an intense sibling rivalry. The younger sister became rowdy, noisy, and aggressive in an attempt to attract more parental attention, which led to frequent fights between her and Brian, who wanted the house to be peaceful, quiet, and hassle-free because his pain was so much worse when he had to feel angry or fight with his sister. Their mother was constantly intervening, telling the younger sister to withdraw from the area, and generally supporting Brian's complaints.

Brian avoided school as much as possible at the beginning of his symptoms. The pain state legitimized his truancy, and the varied treatments he received supplied the power of social sanction. Ultimately, he became totally dysfunctional.

Brian clearly had many of the classic findings of patients demonstrating illness persistence. He also narrowly escaped unnecessary TMJ surgery which might have further reinforced his pain needs.

ECONOMIC AND ETHICAL POLICY ISSUES

The judgments and recommendations on specific economic and ethical issues related to the care of the chronic pain patient have as their foundation the following fundamental principles: (1) every individual has the primary responsibility to maintain his own health; (2) every individual has the moral and legal obligation to honestly report the nature of his pain problem; (3) the health care industry must dispense its considerable intellectual and financial resources when dealing with chronic pain patients in a responsible and efficient manner (Fig. 3.1).

Proposed are several elements that are considered necessary for a national strategy to deal with chronic pain:

1. Improving the education and the understanding of all health care practitioners on pain-related issues (Fig. 3.2).

Reducing the unifocal view of the pain patient by deemphasizing specialty care. Establishing multispecialty pain centers responsible for (a) the further diagnosis and treatment of the unsuccessfully managed pain patient; (b) advising compensation boards on the severity of injury and the degree of functional impairment; (c) clinical research on diagnostic, therapeutic, social, and economic issues related to pain.

2. Policies and programs at all levels of pain issues should encourage pain relief, gainful employment, and economic efficiency.

Creation of a nongovernmental agency that automatically

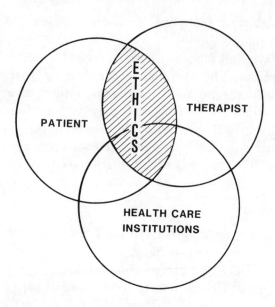

Figure 3.1. The moral and ethical considerations of chronic pain are a shared responsibility.

reimburses costs of patient care and basic income losses to the patient for any accident, irrespective of fault.

Eliminate all legal suits for damages thus obviating the litigious issues related to recovery from pain and disability.

Return to all victims of accidents a significant part of the loss suffered. Establishing criteria for reimbursement of symptomatic treatment regimens and periodic review mechanisms to evaluate the success of the therapy.

TEACHING MEDICAL ETHICS

Socrates and Protagoras centuries ago discussed whether virtues like courage and temperance could be taught (Plato, Meno, Protagoras). Suspicious of Sophists' claims to teach virtues for fees, Socrates argued that if virtues could be taught, teachers of virtues would be universally recognized. Protagoras countered powerfully that virtues could and, indeed, are taught by parents, friends, spouses, early childhood stories, and

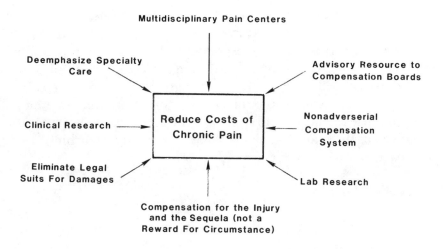

Figure 3.2. Elements of a national strategy to deal with chronic pain.

colleagues. Where Socrates appeared to argue that no one teaches virtues, Protagoras argued that everyone teaches them (Pence, 1983).

Kennan, Brown, Pontell, and Gilbert (1985) surveyed medical students at the University of California, Irvine, California College of Medicine regarding their views on the Medicare and Medicaid programs and on the problem of fraud and abuse in these government medical benefit programs. The students were asked their views on four issues: (1) the quality of various aspects of Medicare and Medicaid; (2) the seriousness and prevalence of physician fraud and abuse in the programs; (3) the punishment that should be given to violators; and (4) the causes and prevention of fraud and abuse in Medicare and Medicaid. They viewed fraud and abuse as serious but not as being widespread. They believed that physicians who violate program regulations are not likely to be punished by official agencies. They favored moderate penalties for violations. Explanations offered by the students for fraud and abuse focused on physicians' attitudes and motivations, as well as on the structure of the Medicare and Medicaid programs.

The information obtained in this study suggests the attitudes and the feelings of the respondents but does not provide sufficient, irrefutable data concerning the ethical attitudes of students overall. It does, however, highlight the growing need for health profession students to have formal training in ethics to enhance their ability to cope with the complex medical moral issues of the day. Johnson (1983) described a teaching approach.

Teaching Aims

The Nature of Medical Ethics. Students must learn how to make difficult decisions.

Awareness of the Problems. Major medical controversies such as abortion, euthanasia, and access to health care are highly visible issues that attract a broad spectrum of views. Ethical problems associated with chronic pain issues are far less dramatic, but of substantial importance. There would be far less inappropriate and ineffectual care dispensed to the pain patient if pain therapists adhered to the principles of truth telling and promise keeping and respecting the dignity of the individual.

The Mechanisms of Decision Making. Students must be taught to analyze problems and how to make decisions. They must be able to distinguish between moral and technical questions.

Information on Existing Ethical Guides and Safeguards. Pain clinics, for example, should establish a rigorous code of patient care and therapist behavior that will eliminate quackery and fraudulent practice; more precisely, acceptable treatment programs for the perplexing chronic pain patient that will have the patient's needs as the primary focus.

The Underlying Basis of Ethics

This, in some ways, is the most important part because ethics must have its basis in a conviction of what is right and wrong. To analyze a problem is not to solve it and after the analysis, if we are to speak of right and wrong, we must know by what standard the right and wrong is being judged. It is, therefore, an important part of teaching to question the basis of accepted practice and to ask why doctors do what they do [Johnson, 1983, p. 6].

Methods

Many health care students in the beginning of their training are more idealistic about patient care than their teachers. These ideals should be maintained by showing students that a harmony can be developed concerning the needs of the patient, the needs of the therapist, and the needs of the health care institutions. We strongly urge a teaching format of small discussion classes held early in the curriculum. Students should demonstrate both written and "mock situation" competency. Satisfactory completion of these exercises should be a prerequisite to advancement.

Summary

The dilemmas that the chronic pain patient presents to the health care system are multifactorial and often without simple solutions. Added to these problems are very complex economic, social, and ethical issues. Patients want to believe that traditional or nontraditional health care therapies will help. Therapists also want to believe that their treatments help, especially when used "their way." Symptomatic treatment of complicated chronic pain states is encouraged by a multibillion dollar health care industry that shields patients from direct costs and offers profits to the care provider. Chronic pain is a disease that affects patients genuinely seeking relief of their discomfort which makes them vulnerable to quacks and misguided therapists. Relief, if not the cure of pain, may be discouraged by secondary gain needs.

More effective treatment programs must be developed for the chronic pain patient. Several studies (Newman, Seres, Yospe, and Garlington, 1978; Herman and Baptiste, 1981; Seres, Painter, and Newman, 1981) of back and extremity injuries have found that the greater the period of time the patient has been unemployed, the lower the probability that the patient will return to work. Based on such data, at least one chronic pain program (Catchlove and Cohen, 1982) has included a direct instruction to return to work as part of its treatment program. Ninety percent of these patients were still working after an average follow-up of 9.6 months.

Results of return-to-work policies suggest that it would be valuable to redirect attention away from the deleterious effects of the "compensation neurosis" and toward the roles of activity and employment in the treatment and rehabilitation of chronic pain patients (Dworkin, Handlin, Richlin, Brand, and Vannucci (1985). White (1966, 1969) concluded "Perhaps effective placement of these unfortunate workmen in jobs which are within the limitations imposed by the pain would maintain morale, avoid concentration of their attention on their complaints and, while keeping up reasonable bodily activities, allow passage of sufficient time for the condition to subside" (1966, p. 56). The New Zealand compensation/disability/rehabilitation system on the surface appears to have considerable merit eliminating adversarial relationships among employer, insurer, and claimant, facilitating rehabilitation and imposing substantial penalties for refusal of alternate employment are reasonable goals for the United States system to consider.

The education and the understanding of all health care providers on pain related issues must be improved.

The moral attitudes of students should be developed by formal training in ethics to enchance their ability to cope with the complex issues involving the pain patient.

REFERENCES

Ackrill J.L. (1974), Aristotle on eudaemonia. *Proc. Brit. Acad.*, 60: Aristotle. Nicomachean ethics, trans. W.D. Ross. Oxford: Oxford University Press, 1925.

Beals, R.K., & Hickman, N.W. (1972), Industrial injuries of the back and extremities. *J. Bone Jt. Surg.*, 54A: 1953–1609.

Bonica, J.J. (1974), New progress against pain. *U.S. News and World Report*, Washington, DC, December.

———(1982), The nature of the problem. In: *Management of Low Back Pain*, eds. H. Carron & R. McLaughlin. Boston: John Wright—PSG, pp. 1–15.

Brena, S.F., & Chapman, S.L. (1981), The "Learned pain syndrome," Decoding a patient's pain signals. *Postgrad. Med.*, 69:55–62.

Carron, H., DeGood, D.E., & Tait, R. (1985), A comparison of low back pain patients in the United States and New Zealand: Psychosocial and economic factors affecting severity of disability. *Pain*, 21:77–89.

Catchlove, R., & Cohen, K. (1982), Effects of a directive return to work approach in the treatment of workmen's compensation patients with chronic pain. *Pain*, 14:181–191.

DeVaul, R.A., & Faillace, L.A. (1978), Persistent pain and illness insistence—A medical profile to surgery. *Amer. J. Surg.*, 135:828–833.

Dworkin, R.H., Handlin, D.S., Richlin, D.M., Brand, L., & Vannucci, C. (1985), Unraveling the effects of compensation, litigation, and employment on treatment response in chronic pain. *Pain*, 23:49–59.

Dyer, A.R. (1985), Ethics advertising and the definition of a profession. *J. Med. Ethics*, 11:72–78.

Fitzgerald, F.T. (1983), Science and scam: Alternative thought patterns in alternative health care. *New Eng. J. Med.*, 309:1066–1067.

Glymour, C., & Stalker, D. (1983), Engineers, cranks, physicians, magicians. *N. Eng. J. Med.*, 308:960–964.

Greenhoot, J., & Sternbach, R.A. (1974), Conjoint treatment of chronic pain. In: *Advances in Neurology*, Vol. 4, ed. J. Bonica. New York: Raven Press, pp. 595–603.

Habgood, J.S. (1985), medical ethics—A Christian view. *J. Med. Ethics*, 11:12–13.

Haffner, M.E., (1986), Health fraud: A growing problem. *Military Med.*, 151:374–379.

Herman, E., & Baptiste, S. (1981), Pain control: Mastery through group experience. *Pain*, 10:79–86.

International Association for the Study of Pain (1979), Pain terms: A list with definitions and notes on usage. *Pain*, 6:249–252.

Johnson, A.G. (1983), Teaching medical ethics as a practical subject: Observations from experience. *J. Med. Ethics*, 9:5–7.

Kelsey, J.L., White, III, A.A., Pastides, H., & Biske, Jr., G.E. (1979), The impact of musculoskeletal disorders on the population of the United States. *J. Bone St. Surg.*, 61A:959–964.

Kennan, C.E., Brown, G.C., Pontell, H.N., & Gilbert, G. (1985), Medical students' attitudes on physician fraud and abuse in the Medicare and Medicaid programs. *J. Med. Ed.*, 60:167–173.

Livingston, W. (1943), *A Physiologic Interpretation of Causalgia and Its Related States.* London: Macmillan.

Mackenzie, M.M. (1985), Plato's moral theory. *J. Med. Ethics*, 11:88–91.

Marbach, J.J., & Lund, P. (1981), Depression, anhedonia and anxiety in temporomandibular joint and other facial pain syndromes. *Pain*, 11:73–84.

Marciani, R.D., Haley, J.V., Moody, P.M., & Roth, G.I. (1986), Anxiety and depression inventories in the evaluation of facial pain patients. *Case Reports and Outlines, 68th Annual Meeting and Scientific Sessions AAOMS New Orleans*, p. 112. American Association of Oral and Maxillofacial Surgery.

Marciani, R.D., Haley, J.V., Moody, P.M., & Roth, G.I. (1987), Identification of patients at risk for unnecessary or excessive TMJ surgery. *Oral Surg. Oral Med., Oral Path. J.*, 64:533–535.

———Humphries, L.L., Maxwell, E.N., Costich, J.F., Weigert, H.T., & Engleberg, J. (1985), Chronic pain: Economic, psychosocial, ethical, preventive and medical aspects. *S. Med. J.*, 78:719–724.

Melzack, R., Katz, J., & Jeans, M.E. (1985), The role of compensation in chronic pain: Analysis using a new method of scoring the McGill pain questionnaire. *Pain*, 23:101–112.

Merskey, H. (1980a), Pain and personality. In: *The Psychology of Pain*, ed. R. Sternbach. New York: Raven Press, pp. 111–127.

———(1980b), The role of the psychiatrist in the investigation and treatment of pain. In: *Pain*, ed. J. Bonica. New York: Raven Press, pp. 249–260.

———Spear, F.G. (1967), *Psychological and Psychiatric Aspects*. Bailliere, Tindall & Cassell, London.

Miller. J.H. (1976), Preliminary report on disability insurance. Subcommittee on Social Security of the Committee of Ways and Means, U.S. House of Representatives, 94th Congress, WMCP, 94–131, pp. 1–61.

Mitchell, S.W. (1965), *Injuries of Nerves and their Consequences*. New York: Dover Publications.

Moss, R.A., & Adams, H.E. (1984), The assessment of personality, anxiety and depression in mandibular pain dysfunction subjects. *J. Oral Rehab.*, 11:233–235.

Newman, R.I., Seres, J.L., Yospe, L.P., & Garlington, B. (1978), Multidisciplinary treatment of chronic pain: long-term follow-up of low-back pain patients. *Pain*, 4:283–292.

Pence, G.E. (1983), Can compassion be taught? *J. Med. Ethics*, 9:189–191.

Phillips, D. (1986), Health fraud in Arkansas. *J. Ark. Med. Soc.*, 83:221–223.

Plato, Meno. Protagoras. In: *Collected Dialogues of Plato*, ed. E. Hamilton & H. Cairns. Princeton, NJ: Princeton University Press, 1961.

Plato. (1945), *The Republic*. New York: Oxford University Press.

Price, A.W. (1985), Aristotle's ethics. *J. Med. Ethics*, 11:150–152.

Schwartz, R.A. (1974), Personality characteristics of unsuccessfully treated MPD patients. *J. Dent. Res.*, 53B:127.

Seres, J.L., Painter, J.R., & Newman, R.I. (1981), Multidisciplinary treatment of chronic pain at the Northwest Pain Center. In: *New Approaches to Treatment of Chronic Pain: A Review of Multidisciplinary Pain Clinics and Pain Centers*, ed. L.K.Y. Ng. NIDA Res Monogr. 36. Rockville, MD. Department of Health and Human Services, pp. 92–111.

Shipman, W.G. (1973), Analysis of MMPI test results in women with MPD syndrome, *J. Dent. Res.*, 82B:79.

Sider, R.C., & Clements, C.D. (1984), Patient's ethical obligation for their health. *J. Med. Ethics*, 10:143–146.

Singer, J.W. (1978), It isn't easy to curb the ailments of the disability insurance program. *Nat. J.*, May 6:715–719.

Spangfort, E.V., (1972), The lumbar disc herniation, a computer—aided analysis of 2504 operations. *Acta Orthop. Scand.*, 1422, Suppl.:1–95.

Sternbach, R.A., (1968), *A Psychophysiological Analysis*. New York: Academic Press.

———(1974), *Pain Patients: Traits and Treatment*. New York: Academic Press.

———Timmermans, G. (1975), Personality changes associated with reduction of pain. *Pain*, 1:177–181.

Walters, A. (1961), Psychogenic, regional pain: alias hysterical pain. *Brain*, 84:1–18.

White, A.W.M. (1966), Low back pain in men receiving workmen's compensation. *Can. Med. Assn. J.*, 95:50–56.

———(1969), Low back pain in men receiving workmen's compensation: a follow-up study. *Canad. Med. Assn. J.*, 101:61–67.

Wilensky, H. (1964), The professionalization of everyone? *Amer. J. Sociol.*, 70:137–158.

Wintz, J. (1987), Economic justice for all. In: *Catholic Update*, CU 0187. Cincinnati: St. Anthony Messenger Press.

Woodforde, J.M., & Merskey, H. (1972), Personality traits of patients with chronic pain. *J. Psychosom. Res.*, 16:167–172.

4

Ethnic Factors Influencing Pain Expression: Implications for Clinical Assessment

VICKIE J. REID, M.A. AND
JOSEPH P. BUSH, PH.D.

Pain is the most common symptom of disease and injury and the most frequently reported reason for seeking medical services (Wolff and Langley, 1967). Diagnosis and treatment of illness and injury are based in large part on the patient's pain report and behavior. Differences in patients' expressions and reactions to pain are a source of interest and concern to investigators across disciplines—psychologists, biologists, physicians, anthropologists, and educators. Physicians and researchers have long suggested that blacks, Jews, Italians, and Puerto Ricans complain more, become overly emotional, and exaggerate symptoms more than groups of Anglo-Saxon and Irish descent (Zborowski, 1952; Zola, 1966), and in general have nonadaptive ways of expressing pain. Several investigators have concluded that these differences are due to variations in exposure to models of pain behavior that embody cultural expectations and meanings attached to pain (Chapman and Jones, 1944; Zborowski, 1952; Zola, 1966). Others have averred that these intergroup differences are due to biological or genetic factors (Woodrow, Friedman, Siegelaub, and Collen,

1972), while others have contended that no real interethnic differences exist (Merskey and Spear, 1964; Flannery, Sos, and McGovern, 1981). Few researchers, however, have investigated the clinical significance of any such differences which may exist either in terms of quality of pain management rendered nor with respect to implications for improving practice in working with minority individuals presenting with pain complaints.

Although there is an abundance of research investigating other factors that influence pain expression, such as age (Sherman and Robillard 1960; Schuderman and Zubek 1962; Abu-Saad, 1984); gender (Notermans and Tophoff, 1967; Goolkasian, 1985); personality (Parbrook, Dalrymple, and Steele, 1973); family response (Vernon, 1974); and socioeconomic status (Larson and Marcer, 1984); there is a paucity of information on the influence of ethnicity (Zborowski; 1952, 1969). Moreover, the few existing studies in this area have yielded equivocal results as to the relevance of ethnic–cultural factors for pain expression, and are plagued with a number of methodological flaws. Despite these problems in the existing research literature and the absence of compelling evidence to the contrary, the prevalent clinical assumptions that blacks, Jews, and Italians exaggerate and complain more about pain symptoms continue. These assumptions are not value-free; describing a group as prone to emotionality and exaggeration is generally a pejorative attribution in scientific and professional circles. For these reasons a critical review of the literature on ethnicity and pain is overdue.

Over the centuries there have been several major theories of pain which have supplanted one another. First, pain was regarded as a passion of the soul, not as a sensation. Aristotle, credited as the first to propose the doctrine of the five senses, did not include pain among them. According to Aristotle (cited in Wolf and Wolff, 1953, pp. 3–4), pain is rather a "passion of the soul" (p. 3), the opposite of pleasure, and has to do with the heart rather than with the nerves and senses. Many subsequent philosophers and scientists have argued against Aristotle's classification and conceptualization of pain, and shifted pain from the category of passion to the category of sensation. In 1794, Erasmus Darwin proposed that pain is the "intensified stage of any sensation" (cited in Wolf and Wolff, 1953, p. 4). In 1858, Schiff (cited in Wolf and Wolff, 1953, pp. 4–5), credited with the first systematic studies of pain, disagreed with early theorists. He argued, based on his studies of the spinal columns of dogs, that pain should be thought of as a distinct sensory process and not as the intensification of other sensations. This notion was further developed in 1884 by Blix (cited in Wolf and Wolff, 1953, p. 5) and by Goldscheider (cited in Wolf and Wolff, 1953, p. 5), who formulated the specific sense theory of pain. They claimed to have discovered specific areas on the skin surface that are sensitive to specific stimuli and yield only specific sensations. According to Blix and Goldscheider, regardless of the intensity of stimulation by other media, each surface area can yield only its own specific qualities of sensation, of which pain is one. Therefore, the intensity of stimulation may be related to perceived levels of pain intensity, but it is the medium and site of stimulation which are important in causing a sensation to be experienced as pain.

Today most researchers agree that "pain is a psychophysiological experience" (Weisenberg, Krendler, Schachat, Werboff, 1975, p. 123). Note that modern thinking has returned in part to Aristotle's notion, in rejecting a purely physical explanation. Pain has moved, at least in part, beyond the realm of sensation and does appear to involve "passions" in essential ways. Pain does not have a one-to-one relationship with tissue damage, but is a multidimensional construct mediated by a number of factors. These factors include intensity of stimulation, anatomical site of stimulation, the physical and psychological state of the organism, the meaning and context of the pain experience, and the way the patient has learned to label and communicate his or her pain (Weisenberg et al., 1975).

This increased appreciation of the complexity of pain has not yet resulted in commensurate increases in the sophistication and precision with which researchers and clinicians measure and discuss pain. Pain may be described in terms of the individual's phenomenological subjective experience ("pain experience" or "pain perception"), or in terms of the total organismic response—including but not limited to subjective awareness ("pain response"). A potentially more precise construct, "pain sensation," refers to the objective sensory detection of painful stimuli. This construct, however, is highly refractory to measurement and is probably inappropriate given current notions of pain as a psychophysiological construct. The more suitable term, *nociception*, refers to the body's neurophysical response to tissue damage (Degenaar, 1979). Pain may also be operationalized as the individual's verbal or nonverbal acknowledgment of pain experience along with his or her description of its intensity, quality, and temporal characteristics ("pain report"). Alternatively, pain may be operationalized as the entire repertoire of observable behaviors occurring in association with presumably painful stimuli, including, but not limited to, pain report ("pain expression").

Authors have not been consistent in specifying which of these or other pain-related constructs they are using when discussing pain. Furthermore, even when they do use more explicit language, it is not always clear that they are defining their terms consistently with other authors. Adding further to the complexity of this issue, *pain behavior* is another construct, different from any of the above, appearing with increasing frequency in the literature. This term is usually used to refer to a class of behaviors commonly associated with pain expression, such as grimacing, moaning, or limping. This conceptualization of pain behaviors as phenomena separate from but related to pain sensation has been useful in chronic pain populations, and may be particularly relevant in research on interethnic pain differences. That is, the "prevalent clinical assumptions" previously referred to regarding maladaptive modes of pain expression in certain ethnic groups may be operationalized as pain behaviors disproportionate to pain experience.

With the current usage of terms such as *ethnicity* and *culture*, one would also expect clearer definitions of these terms. Ethnicity involves far more than race, including traditions, values, and norms. Unfortunately, ethnicity has been defined most often in the pain literature by observed race or self-reported race, as a unidimensional categorical variable. Furthermore, little or no rationale is typically given for selection of included categories, resulting in a mixing of categories at varying levels of comprehensiveness. For example, ethnic categories constituting the ethnicity variable in a given study might include blacks, Jews, Irish Americans, Italian Americans, and "other." A single individual could easily fit into several, or conceivably even all of these categories. Clearly, in any study utilizing statistical procedures based upon analyses of relative proportions of between-group and within-group variance, this constitutes a potentially serious flaw, because the relative amount of heterogeneity within any group is influenced not only by true population variance but also by the experimenter's inconsistencies in defining categories.

Lipton and Marbach (1984) conducted one of the few studies which tried to operationalize and quantify ethnicity or ethnocultural factors. In this study, patients were categorized based on race, religion, and country of origin. In addition, however, the investigators also examined social assimilation, acculturation, and subjects' levels of psychological distress with their ethnocultural status, in an attempt to understand the relevance of ethnicity to pain expression. They operationalized social assimilation as degree of social integration and interaction with members of the dominant culture, while acculturation was defined as subjects' levels of acceptance of the values, life-style, and language of the dominant culture. This approach closely resembles techniques which have been used in the development of "culture-fair" procedures for intellectual assessment (Mercer, 1979). Unfortunately, this study is quite unusual in its sophistication in dealing with ethnicity; most researchers continue to define race categories quite casually and to confuse race with ethnicity.

In addition to these definitional complications, research on the relationship between ethnicity and pain has been plagued by several recurrent methodological flaws. These include method variance in measuring pain response (which may be confounded with ethnic variables), and failure adequately to account for socioeconomic status. Finally, a particular problem rarely addressed in the literature concerns examining intragroup variability. Lipton and Marbach (1984) claim that intragroup variability is as important as intergroup variability. When only intergroup differences in pain expression are recognized, practitioners' diagnostic and treatment decisions, as well as their manner of interaction with the patient, may be influenced by stereotyped expectations regarding the patient's pain expression based upon ethnic group membership. Appreciation of intragroup variability is needed to counteract the tendency toward stereotypic responding by physicians, thereby enabling more optimal care for pain sufferers.

INTERGROUP VARIABILITY IN PAIN EXPRESSION

Chapman and Jones (1944) compared the pain reports of blacks with those of whites in an experimental situation. There were thirty-six subjects (eighteen whites and eighteen blacks) matched for age and sex. Subjects' ethnic origin was determined by self-report and observed skin color. Participants in the study received radiant heat stimulation to the forehead; this technique was developed by Hardy, Wolff, and Goodell (1940). Subjects' pain thresholds (i.e., first report of feeling pain or discomfort) and pain tolerance (i.e., first request either verbally or nonverbally for stimulation cessation) were recorded. Chapman and Jones reported that blacks had lower pain thresholds and pain tolerance levels than whites, as operationalized in this study. An additional group of thirty Russian, Italian, and Jewish subjects (not specified in what proportions) were administered the same radiant heat technique. These Russian, Italian, and Jewish subjects showed pain thresholds and tolerance levels similar to those of blacks. The only difference noted by Chapman and Jones between the added patients and blacks was that these patients complained loudly whereas blacks did not. Chapman and Jones concluded from these findings that differences in pain sensitivity and pain tolerance do exist between ethnic groups and that these differences are due to cultural differences in learned pain responses.

Several methodological problems are apparent in this early study of ethnic factors associated with pain report. Perhaps most obviously, Chapman and Jones failed to measure socioeconomic status, which has been shown since the time their study was published to be related to pain expression (Klee, Ozelis, Greenberg, and Gallant, 1959; Merskey, 1965) and is of course perennially confounded with ethnic differences. More generally, Chapman and Jones failed to examine any dimensions of intragroup variability in pain reports, utilizing only a simple, one-predictor univariate design. Furthermore, the interpersonal context in which pain report was measured (including experimenter race) was not considered. Finally, the authors do not present any empirical evidence for their attribution of observed ethnic variability in pain expression to learned cultural differences.

Zbrowski (1952) conducted what is probably the most widely cited study on cultural factors and pain. He hypothesized that patterns of pain expression are learned as part of one's cultural heritage. He sought to determine differences among the patterns of pain expression, attitudes, beliefs, and the meanings associated with pain by members of distinct ethnic groups. Zbrowski observed the pain reports of four ethnic groups: Irish, Italian, Jewish, and Old American (whom Zbrowski described as Caucasians whose grandparents were born in the United States). In Zbrowski's study, 146 male lower back pain patients participated. Subjects ranged in age from twenty to sixty-four years and were inpatients at a Veterans Administration Hospital in New York City. Ethnicity was determined by the observed race of the patient. Criterion for selection was the presence of some type of pain in the patient. Subjects were observed during a physical examination and interviewed following the examination. Physicians were also interviewed regarding patient pain behaviors. No standard questionnaires were employed. According to Zbrowski, Italian and Jewish patients used emotional descriptions of their pain experiences more frequently than Irish and Old American subjects. They tended to show pain freely by crying, complaining, frequently moaning and groaning, and by being more demanding about procuring pain relief. Irish and Old Americans, in contrast, tended to minimize their expression of pain, were more behaviorally withdrawn when in pain, and preferred to hide their pain expression from others. Zbrowski concluded that interethnic group differences do exist and that these differences are due to different attitudes and beliefs about pain that are a learned part of the patients' heritages.

However, this latter attribution was apparently based on clinical observation rather than on any systematic empirical investigation of specific ethnocultural factors. Although Zbrowski mentioned several other factors such as age, gender, underlying pathology, and socioeconomic status that could have accounted for some of the intergroup variability in patients' pain behavior, he failed to control for these factors in his research design. Further, Zbrowski failed to employ questionnaires that could be statistically tested or to use any other quantitative methods in the measurement of his dependent variables and in evaluating the significance of his findings.

Sternbach and Turskey (1965) conducted a follow-up of this study by examining the responses to experimentally induced pain (electric shock) of housewives falling into each of the same four ethnic groups. They found that the Old Americans were different from all other groups in showing more rapid and complete electrodermal habituation across repeated stimulus presentations. The authors interpreted these findings as consistent with the idea that culturally transmitted beliefs and attitudes regarding pain and its expression can exert a moderating influence on physiological reactivity. These interesting findings emphasize the importance of the individual's understanding of the "meaning" of his pain as well as of the interpersonal context in which pain expression occurs. The attitudes presumed to account for these intergroup differences are aspects of more general cultural values and norms regarding interpersonal interactions, self-control, and interdependency. Clearly, the individual's perception of the interpersonal context will thus be likely to affect pain expression; pain expression will differ between ethnic groups to the extent that they systematically differ in their perceptions of these interpersonal contexts. Based upon this premise, it is quite likely that perceptions would be influenced by ethnic and socioeconomic dissimilarity between physician (or experimenter) and patient (or subject), but this factor has not been systematically investigated.

Zola (1966) conducted a study in which he found differences among ethnic groups in pain expression after controlling for socioeconomic status. He interviewed 196 primarily lower-class patients on their first visit to a Boston, Massachusetts hospital. He compared Irish Catholic, Italian Catholic, and Anglo-Saxons' pain reports. Zola used an open-ended interview which examined both the patients' self-reports regarding their pain and the patients' families' responses to their pain. Checklists and attitudinal scales were also used to measure pain responses. Zola found that Irish patients tended to deny the presence of pain and any effects of their illness on everyday behaviors. Irish patients also tended to localize their pain to a specific anatomical site and to relate it to a specific malfunction. Among the Italians, according to Zola, pain complaints were more diffuse and were not expressed in terms of specific sites and malfunctions. Rather, pain was described more generally as it interfered with daily life. Italians were more vocal, dramatic, and often irritable in communicating with others about their pain. Zola found that Anglo-Saxons were intermediate between Irish and Italians in terms of acknowledging the presence of pain, and in most cases were more similar to Irish patients in expressing their pain in terms of a specific malfunction. Significantly, Zola also found that pain behaviors of members of higher socioeconomic classes tended to become more similar across groups and thus that socioeconomic status seemed to mediate ethnic influences. Although Zola improved on earlier research by controlling for socioeconomic factors, he too failed consistently to define ethnic categories and to examine other sources of intraethnic variability. Zola also did not consider the importance of interactive context as a source of influence on pain expression which could affect members of various ethnic groups differentially.

Woodrow and his colleagues (1972) studied group differences in pain tolerance associated with age, sex, and race. They hypothesized that differences in pain tolerance exist between ethnic groups and that these differences are due to both cultural and biological factors. In this study, 41,119 persons (34,077 whites, 5,393 blacks, 1,649 Asians) were administered the Automated Multiphasic Screening Examination at testing laboratories in the San Francisco area. Race was determined by skin color. Pain tolerance was determined by placing subjects' Achilles tendons between motor driven rods and applying pressure. The point at which subjects requested cessation of the stimulation was operationalized as tolerance level. To control for age and socioeconomic factors, pain tolerance was recorded in a middle-aged sample (forty to forty-nine years old) of 10, 671 subjects, categorized by race and educational attainment (used as a measure of SES) using the same pain technique previously outlined. Through a comparison of group mean scores, it was observed that white subjects showed significantly higher pain tolerance levels than black subjects, and that blacks in turn showed more pain tolerance than Asians. This same pattern of racial differences in pain report was found across all levels of educational attainment. Woodrow et al. concluded that observed ethnic differences in pain report were not due to socioeconomic differences between groups but rather to real ethnic differences. They further suggested that these differences could be due to biological variation between groups as well as to learned cultural factors. However, there were no methods employed to test possible biological influences on pain report, nor were cultural factors measured in any way. In addition, the validity of findings based upon experimentally induced pain for predicting responses to clinical pain is uncertain at this time.

In an attempt to clarify ethnic and sex influences on pain perception and measurement, Lawlis, Achterberg, Kenner, and Kopetz (1984) studied sixty chronic spinal pain patients who were involved in an inpatient treatment program. Measures were administered during the patients' hospital admission screening evaluations. Over a six-month period, data were collected for all new admissions, until researchers obtained an equal number of men and women in each ethnic group. All subjects were middle or upperclass. Ethnic groups studied were white, black, and Mexican American, though method of determining race was unspecified. Medical histories revealed no differences among groups in terms of prior surgeries. An anxiety score derived from the 16PF was used to indicate psychological predisposition to pain response; all groups were equivalent on these variables. Three types of pain measures were administered. First, an ischemic pain test was administered by tying a tourniquet above each subject's elbow to interfere with circulation. Subjects then were asked to squeeze a ball and to designate when the pain equalled their back pain. The second measure was a self-rating of back pain intensity on a 100-point scale. Finally, patients were rated by two physical therapists involved in their treatment in terms of their pain behaviors. Results showed significant differences in pain expression between sexes and across ethnic groups. More important, the study showed that these differences related to the manner in which pain was measured. Mexican Americans reported higher estimates of pain, but this was not consistent with observation by therapists. Caucasians expressed significantly less spinal pain and also showed lower pain tolerance on the ischemic tests. Blacks, when sex was accounted for, in contrast to other studies did not show consistent differences from other groups on any of the tests of pain. On the numerical pain estimate, no ethnic differences were reported. Thus, Lawlis et al. concluded that since findings were inconsistent across pain measures, observed differences between ethnic groups were probably more a reflection of the manner in which pain was measured rather than of real ethnic differences. The authors further speculated that language differences between groups may also relate to apparent interethnic differences in pain perception and tolerance. Unfortunately, there has been little if any research in this area.

Despite studies which have found evidence of interethnic group differences in pain behavior, several other studies have failed to find such disparities. Merskey and Spear (1964) in a study to examine ethnic differences in pain tolerance and reactions compared the pain reactions of twenty-eight white and eleven Afro-Asian (black Asians) male medical students. Subjects' ethnicity was determined by observed race. A pressure algometer, a simple mechanical device that applies pressure against hard surfaces, such as the shin or forehead, was used as the independent variable. Pressure was exerted until pain responses were obtained. Pain threshold and pain tolerance were recorded for all subjects, with pain threshold defined as the amount of pressure applied when the subject first reports feeling pain and pain tolerance as the amount of pressure applied when the subject requests cessation due to unwillingness to tolerate the pain any longer. The experimenters were particularly interested in the interval between pain threshold and pain tolerance. Verbal and nonverbal pain reactions were also recorded. Results indicated no significant differences between white and Afro-Asian medical students in their pain reports or reaction intervals.

In another study, conducted by Flannery et al. (1981), no differences were found in pain responses of black, Italian, Jewish, and Anglo-Saxon Protestant patients. The study was conducted in a metropolitan hospital in an eastern American city. In this study seventy-five subjects who had just delivered babies were interviewed, their behaviors were observed, and they were given self-report measures. These self-report measures assessed the meanings patients attached to their pain, attitudes about their pain, awareness of pain, report of episiotomy pain, and urogenital anxiety (anxiety over the return of normal biological functioning following delivery). Subjects were drawn from a sample of 1500 mothers between the ages of seventeen and forty years. Fifteen subjects were randomly selected from each ethnic group. Criteria for selection were: Old American Protestants for whom Anglo-Saxon identity was traced for three generations; Irish, Italians, and Jews whose parents had migrated to this country; blacks who were Protestants and whose antecedents were born in this country in the rural south. Both of the subjects' parents had to be from the same ethnic background. Subjects were approached forty-eight hours after delivery and data were collected. The Old Americans served as the control group with whom the other four groups were compared. No statistically significant differences were found on the self-report or behavioral scales. Interestingly, a significant difference was found between blacks, Italians, and Old Americans on the urogenital anxiety scale. Blacks and Italians reported more anxiety than whites. However, when socioeconomic factors were covaried, no significant differences remained.

The research literature regarding the relationship between ethnicity and pain is thus far from conclusive. This literature is laden with methodological flaws and contradictory findings, and is marked by a surprising paucity of sophisticated systematic investigations. Perhaps most conspicuous are the lack of attention to the interpersonal context in which pain expression occurs, and to intraethnic group variability in pain expression.

INTRAGROUP VARIABILITY IN PAIN EXPRESSION

While it is important to identify intergroup differences in pain expression if such exist, it is equally important to recognize intragroup variation. Knowledge of intragroup variation may help to avoid stereotyping an individual based on group affiliation. Often the practitioner and patient have different ethnocultural backgrounds. Recognizing only intergroup differences may influence expectations regarding patients' pain behavior based on ethnic group membership and in turn affect quality of care, diagnosis, and treatment. Awareness of variability within groups is likely to reduce this sort of clinical error. Furthermore, awareness of intragroup differences may offer insight into the dynamics that underlie and accompany observed intergroup differences in pain expression. For example, if ethnic group differences in pain expression exist only at certain socieconomic levels, as reported by Zola (1966), this provides a clue toward identifying the actual factors and mechanisms underlying influences on pain expression.

Unfortunately, there is only one study, conducted by Lipton and Marbach (1984), that adequately examined variation in pain expression within ethnic groups as well as interethnic group differences. A pool of 476 facial pain patients from a large metropolitan hospital was categorized into seven ethnic groups based upon race, religion, and country of origin. The categories were black, Irish, Italian, Jewish, Puerto Rican, white Catholic and white Protestant. A thirty-five-item scale which utilized statements representing the physical experience, behaviors, and attitudes associated with pain, as well as behaviors used to obtain relief, was developed and administered to subjects.

Groups were then subdivided by sociodemographic background, social and cultural assimilation, and level of psychological distress or comfort with ethnocultural status. Sociodemographic background represented age, sex, ordinal position in family, and years of education completed. Ethnicity was identified through self-report. Social assimilation was the extent to which the patient socialized with members of the dominant culture and was primarily measured in terms of an individual's social network differing from his or her national origin. Cultural assimilation referred to the extent to which patients identified their own values, language, and life-style with those of the dominant culture, and was measured by using affective, behavioral, and cognitive scales taken from Suchman's (1964) work.

To determine whether interethnic differences existed in pain expression, the investigators conducted an analysis of variance on thirty-five pain response items. A Duncan's multiple range test was used to determine those ethnic groups which significantly differed. Then, an analysis of covariance was performed on those pain response items for which significant interethnic differences were found. Covariates consisted of variables which previous studies indicated were related to pain expression, such as symptom history, signs elicited on physical, radiographic, and laboratory examinations, as well as social, cultural, and psychological variables. Through multiple regression the most influential variables on intraethnic variation were uncovered. Results indicated that the pain expression reported by black, Italian, and Jewish patients were most similar and that Puerto Rican patients appeared relatively distinct from the other groups. Moreover, results indicated that specific variables which most influenced intraethnic variability differed according to ethnic groups. Degree of medical acculturation (operationalized as degree of familiarity with the social roles, behaviors, and expectations associated with medical institutions and settings, and health knowledge) and social assimilation were most influential for blacks; degree of social assimilation was most important for Irish patients; duration of pain was most important for Italian patients; and level of psychological distress was the most distinguishing factor for both Jewish and Puerto Rican patients. There appears to be as much variability within groups as there is between groups, and awareness of these differences should enable more efficient and accurate clinical interactions with these patients.

SOCIOECONOMIC STATUS

Socioeconomic status has been a term used liberally in the behavioral and social sciences to define a number of different concepts, and has become a vague and potentially misleading construct. Socioeconomic status is typically thought of related to social class, which includes occupation and social prestige. Social class is usually thought of categorically; mention is frequently made of the lower, middle, and upper classes (sometimes including subdivisions within these three classes). Socioeconomic status, however, is usually operationalized as a continuous variable consisting of a weighted combination of scores representing educational level, occupational prestige, and income. Because of the complexity of the term, investigators have operationalized socioeconomic status in a number of different ways. This has resulted in inconsistency in measurement and a possible source of variability in findings regarding the relationship between socioeconomic status and pain expression.

Early studies attempted to show that psychological illness, pathogenic, and nonpathogenic pain complaints were influenced by socioeconomic status (Hollingshead and Relich, 1958; Klee, Ozelis, Greenberg, and Gallant, 1959; Merskey, 1965). Furthermore, these studies suggested that psychogenic pain and somatization are more common among people of lower socioeconomic status. It was believed that poorer people perceive and complain more of pain than people of higher socioeconomic status. To the extent that this is true, it is critical to include socioeconomic status when examining interethnic differences in pain expression, since it and ethnicity are perenially confounded. Unfortunately, among the studies that have examined the relationship between pain expression and ethnicity, few have measured socioeconomic status, and among these the findings have been inconsistent.

In the aforementioned study by Zola (1966), socioeconomic factors were found to mediate the relationship between ethnicity and pain expression. Zola found that as subjects' socioeconomic status became more similar, so did their pain expression. In another previously cited study, however, Woodrow et al. (1972) found that socioeconomic status was not a significant factor in the relationship between ethnicity and pain expression. The inconsistency between these studies may be attributable to differences in the measurement of socioeconomic status. In the study conducted by Zola, socioeconomic status was measured by occupation, whereas in the study conducted by Woodrow et al., socioeconomic status was measured by educational level. For many people educational status does not closely coincide with occupational status.

Interestingly, in a study conducted by Larson and Marcer (1984) it was found that lower socioeconomic groups preferred to complain of pain rather than of stress. These authors concluded that observed socioeconomic differences in pain expression are mostly an artifact of language (semantic) and communication differences. Thus, more precise delineation of the interaction of socioeconomic factors with ethnicity in terms of pain expression will require more rigorously controlled multifactorial research in which socioeconomic status is operationalized consistently.

ETHNICITY

Another inconsistency that has recurred in the literature is the classification of ethnicity. Under what criteria are individuals classified as white, black, Hispanic, and so on? In the early 1900s, ethnicity was not recognized as separate from race. Methods used to distinguish race were primarily physiognomic. In *Davenport's Guide to Physical Anthropometry and Anthroposcopy* (Davenport, 1927) as well as other sources (Sullivan, 1928), it was recommended that lip thickness measured by calipers was the best method of distinguishing race. Today, although our preferred methods of measurement are usually more sophisticated, there is still much inconsistency and little attention to validity issues.

Most commonly, visual observation of skin pigmentation or self-report is used to establish subjects' ethnicity. However, ethnicity is a complex, multifaceted construct and casual observations can often be misleading. Ethnicity has been defined as "the values, traditions, customs, and sometimes language which make a particular group distinguished from another" (Lipton and Marbach, 1984). While observed race may serve as a rough classifier of ethnicity, other factors beyond race are critical.

Of the studies that have examined the relationship between ethnicity and pain, few have tried to operationalize ethnicity in a rigorous and consistent manner. For example, some studies combine all Caucasian subjects into one group whereas others subdivide this group; the same is true for Asians and Hispanics. Thus, it becomes increasingly difficult to know which ethnic groups are being investigated. Perhaps with consistent and operationalized classification the relationship between ethnicity and pain expression will become more lucid.

PAIN ASSESSMENT

Diagnostic classification and labeling have at times been used to preserve social inequities and disenfranchisement of ethnic minorities. Diagnoses often carry pejorative implications and suggest limitations in capacity for responsible autonomous functioning. Given the greater vulnerability of minority groups, any important classification system is inherently susceptible to intentional or inadvertent abuse of this sort. The ultimate goal of assessment should be facilitation of optimal treatment choice. Unfortunately, however, assessment historically has been used to legitimize exclusion, discrimination, and inaccurate categorization of certain groups. Assessment methods utilized in the task of pain assessment should be developed with cognizance of these issues.

Differences between minority and white populations have been found with traditional assessment instruments, particularly mental abilities tests (Potthoff, 1966) and personality measures (Gynther, 1979). Minorities have often been labeled as genetically inferior due to their receiving lower scores

(Strong, 1913; Jensen, 1966) or as pathological because of deviation in personality scores. On the other hand, some researchers have indicated that these interethnic differences are due in some part to psychologists relying on tests that are culturally biased (Anastasi, 1982). This is a much debated issue, particularly in the area of mental and vocational aptitude testing.

Most investigators of test bias conclude that many psychological tests do not measure the same attributes across populations. While in some populations these measures are valid, in other populations their validity is questionable, in terms of measuring the attributes which they purport to measure. For example, IQ tests may not measure intelligence with black and Hispanic populations but rather may measure familiarity with white middle-class standards (Kagan, Moss, and Siegel, 1963; Lesser, Fifer, and Clark, 1965). Other investigators believe that biased items are not responsible for test differences (Flaugher and Schrader, 1978) but that differences in test scores reflect the effects of unequal environments and unequal opportunity (Flaugher, 1978; Green, 1978).

Other problems are due to deficiencies in test standardization. Not until recently have the norming samples of mental and personality tests consistently included proportional minority representation. Wechsler (1944) warned clinicians that the Wechsler-Bellevue norms were developed exclusively for the white population. However, the Wechsler-Bellevue, as well as other inadequately standardized techniques, have been widely used to assess intelligence across various ethnic populations, despite these warnings. Examples include the Peabody Picture Vocabulary Test (Dunn, 1965), as well as widely used personality measures such as the MMPI (Hathaway and McKinley, 1967). If the standardization sample is not representative of the subjects the test is used with, then the degree of confidence in test results becomes greatly reduced (Groth-Marnat, 1984).

Cultural bias might also be present in test items, even when an appropriate norming population was utilized in test standardization. Test items often call upon certain attitudes, skills, or facts reflected in white middle-class traditions, values, and customs. Hence, familiarity with white middle-class traditions will increase the likelihood of an accurate response. Other ethnic group members are thereby likely to be placed at a disadvantage relative to middle-class whites in terms of responding correctly to these items.

Previous researchers have often obtained different findings between ethnic groups on the same construct, based on the instrument used in assessment. Particularly in mental testing, changes in the method of assessment have often produced different results when minority groups are assessed (Dove, 1968; Long and Anthony, 1974; Andre, 1976). To assess intelligence in black children, Williams (1972) created the Black Intelligence Test of Cultural Homogeneity (BITCH). Items were chosen based on familiarity with black traditions and information about the inner city. When used comparatively with whites, it was found that white children scored significantly lower than black children on this test (Andre, 1976). This test as well as others designed to measure "black intelligence" have been critized for measuring the degree of familiarity an individual has with a particular environment rather than intelligence (Cronbach, 1978). Hence, this is the same criticism that others have suggested regarding traditional IQ tests. Pain assessment could also be susceptible to various sources of test bias. Ethnic group differences in assessment results may be related to the manner in which the pain is assessed. Evidence for variance in pain expression due to manner of assessment exists in the research literature (Lawlis et al., 1984).

Scott, Donnelly, Gallagher, and Hess (1973) also found that the method of assessment was crucial to information reported by the patients. Indirect methods increased the likelihood of the client reporting useful information, and interviews were rated as more effective. Nondirective questioning that allowed patients to participate actively in the interview increased the likelihood that important social, emotional, as well as medical information would be communicated.

In this study, medical students were trained, between their first and second interview, to use an indirect interviewing style. A number of specific behaviors were used to rate interviewing style. Students were then given self-instructional programmed booklets which were used as a part of the training. Viewing of videotapes allowed students to focus even more sharply on their interviewing styles. Results showed that as students used more of an indirect interviewing style they increased the likelihood of receiving important medical, social, and emotional information.

Thus, the choice of method of assessment is crucial when working with minority individuals. Responses to different methods of assessing pain are not always uniform and observed differences may be related to the manner in which pain is assessed, due to biases in test construction and/or the lack of minority representation in standardization. Sophistication and refinements developed in the mental testing area in response to these concerns should be applied to pain assessment.

INTERPERSONAL INTERACTIONS AND PAIN EXPRESSION

Several variables have been considered in terms of their interaction with ethnicity (e.g., sex and socioeconomic factors) in their influence on pain expression, but little if any attention has been given to the interpersonal relationship as a mediator of interethnic group variability. In other helping professions— clinical psychology, counseling, and psychiatry—the relationship between client and practitioner has been shown to be crucial to the disclosure and resolution of problems (Rogers, 1962). Pain expression usually takes place in an interpersonal context insofar as diagnosis and treatment are often based in large part on the patient's disclosure of pain through report and behavior. Thus, the relationship between physician and patient would seem to be as crucial as in other helping professions, yet there has been little research on this topic in the medical literature (Korsch, Gozzi, and Francis, 1968; Scott, Donnelly, Gallagher, and Hess, 1973) nor has this relationship been sufficiently emphasized in medical training programs. Furthermore, ethnic differences between client and practitioner add another dimension to this relationship which is an essential consideration when examining ethnic differences in pain expression. Even otherwise comprehensive current textbooks in behavioral medicine devote little or no attention to this aspect of pain expression (Levine, Carey, and Crocker, 1983; Feuerstein, Labbé, and Kuczmierczyk, 1986). Because of the sparsity in medical research on this topic, information needs to be borrowed from other areas to investigate this.

Establishment of rapport in relationships depends upon such factors as active listening, empathy, unconditional positive regard for the client, and congruency on the part of the practitioner (Rogers, 1962). These features enhance the relationship and thereby increase communication between patient and practitioner. Without these features, patients may feel uncomfortable, misunderstood, and dissatisfied with treatment (Korsch et al., 1968; Duff, Rowe, and Anderson, 1972). If a patient does not feel comfortable with the relationship, accurate expression of pain and disclosure of other vital information is not likely to occur.

The physician–patient relationship has long been regarded as an important component of good medical practice (Engel, 1972). Although a common goal of the medical profession is to help doctors learn to interact effectively with their patients, this is neither a major focus of instruction nor of research. Historically, treatment of minorities by helping professionals has been appreciably different than treatment of their white counterparts. This has negatively affected the quality of these relationships. Studies from the clinical psychology and counseling literatures reveal that minorities, particularly blacks, are far more likely to be given drugs in lieu of psychotherapy, are seen for shorter periods of time, are more often seen by inexperienced therapists, and are apt to be diagnosed as having more severe disorders than Caucasian clients (Brill and Storrow, 1960; Gross and Herbert, 1969; Cannon and Locke, 1976; Jones, 1978). Yamamoto, Jones, and Palley (1968) looked at 594 consecutive new patients at an outpatient psychiatric service in Los Angeles. Records were reviewed to determine which patients were offered therapy, and if so for how long; all therapists were white. A survey of patients' attitudes was administered at the end of the study period, along with therapist questionnaires. Number of visits, sex, and race of the patient were recorded. Results indicated that whites were more often offered therapy, were seen longer, and were viewed as the most "popular" patients.

Even though attention has been called to these inequities, differential treatment of minority patients appears to persist and is contrary to the establishment of positive relationships between the patient and practitioner. Thus, interactional factors associated with poor relationships may interfere with accurate reporting and may account for some of the variability in pain expression between different ethnic groups. Expectation of ethnic bias in treatment and negative experiences in interactions with white practitioners may make minority patients distrustful of white professionals. Some ethnic group members may amplify or inhibit expression of their pain as a function of these factors.

Frequently, physicians are placed in training centers where they have different racial and socioeconomic backgrounds from the patients they are treating. In most American training hospitals the physician is likely to be white and upper middle class. Racial differences are thus further complicated by class differences. When the patient is culturally, ethnically, and/or socioeconomically dissimilar to the physician, this adds another dimension to the physician–patient relationship which may impact on pain expression.

According to Levy (1985) people who share similar cultural patterns, experiences, and values are more likely to feel comfortable with, and to understand, each other. Similar cultural experiences may serve to increase the chance of a positive relationship. This belief finds roots in the social influence theory proposed by Simons, Berkowitz, and Moyer (1970). These investigators postulated that attractiveness, influence, and source credibility are associated with the degree of similarity between the source and the receiver of communications. It was therefore assumed that people would prefer providers who were similar to those who were not. Many studies have been conducted on the topic of patient–practitioner similarity (Mendelsohn, 1966; Mendelsohn and Rankin, 1969; Grantham, 1973; Atkinson, 1983) and have found support for the hypothesis that patient–practitioner similarity positively affects treatment, diagnosis, relationship, and patient satisfaction.

In a widely cited study by Grantham (1973) thirty-seven black college students in a special program for the "disadvantaged" were used to investigate the influence of counselor–client similarity on satisfaction, self-disclosure, and the therapeutic relationship. Similarity was the independent variable, operationalized as including language, sex, and race. Self-disclosure and satisfaction were the dependent variables, and were measured by outcome questionnaires (Mendelsohn and Geller, 1963; Mendelsohn, 1966; Mendelsohn and Rankin, 1969). Facilitative conditions were defined by the counselors' respect, empathy, and positive regard and were rated by the subjects (Carkhuff, 1969). A multivariate analysis of covariance was computed, using sex and facilitative conditions as covariates. Results indicated that clients preferred counselors similar to themselves, and disclosed more with these counselors.

Others have contended that similarity between patient and practitioner has little bearing on client comfort and self-disclosure, but rather that practitioner warmth, empathy, and positive regard are the key factors. As long as these dynamics are perceived by the client, a positive relationship will be established. The degree to which practitioner–client similarity facilitates the establishment of a therapeutic relationship has been a longstanding debate which probably will continue. When practitioner–client dissimilarity creates cultural and communication barriers that block the establishment of a therapeutic relationship, effective health care is seriously compromised.

Interpersonal barriers between members of different ethnic groups, particularly blacks and whites, have strong societal roots. Vontress (1969) identified some specific cultural barriers. These include language, racial attitudes, and familiarity with medical institutions and settings. Health care providers are as prone to perpetuate these barriers as are other individuals; minority patients as well may interact with the nonminority practitioner on the basis of negative stereotypical preconceptions. These barriers may predispose minority patients to distrust white professionals, and may foster negative countertransferance in the medical professional.

Another barrier cited by Vontress (1969) is language.

Minority individuals often use nonstandard English. In addition, they may use fewer adjectives, modifiers, and adverbs (Bernstein, 1964) which qualify expression of subtle nuances of sensation and feeling, whereas middle-class whites tend to communicate with abstractions and words that specify feelings. Verbalization of feelings is essential in pain expression. White physicians may be left helpless unless they can understand what the patient means while at the same time obtaining the information they need and maintaining a positive interaction.

Unfamiliarity with the setting may also create barriers to the relationship. White middle-class patients are more likely to have many contacts with professionals in their day-to-day lives than lower-class patients. Thus, professional roles and the functions within these roles are more clear to middle-class than to lower-class patients. This ambiguity may disrupt the development of effective relationships between physician and patient, to the extent that each has expectations of the other that the other does not understand, accept, or meet. Each may then be likely to attribute the other's "discrepant" behaviors to undesirable ethnic stereotypes, such as stupidity, irresponsibility, arrogance, or insensitivity, or to racism on the part of the other. Greater cultural sensitivity by professionals is necessary to counterbalance the cultural barriers that may interfere with a positive physician–patient relationship and may account for much of the interethnic group variability in pain expression.

Hence, the potential for barriers exist when people who are different interact. Racial differences are often compounded by class differences. When a physician and patient interact there exists the possibility that these differences may become barriers. Both the physician and patient can enter the interaction with preconceived notions and stereotypes that can impede the relationship. However, it is incumbent upon the physician, as the helping professional, not to allow these differences to become barriers and not to allow the care they provide to be thereby compromised.

It may be the case that pain expression is affected by the quality of the physician–patient relationship and that discrepancies in the literature on interethnic variability and pain expression are related to this. Historically, minorities, typically lower socioeconomic level minorities, have received poorer services from helping professionals than their ethnic majority counterparts. Past treatment and experiences as well as negative expectations may serve as obstacles to the establishment of positive relationships between physician and patient. This, coupled with the dissimilarities prevalent in most medical training centers between physician and patient, further complicates the issue. Minorities often come in distrustful of white physicians, while doctors may respond to the patient with stereotypical racial attitudes, creating barriers in the interpersonal relationship. To the extent that a minority patient anticipates or perceives communication problems and perhaps insensitivity or malevolence on the part of a white physician, he may amplify his expression of pain, both out of frustration and out of an intensified effort to communicate his need for medical assistance to that practitioner. Cultural sensitivity on both the doctor's and the patient's parts can serve to counterbalance interpersonal obstacles and to enhance positive relationship which in turn would improve open and accurate pain expression on patients' parts and accurate evaluations on doctors' parts. Hence, the interpersonal context seems likely to influence how pain is expressed, addressed, managed, and treated.

CONCLUSION

Throughout the research literature there are many discrepant findings regarding the relationship between ethnicity and pain expression. There are as many studies that have found differences as there are those that have not. The main problems with many previous investigations were lack of consistency when defining particular ethnic categories and socioeconomic status, failure even to consider socioeconomic status, and failing to look at intragroup as well as intergroup variability in pain expression. Other problems involve inadequately explained method variance in pain assessment, ambiguities in the operationalization of pain, utilization of simplistic univariate research designs, and failure to appreciate the influences of interpersonal context on pain expression.

Research that examines the interpersonal component when investigating the influence of ethnic differences on pain expression may add to our understanding of these phenomena. Investigators should carefully and explicitly operationalize pain, socioeconomic status, and ethnicity (which is more than just race). Further, research designs that include consideration of within-group variation in addition to between-group differences may offer some insight into the nature of these differences. These designs should not only comprehend the multivariate nature of ethnicity and control for socioeconomic status, but should incorporate sophisticated means for evaluating possible interactions between pain assessment context (including examiner race) and ethnicity affecting pain expression.

One of the primary goals for medical professionals who treat pain patients is to appreciate the phenomenological reality of their pain experience and, by doing so carefully, humanely, and personally, enhance health and minimize suffering. Understanding pain expression is crucial for this to occur. It seems likely that characteristics of the physician–patient relationship can cause variation in pain expression and might account for many of the inconsistent findings on ethnicity and pain expression throughout the literature.

REFERENCES

Abu-Saad, H. (1984), Cultural components of pain: The Asian-American child. *Child. Health Care*, 13:11–14.

Anastasi, A. (1982), *Psychological Testing*, 5th ed. New York: Macmillan.

Andre, J. (1976), Bicultural socialization and measurement of intelligence. *Diss. Abst. Internat.*, 36B:3675–3676.

Atkinson, D. (1983), Ethnic similarity in counseling: A review of the research. *Counsel. Psychol.*, 11:79–92.

Bernstein, B. (1964), Social class, speech systems, and psychotherapy. In: *Mental Health of the Poor*, ed. F. Reissman, J. Cohen, & A. Pearl. New York: Free Press, pp. 194–204.

Brill, N., & Storrow, H. (1960), Social class and psychiatric treatment *Arch. Gen. Psychiat.*, 3:340–344.

Cannon, M., & Locke, B. (1976), Being Black is Detrimental to One's Mental Health:

Myth or reality? Paper presented at W.E.B. Dubois Conference on the Health of Black Populations, Atlanta, GA.

Carkhuff, R. (1969), *Helping and Human Relations: A Primer For Lay and Professional Helping, Vol. 2.* New York: Holt, Rinehart & Winston.

Chapman W., & Jones P. (1944), Variations in cutaneous and visceral pain sensivitivity in normal subjects. *J. Clin. Investig.*, 23:81–91.

Cronbach, L. (1978), Black Intelligence Test of Cultural Homogeneity: A Review. In: *The Eighth Mental Measurements Yearbook*, Vol. 1, ed., O.K. Buros. Highland Park, NJ: Gryphon Press.

Davenport, C. (1927), *Davenport's Guide to Physical Anthropometry and Anthroposcopy.* Cold Spring Harbor, NY: Eugenics Research Association.

Degenaar, J. (1979), Some philosophical considerations on pain. *Pain*, 7:281–304.

Dove, A. (1968), Taking the chitling test. *Newsweek*, 72:51–52.

Duff, R., Rowe, D., & Anderson, F. (1972), Patient care and student learning in a pediatric clinic. *Pediatrics*, 59:839–845.

Dunn, L. (1965), *Expanded Manual For the Peabody Picture Vocabulary Test.* Circle Pines, MN: American Guidance Service.

Engel, G. (1972), Must we precipitate a crisis in medical education to solve the crisis in health care? *Ann. Intern. Med.*, 76:487–492.

Feuerstein, M., Labbé, E., & Kuczmierczyk, A. (1986), *Health Psychology: A Psychobiological Perspective.* New York: Plenum Press.

Flannery, R., Sos, J., & McGovern, P. (1981), Ethnicity as a factor in the expression of pain. *Psychosom.*, 22:39–50.

Flaugher, R., (1978), The many definitions of test bias. *Amer. Psychol.*, 33:671–679.

Flaugher, R., & Schrader, W. (1978), *Eliminating Differentially Difficult Items as an Approach to Test Bias.* Princeton, NJ: Educational Testing Service.

Goolkasian, P. (1985), Phase and sex effects in pain perception: A critical review. *Psychol. Women Quart.*, 9:15–28.

Grantham, R. (1973), Effects of counselor sex, race, and language style on black students in initial interviews. *J. Counsel. Psychol.*, 20:553–559.

Green, B. (1978), In defense of measurement. *Amer. Psychol.*, 33:664–670.

Gross, H., & Herbert, M. (1969), The effects of race and sex on variation of diagnosis and disposition in a psychiatric emergency room. *J. Nerv. & Ment. Dis.*, 148:638–642.

Groth-Marnat, G. (1984), *Handbook of Psychological Assessment.* New York: Van Nostrand Reinhold.

Guthrie, R. (1976), *Even the rat was white: A historical view of Psychology.* New York: Harper & Row.

Gynther, M. (1979), Ethnicity and personality: An update. In *New Developments in the Use of the MMPI*, ed. J. Butcher. Minneapolis: University of Minnesota Press, pp. 454–484.

Hardy, J. Wolff, H., & Goodell H. (1940), Studies on pain. A new method for measuring pain threshold: Observations on the spatial summation of pain. *J. Clin. Invest.*, 19:649–657.

Hathaway, S., & McKinley, J. (1967), *Minnesota Multiphasic Personality Inventory: Manual For Administration and Scoring.* New York: Psychological Corporation.

Hollingshead A., & Relich F. (1958), *Social Class and Mental Illness: A Community Study.* New York: John Wiley.

Jensen, A. (1966), How much can we boost IQ and scholastic achievement? *Harvard Ed. Rev.*, 39:1–123.

Jones, E. (1978), Effects of race on psychotherapy process and outcome: An exploratory investigation. *Psychother.: Theory, Res. & Pract.*, 15:226–236.

Kagan, J., Moss, H., & Siegel, E. (1963), Psychological Significance of Styles of Conceptualization. *Monographs of the Society for Research in Child Development*, 33:73–124.

Klee, G., Ozelis, S., Greenberg, I., & Gallant, L. (1959), Pain and other somatic complaints in a psychiatric clinic. *MD State Med. J.*, 8:188–191.

Korsch, B., Gozzi, E., & Francis, V. (1968), Gaps in doctor–patient communication. *Pediatrics*, 42:855–862.

Larson A., & Marcer D. (1984), The who and why of pain: Analysis by social class. *Brit. Med. J.*, 228:883–885.

Lawlis, F., Achterberg, J., Kenner, L., & Kopetz, K. (1984), Ethnic and sex differences in response to clinical and induced pain in chronic spinal pain patients. *Spine*, 9:751–754.

Lesser, G., Fifer, G., & Clark, D. (1965), Mental Abilities of Children From Different Social-class and Cultural Groups. *Monographs of the Society for Research in Child Development*, 30: serial no. 102.

Levine, M., Carey, W., & Crocker, A. (1983), *Developmental Behavioral Pediatrics*. Philadelphia: W.S. Saunders.

Levy, D. (1985), White doctors and black patients: Influence of race on the doctor–patient relationship. *Pediatrics*, 75:639–643.

Lipton, J., & Marbach, J. (1984), Ethnicity and the pain experience. *Sci. Med.*, 19:1279–1297.

Long, P., & Anthony, J. (1974), The measurement of mental retardation by a culture-specific test. *Psychol. in the Schools*, 11:310–315.

Mendelsohn, C. (1966), Effect of client personality and client-counselor similarity on the duration of counseling: A replication and extension. *J. Counsel. Psychol.*, 13:228–234.

———Geller, M. (1963), Effects of counselor–client similarity on the outcome of counseling. *J. Consult. Psychol.*, 10:71–77.

———Rankin, N. (1969), Client–counselor compatibility and the outcome of counseling. *J. Abnorm. Psychol.*, 74:157–163.

Mercer, J. (1979), *System of Multicultural Pluralistic Assessment: Technical Manual*. New York: Psychological Corporation.

Merskey, H. (1965), Psychiatric patients with persistent pain. *J. Psychosom. Res.*, 9: 299–309.

———Spear, F. (1964), The reliability of the pressure algometer. *Brit. J. Soc. & Clin. Psychol.*, 3:130–136.

Notermans, S., & Tophoff, M. (1967), Sex differences in pain tolerance and pain apperception. *Psychiat. Neurol. Neurochirog.*, 70:23–27.

Parbrook, G., Dalrymple, D., & Steele, D. (1973), Personality assessment and postoperative pain and complications. *J. Psychosom. Res.*, 12:277–285.

Potthoff, R. (1966), *Statistical Aspects of the Problem of Biases in Psychological Tests*. Chapel Hill, NC: University of North Carolina Institute of Statistics Mimeo Series.

Rogers, C. (1962), The interpersonal relationship: The core of guidance. *Harvard Ed. Rev.*, 32:416–429.

Schuderman, E., & Zubek, J. (1962), Effect of age on pain sensitivity. *Percept. & Motor Skills*, 14:295–305.

Scott, N., Donnelly, M., Gallagher, R., & Hess, J. (1973), Interaction analysis as a method for assessing skill in relating to patients: Studies on validity. *Brit. J. Med. Ed.*, 7:174–178.

Sherman, E., & Robillard, E. (1960), Sensitivity to pain in the aged. *Can. Med. Assn. J.*, 88:944–955.

Simons, H., Berkowitz, W., & Moyer, R. (1970), Similarity, credibility, and attitude change: A review and a theory. *Psycholog. Bull.*, 73:1–16.

Sternbach, R., & Turskey, B. (1965), Ethnic differences among housewives in psycho-physiological and skin potential responses to electric shock. *Psychophysiol.*, 1:241–246.

Strong, A. (1913), Three hundred fifty white and colored children measured by the Binet-Simon measuring scale of intelligence. *Pedagog. Sem.*, 20:485–545.

Suchman, E. (1964), Sociomedical variations among ethnic groups. *Amer. J. Sociol.*, 70:319–331.

Sullivan, L. (1928), *Essentials of Anthropometry: A Handbook For Explorers and Museum Collectors*, rev. ed. New York: American Museum of Natural History.

Vernon, D. (1974), Modeling and birth-order and response to painful stimuli. *J. Person. & Soc. Psychol.*, 29:794–799.

Vontress, C. (1969), Cultural barriers in the counseling relationship. *Personnel & Guid. J.*, 10:11–17.

Wechsler, D. (1944), *The Measurement of Adult Intelligence*. Baltimore: Williams & Wilkins.

Weisenberg, M., Krendler, M., Schachat, R., & Werboff, J. (1975), Pain: Anxiety and attitudes in black, white, and Puerto Rican patients. *Psychosom. Med.*, 37:123–133.

Williams, R. (1972), The BITCH-100: A culture-specific test. Paper presented at the meeting of the American Psychological Association, Honolulu, Hawaii.

Wolf, S., & Wolff, H. (1953), *Headaches, Their Nature and Treatment*. Boston: Little, Brown.

Wolff, B., & Langley, S. (1967), Cultural factors and the response to pain: A review. *Amer. Anthropol.*, 69:494–501.

Woodrow, K., Friedman, G., Siegelaub, M., & Collen, M. (1972), Pain tolerance: Differences according to age, sex, and race. *Psychosom. Med.*, 34:548–555.

Yamamoto, J., Jones, Q., & Palley, N. (1968), Cultural problems in psychiatric therapy. *Arch. Gen. Psychiat.*, 19:45–49.

Zborowski, M. (1952), Cultural components in responses to pain. *J. Soc. Issues*, 8:16–30.

——(1969). *People in pain*. San Francisco: Jossey-Bass.

Zola, I. (1966), Culture and symptoms: An analysis of patients' presenting complaints. *Amer. Sociol. Rev.*, 31:615–630.

5

Compensation and Litigation in Disabled Pain Patients

JAMES C. NORTON, PH. D.

INTRODUCTION

Historically, persons unable to work or to provide for themselves have been treated in a variety of ways, depending on the particular era and culture into which they were born. Such persons are subject to both the response of individuals to their condition and to whatever provisions are made for them by the social group. Thus an aged and infirm parent might or might not be cared for by his children, and such caring behavior might or might not reflect widely held religious or cultural values. Should the children fail to care for the parent, there might or might not be social structures in place to provide that care.

Without attempting to survey the variety of experiences the disabled have faced historically and continue to face throughout the world, it is worth making the point that our contemporary American approach to such people represents a new development in ways of relating to the disabled. Though it is admittedly an oversimplification, three paradigmatic approaches might be identified: neglect–rejection, charity–largesse, and entitlement.

The first is, operationally, survival of the fittest, in which the disabled person may be viewed as an object of pity, contempt, or indifference, but in which there is lacking a sense of either personal or social obligation to care for him. The second entails a moral or ethical imperative to care for the disabled which may reflect various value systems, and which may be seen as a family obligation, an obligation of a group bearing some other relationship to the disabled, or a duty of the social group as a whole. Operationally it relies on the largesse of the well, that is, the disabled may or may not be cared for, depending on the discretionary caring–giving of the well. There is, in this paradigm, a shared societal notion that the well *ought* to care for the disabled, but not that they *must*. Entitlement, the last paradigm, removes the discretionary aspect by making disability a legally defined status with certain rights, including care, attached. Thus, once one is defined as disabled, caring is a matter of legal necessity, not dependent on the goodwill of individuals. Since entitlement entails matters of law, the disabled person may have to relate to the legal system as a consequence of his status.

The present situation in our country represents a mixture of the charity and entitlement models. The systems and procedures to be discussed shortly, Social Security and Workers' Compensation, are entitlement programs reflecting a social commitment to care for certain categories of the disabled. Yet there also are many private organizations and individuals offering services to categories of disabled persons, funded by discretionary giving. Many of these are organized around more or less specific age and/or diagnostic groups and have regional or religious preferences. A disabled American thus may be entitled to certain services as a matter of law, and/or be eligible for certain services at the charitable discretion of various private bodies.

There are important and obvious psychological differences among these three paradigms from the point of view of the disabled person. The charity and entitlement situations are of particular interest since, as noted, disabled people in our country may experience either or both. Put simply, charity may put the patient in a supplicant posture and engender feelings of gratitude and indebtedness. Entitlement puts the patient in a petitioner posture in which, if he meets certain objective criteria, certain things will happen as a matter of course. Feelings of gratitude are neither necessary nor appropriate.

As we turn to an examination of the disability compensation systems and the psychological problems both disability status and coping with such systems may engender, it is well to keep in mind that the conceptual distinction between charity and entitlement programs may not be entirely clear in the minds of the patient, his family, or the workers in the disability systems. If an award is viewed by one person as a gift given out of the charity of the giver, yet seen by another as a legal right of the receiver, these represent very different evaluations of the event, and would be expected to lead to very different behavioral expectations and subjective experiences.

Included among those experiencing disability determination or litigation are patients experiencing pain. The legal status of such patients may affect their pain experience, alter their behavior in reaction to their pain, and affect in a variety of ways the way they relate to health care providers. Patients who have been disabled also face a host of changes in life circumstances which may have profound psychological effects. The purpose of the present chapter is to outline the types of proceedings most frequently encountered by pain patients, and to explore some ways in which these circumstances may affect the medical evaluation and treatment processes. We will look as well at some of the psychological implications of disability and how they might affect pain management efforts.

Let it be emphasized at the outset that most patients experiencing pain are not involved in either litigation or disability controversies and hence are not the concern of the present chapter. Those patients who are involved in such proceedings, moreover, do not represent an etiologically random sample of pain patients; that is, the circumstances giving rise to pain syndromes among potential litigants are often different from those giving rise to pain syndromes not leading to legal questions or action. This relative specificity in etiology, usually traumatic injury, must be borne in mind in comparing pain patients with regard to such variables as the quality of the pain experience and complaints, the modes of coping with pain, or the response to treatment.

The legal issues in which pain patients might be involved show some jurisdictional variability, as is true of most legal matters, but the general areas within which legal questions concerning pain are contested are similar throughout the United States. In general, patients become involved in controversy in one of three arenas. First, they may claim disability and therefore compensation from the Social Security Administration (SSA). Second, they may claim disability following a work-related injury and therefore seek compensation through the Workers' Compensation mechanism. In either of these cases, if their claims are denied, they may end up in court. Finally, they may claim pain following injury sustained due to the negligence of some named party or parties, and therefore seek compensation from these parties or, more usually, their insurers. In addition to these three mechanisms, private disability insurance policies are offered by some employers as optional benefits, or they may be purchased individually from insurance brokers. Such policies affect a relatively small proportion of the work force, vary in benefits and eligibility requirements and are entirely voluntary. They will not be discussed here. In order to understand what patients involved in disability proceedings are experiencing, providers should have some awareness of their nature: what are the time frames, who are the participants, how are decisions reached and amounts determined?

To summarize, the contemporary entitlement paradigm of disability involves persons claiming disability via legal processes by virtue of their status. Pain patients may be among such persons.

Types of Disability Determination and Areas of Litigation

The Social Security Administration (SSA) Disability Mechanism

The Social Security Administration provides disability benefits under two general programs. One is the basic Social Security Insurance program which funds retirement benefits in amounts roughly based on years of work and level of earnings. Thus, if a patient who has participated in Social Security becomes disabled, he is eligible to apply for these benefits. Such benefits are in addition to Workers' Compensation payments, to be discussed later, but may be reduced should the combined Workers' Compensation and SSA benefits exceed 80 percent of previous earnings (Price, 1984). In addition, Supplemental Security Income (SSI) provides funds which come from general revenues and are not part of the Social Security Trust Fund (Trout and Mattson, 1984) Supplemental Security Income is not based on past earnings, but rather is keyed to the patient's current economic need. For persons under sixty five, both of these programs require a determination of disability. In the following paragraphs, the general criteria for disability will be described, followed by an outline of the needs tests for SSI, and concluding with a look at the appeals process. The discussion should not be taken to be a definitive guide to the SSA. The purpose is rather to help the reader understand what the system is like in order that he might appreciate what his patient may be facing.

For SSA purposes, "disabled" means that the patient is either terminally ill or that he has a physical or mental impairment that prevents him from doing any gainful work for at least twelve months. This judgment is made in each case by the Disability Determination Service (DDS) in the state where the patient resides. The mechanism is basically as follows: The patient who is claiming disability contacts the SSA office nearest him and is given forms to fill out and brochures to read with instructions. He then submits his medical record to the DDS for determination of his status. This determination is made by a team consisting of a disability examiner and a physician who usually is a private practitioner who does DDS work part time. The DDS physician does not examine the patient, but rather relies on the evidence submitted by the patient's physician. Additional studies may be requested by DDS and are paid for by the government. If the claim is approved (i.e., the patient is declared disabled), the rate of pay is calculated for Social Security benefits. Payment begins and continues at least until the case is reviewed, which may occur as early as six months or as late as seven years, depending on the patient's type of illness. At that time, if another determination of disability is made, payment continues until at least the next review, and this process can go on indefinitely. If, at any of these examination points, a decision is made that the patient is not disabled, he has the right to appeal.

If a patient is disabled for SSA purposes, he may be eligible for SSI as well. Supplementary Security Income is directed toward persons with very limited means and in applying for it, the patient must demonstrate his need. To be eligible for SSI in 1987, a disabled person must have had resources valued at less that $1700 if he was single or $2700 if married. The resources calculation excludes the individual's primary dwelling and its effects up to a value of $2000, his car if worth less than $4700, his burial plot and burial funds up to $1500. Income limitations also are stringent. Income for SSI purposes is broadly defined to include "anything received that can be used to meet needs for food, clothing or shelter." Both earned (e.g., wages) and unearned (e.g., interest) are included, and the aggregate must be less than approximately $350 per month if single and $500 per month for a married couple. These income limitations are calculated based on a number of deductions; that is, such things as need-based state assistance, homegrown produce, and food stamps are not included. Supplemental Security Income brochures include twenty seven exclusions to be used in calculating income. As with disability determination, SSI eligibility is periodically reviewed, and adverse rulings from the patient's point of view can be appealed.

TABLE 5.1

APPEALS STEPS IN SSA/SSI

	Approximate Time to Process	Time Allowed to Appeal
File Claim	2–3 months	60 days
Reconsideration: Case Review, or Informal Conference, or Formal Conference	3 months	60 days
Hearing Before Administrative Law Judge	3 months	60 days
Appeals Council Hearing	Depends on backlog	60 days
Suit in Federal District Court	Depends on backlog	

The appeals processes are similar in SSA and SSI and consist of four steps or levels of review. The first is Reconsideration, which must be requested in writing within sixty days of notice of the original determination. This sixty-day requirement applies to all four appeals steps. Patients who are already receiving checks may continue to receive them during Reconsideration and during the next level of appeal, Hearing, but they must file the request within ten days and sign a request for continued payment. Patients may be required to reimburse the government for continuing payments if they lose their case on appeal. Patients who are turned down on initial application cannot be paid during the appeals process, and patients who lose at the Hearing level are not paid during the following Review and Court levels.

Reconsideration may proceed in one of three ways, depending in part on the nature of the grounds for appeal and in part on the wishes of the patient. Case Review involves a reexamination of the patient's file by someone not involved in the preceding determination. The patient has a right to examine his file and may add relevant information. In Informal Conference, the patient may be present at the review and may call witnesses to support his claim. In Formal conference, the patient may require that reluctant persons appear and be questioned regarding his case. In each of these situations the patient may be represented by someone he chooses, usually an attorney.

If the patient is turned down on Reconsideration, he may request a Hearing by an administrative law judge. The patient and/or his representative may be present at this hearing and may be questioned by the judge. Witnesses may be called by the patient and the judge may examine them. If the patient chooses not to be present, the judge will base his decision on the patient's file. The patient is informed of the outcome by mail, and this is done after each appeal proceeding.

Review by the Appeals Council is the next step for unsuccessful applicants, but the Appeals Council is free to decide whether or not to review the case. If the case is accepted for review, the patient may or may not appear with or without his representative. If the patient loses again at this level, or if the Council refuses to hear the case, the patient may file suit in Federal District Court. At this point, the patient has essentially left the SSA arena and entered the judicial one in which very different rules and procedures apply.

The foregoing is a general outline of the SSA process for determination of disability and eligibility for SSI. With regard to the latter, satisfaction of the needs test is all that is necessary, and medical or psychological input is not relevant. It is worth remembering, however, that from the patient's point of view, the process may be complicated and intrusive, depending on the helpfulness of the particular SSA official with whom he is working. As regards the disability determination, however, there is considerably more room for difficulty, particularly in the area of pain.

Under current SSA policy, pain may be considered in determining disability only if it is attributable to a medically determinable physical or mental impairment, yet there are many patients who experience pain for which no present diagnosis is reached, for example, pain persisting long after healing of a traumatic injury (Fordyce, 1986). In hearings pursuant to revision of the Social Security law, Congress noted that there was considerable jurisdictional variability in appeals cases involving pain and mandated that a commission be appointed by the Secretary of Health and Human Services to study the evaluation of pain in determining disability (The Social Security Disability Benefits Reform Act of 1984). The report of the commission highlights the complexity of these issues and will be discussed further in later sections (Commission on the Evaluation of Pain, 1987). Suffice it here to note that patients with pain present evaluators with complex problems. Such complexities give rise to differences of opinion and differences of opinion lead to appeals. Once the appeals process is begun, time frames may become lengthy, depending on caseloads in the particular office, the skill of the patient in understanding just what is required and doing it properly, and so on. People who work with such patients can cite instances of the SSA procedures running on for months. If the case finally ends up in Federal Court, given the backlog in many jurisdictions, months become years.

Workers' Compensation

Workers' Compensation is a program to compensate workers for on-the-job injuries. It is mandated by law in all fifty states, but there is variation among states as to procedures, who is covered, and what is paid. The program in Kentucky is described here as an example, but the reader should be aware that the experience of the patient in his state may differ (Kentucky Workers' Compensation Law, 1982). Even for Kentucky, furthermore, the following should not be taken as a definitive procedural guide, but rather as an introduction.

Workers' Compensation offers several forms of help to injured workers. The program insures coverage for medical care for work-related illness or injury. In cases where there is temporary total disability, the program offers wage supplementation for the period of disability. If disability is permanent, a lump sum payment may be negotiated, based on the degree of disability, or the worker may receive wage supplementation for a period based upon his life expectancy. Disability may also be total or partial; that is, the patient may be totally unable to work, or his capacity to work may be limited. The payment source is, in most cases, an insurance company, though it is possible, with approval of the Workers' Compensation Board, for an employer to self-insure.

TABLE 5.2

CATEGORIES OF WORKERS' COMPENSATION AWARDS

1. Medical care at the time of injury or illness.

2. Continuing medical care necessitated by the injury or illness.

3. Compensation for lost wages limited to 2/3 of average earnings or a state formula determined maximum, whichever is less.

4. Compensation for partial disability.

5. Death Benefits to cover burial and to support dependents not to exceed the amount the recipient would have received had he survived.

Certain categories of workers are excluded in various states. Under Kentucky law, for example, domestic workers in homes employing fewer than two people, agricultural workers, employees of the Federal Government, or people working for aid and sustenance, such as people at welfare missions, are excluded. The proportion of the workers covered varies among the states with over half the states covering over 85 percent and four states covering less than 70 percent, as of 1980 (Price, 1984). The law applies to all employers meeting state established minimum numbers of employees. All who meet the requirement must have insurance or be declared eligible for self-insurance. The assets of an uninsured employer may be garnished to cover Workers' Compensation claims.

The procedure for obtaining both medical and wage benefits is the same and begins with the injured worker informing his employer of a work-related injury. To be eligible for total disability benefits, he must be totally unable to work for at least seven days after informing his employer of the injury. He is then paid wage supplements on regular paydays at a rate of 66⅔ percent of his weekly wage, not to exceed a maximum figure based on statewide wage rates ($322.19 in 1987 in Kentucky). This continues as long as the person is totally disabled and includes the first seven days if his disability lasts for two weeks or more. Medical bills related to the disabling injury are also paid by the employer or his carrier.

Workers' Compensation also allows for partial disability, but only on a permanent basis. Partial disability is expressed as a percentage of the worker's body and this percent is then applied to what he would be paid were he totally disabled, to calculate his weekly wage supplement. This may be paid for a period of up to 425 weeks in Kentucky. As in total disability, the employer is responsible for medical expenses. Compensation for partial disability shows variation among the states and by age of workers within some states (Price, 1984).

At the time the worker reports a work-related injury or illness, or at any time thereafter, the employer or his carrier may refuse to pay. When this happens, the worker may either accept this decision or file a claim. To file a claim, the worker need not have an attorney. The Workers' Compensation Board usually recommends that he seek representation, however, since there is no doubt that the employer or his carrier will be represented by competent attorneys. To file a claim, the worker fills out forms and submits his medical records and anything else he feels is relevant to show that his injury is work related and disabling. Both he and the employer have sixty days to provide evidence for the file. After it is submitted to the Board, the employer has thirty days to add information, then the worker has fifteen days to add rebuttal. These materials consist in the main of records and deposed testimony of experts. At the end of this period, the worker has fifteen days to submit a brief synopsis of his position, then the employer has fifteen days to submit his, and the worker has five days to rebut. During any of these steps, either side may seek and be granted a continuance or delay. After all these materials are in hand, the Board makes a decision which is conveyed to the parties. This may take six weeks or more, if the medical questions are complicated.

The appeals process for Workers' Compensation may begin with a petition for reconsideration. This must be filed within fourteen days of the notice of the Board's decision. Reconsideration is limited to correcting patently obvious error in the original award; for example, some important piece of evidence was not noted. The Board cannot, on reconsideration, alter its opinion on the merits of the case. The Board will act on the petition within ten days. The next step in the appeals process is to the Circuit Court and must be filed within twenty days of the preceding Board ruling. A judge decides the case based on the briefs submitted by both sides and based on the original record. No new information may be submitted here or later in the appeals process; that is, appeals look only at whether or not the Board acted rightly, given the information in the file. The time involved here depends on the backlog in the particular jurisdiction, and this is true also of the next level of appeal, the Court of Appeals.

The decision of the Circuit Court may be appealed to the Court of Appeals within thirty days of the decision. The Court of Appeals action may be a long time in coming, given the volume of work in many jurisdictions. Appeal from the decision of the Court of Appeals is to the Supreme Court of Kentucky, who may or may not decide to hear the case. There is no further appeal of either the ruling of the Supreme Court, should they agree to hear the case, or of their decision not to hear the case.

There is considerable variability among the states in the appeals process for Workers' Compensation. In Illinois, for example, the initial hearing is before an arbitrator. Appeal of his ruling is conducted before a member of the Illinois Industrial Commission, a body roughly analogous to the Workers' Compensation Board in Kentucky. This procedure is termed a Hearing on Review and its ruling may be appealed to the Commission whose three members include the person who conducted the Hearing on Review. Appeal of the Commission's ruling is to the Circuit Court. Subsequent appeal in Illinois is to a special panel of the Appellate Court which hears Workers' Compensation cases. The Illinois Supreme Court may or may not hear an appeal of the Appellate ruling. This is a fairly recent change in Illinois. Until the early 1980s, hearing of Workers' Compensation appeals at the Supreme Court level was a matter of right. The appeals process in Illinois can be very lengthy. It is not uncommon for two or more years to pass between appeal of a Hearing on Review finding and actually appearing before the Commission, so deep is the backlog of cases. A claimant who proposes to pursue the full gamut of appeals faces many years of unresolved litigation.

The filing of a Workers' Compensation claim and the process of appeal can be laid out as above with relative simplicity. The actual experience of pursuing one of these claims, however, may be very complex and lengthy. The help of an attorney is a virtual necessity, the cost of which must be borne by the claimant. Since the disabled worker is usually short of funds, the contingency mechanism is frequently employed; the attorney collects a fee based upon a percentage of what the worker finally receives. In Kentucky, as of 1987, this amount is limited to 20 percent of the first $25,000 of the award and 15 percent of the amount thereafter, the total fee not to exceed $6500. This is true whether the settlement is lump sum or continuing, and the amount is deducted from what the patient–client receives. In the case of the continuing payment, the fee is based on a calculation of what the total amount will be depending on the percentage of disability and its duration. The attorney is paid at the time of settlement, while the patient's payments are ended sufficiently early to cover the fee.

This then is how Workers' Compensation operates in one state. As noted above, states differ in important respects and thus the patient–client's experience may be quite different from what has been described here. The point to be emphasized, however, is that the process may be protracted and complex from the patient's point of view.

Tort Liability

Tort liability proceedings are what most people are thinking of when they speak of "filing suit." The essential element is an assertion that one party, the plaintiff, has been wronged by another, the defendant. A civil action or lawsuit is the procedure through which such conflicts are ultimately resolved. When pain patients are plaintiffs, most frequently they are claiming damages following accidental traumatic injury which they claim is due to the defendant's negligence. Motor vehicle accidents are examples, as are cases where injury is claimed as being due to faulty products. In these proceedings, the defendant for all practical purposes is almost always an insurance company, rather than the driver or manufacturer. The legal confrontation thus will involve the plaintiff and his attorney and the insurance company and its attorney or, more fre-

quently, attorneys, as insurance companies are usually represented by large firms specializing in such defense work.

If a tort action involves a patient–client's claim that he has
pain due to the defendant's negligence, there are two issues
being raised. First, there is the question of liability—whether or
not the defendant is, in fact, responsible for the injury. Second,
there is the question of damages—whether or not the injury, in
fact, occurred, whether the claimed effects of the injury are
real, and what is reasonable compensation for those effects. If
a tort procedure actually goes to trial, the plaintiff must
establish that both circumstances obtain, if he is to recover from
the defendant. In such a trial, the standard applied is that of
the preponderance of evidence. That is, unlike in a criminal
proceeding, where the culpability of the defendant must be
proved beyond a reasonable doubt, tort liability requires only
that a preponderance of evidence indicates that the damage to
plaintiff is real and due to the defendant's error, in order for
the court to find for the plaintiff.

Many claims are settled without a trial and without even
the filing of a suit. The patient's claims are agreed to by the
potential defendant's carrier, the patient signs a document
releasing the carrier from any further liability, receives his
settlement, and that's the end of it. Problems arise when the
patient claims impairment, loss, or suffering beyond what the
carrier is willing to recompense, or when the defendant denies
responsibility for the injury. At this point, the patient will
usually consult an attorney. The attorney may then attempt to
settle the issue, or he may file suit.

Once a suit has been filed, a process known as discovery
begins. This means that both sides have a right to obtain
information relevant to the case. For example, both sides have
access to all relevant records. Both sides have a right to question
each other's experts and to examine depositions given by such
experts. The patient may be examined by specialists chosen by
either side. The discovery process is time limited in most
jurisdictions, but there is wide variation among them. Furthermore, the stated limit is not absolute; that is, either side may
request and receive an extension. Also during the pretrial
period, both sides may file motions requesting the court to

pursue various courses of action. The judge's rulings on these motions are among the many grounds for appeal that may be invoked after the trial.

After the discovery process is completed, a date will be set by the court for a pretrial hearing. At this time the judge will hear from both sides the nature of the case and will try to get them to agree to settle it without a trial. There may be repeated pretrial hearings as both sides respond to things the other has brought up. If no agreement can be reached through this procedure, a trial date will be set.

All of this can take an extremely long time. During the discovery phase, particular experts may be unavailable for deposition, or one or the other set of attorneys may be unavailable when the expert is available. Court dockets are backlogged in many jurisdictions such that the initial trial date may be many months after the last pretrial hearing. Should either side seek a delay, the next available date may push the trial into the following year. What all of this means from the patient's point of view is that the issue is unresolved and will remain unresolved for an indeterminate period of time. Furthermore, throughout the pretrial period, as both sides explore the possibility of settling the case, the patient must be informed of each defense proposal and, with his lawyer, must decide whether or not to take it. It is not uncommon for cases to drag on for years, then settle immediately before the trial begins.

The trial procedure itself may take hours, days, or weeks, depending on the complexity of the issues involved. The process of case presentation by the plaintiff and rebuttal by the defense is familiar to all of us from television, if not from experience. From the patient's perspective, what is happening is an effort to convince the judge or jury that his injury and suffering are real and that the defendants are at fault. The task of the defense attorneys in our system is to raise doubts as to the veracity of the plaintiff's claims, and/or to argue against the culpability of the defendant, even granting the plaintiff's claims.

Whatever the outcome of the trial, the result may be appealed. The grounds for appeal are generally limited to judicial or procedural error; that is, the appealing party must argue, not that the jury or judge erred, but rather that they were not properly given the information upon which to base a decision; for example, that relevant data were wrongly ruled as inadmissible by the judge, or that irrelevant matters were included. In any case, should the judgment be appealed, the patient usually faces not months, but years of litigation.

TABLE 5.3

CATEGORIES OF TORT AWARDS FOR DISABLED PATIENTS

1. Medical care at the time of injury or illness.
2. Continuing medical care necessitated by the injury or illness.
3. Compensation for lost wages and other economic losses related to the injury or illness.
4. Compensation for partial disability.
5. Compensation for pain and suffering.
6. Punitive damages.

As regards determination of awards, two general categories are used in most jurisdictions: compensatory and punitive. The former accounts for the vast majority of awards and represents amounts calculated to recompense the plaintiff for what he has lost or suffered as a consequence of the injury. Lost wages would be calculated and projected over his life expectancy, for example, were he totally disabled for life. In addition, his pain and suffering may be given a dollar value and awarded over and beyond his income losses. Medical expenses, actual and/or anticipated may be awarded. Punitive damages, as the name suggests, are awarded in rare cases where the defendant is found to have been grossly negligent and therefore deserving of punishment. The standard for awarding punitive damages is strict; the defendant must be shown to have engaged in willful and wanton conduct which led to the plaintiff's injury. If, for example, a patient is injured as a result of surgery performed while the surgeon was inebriated, or if a worker is injured by a tool the manufacturer knew to be defective, punitive damages might be awarded.

PSYCHOLOGICAL EFFECTS OF DISABILITY AND RE-
LATED LEGAL PROCEEDINGS

Having outlined the proceedings which pain patients may experience, we turn now to an examination of the potential effects of such experiences on patients. It must be noted first, however, that, if a pain patient has sustained a disabling injury, his life has been dramatically altered and this must be borne in mind when approaching a person involved in disability proceedings. First, he has experienced a serious traumatic injury, an event involving physical pain and suffering and associated psychological distress. There may be disfigurement, and limitation on activity is a certitude. The long-term implications of the injury may not be known with certainty. Second, the inability to work has obvious and very serious effects on income, but also on self-image. Work occupies the greatest part of the waking lives of most adults. It is a source of identity in our culture as well as a source of income. The sudden loss of this important role profoundly alters the life of the injured person. Third, and related to the loss of the work role, are alterations in other social roles. The breadwinner may cease to occupy this position in the family. The homemaker similarly may be severely limited in child rearing and other domestic activities. Looking at these factors as a whole, it is clear that the pain patient involved in disability proceedings faces problems that go well beyond pain. Any specific effects of legal proceedings, thus, are superimposed on other more pervasive effects related to the injury and its aftermath. After looking at the possible consequence of legal proceedings, therefore, we will return to these more general effects.

Effects of Legal Proceedings

The potential effects of legal actions are several. First, the fact that they may be lengthy means that, for some patients, the disposition of their financial circumstances may be unknown for a long time. This, like any lingering uncertainty, is, for many people, inherently anxiety arousing. If one is unable to work and, perhaps, unable to pay the rent, the protracted nature of some disability determinations can be excruciating. Second, the issues of litigation may concern argument as to the extent of the patient's disability and/or his suffering. In the most extreme case, it may be suggested that the patient is frankly malingering; that is stating that he is experiencing pain when he is not, or exaggerating the extent to which his pain limits his ability to work. Alternatively, in a tort proceeding it may be argued that the patient's injury and suffering deserve lesser compensation than the patient believes is just. Finally, there is the fact that, for some patients, the proceedings may be difficult to understand. This is especially true in tort cases where the rules which govern the legal process are understood by lawyers, but not by most laymen. The patient thus finds himself in an arena where decisions of great import to his life are to be reached through processes which are complex and, perhaps, beyond his full understanding.

With regard to the sometimes protracted nature of pain-related legal proceedings, there seems little more to say after pointing it out. Lack of resolution is distressing to most people and, the more vitally important the unresolved issue, the greater the distress. This might be seen as a particular instance of the more general phenomenon of perceived lack of control over important events leading to negative feeling states (Miller and Norman, 1979). In legal matters, the course of the process is punctuated by various events; hearings, depositions, perhaps ultimately a trial, possible appeals, and so on. For the person whose livelihood hangs in the balance, each of these events is a potential occasion for anxiety. A practitioner working with such a patient in pain management should be aware of the fact that the patient's experience is colored by these events as they stretch into an uncertain future. Psychological support for the patient and his family may be an important part of treatment beyond what can be done for pain. If the patient's mind "seems to be elsewhere," it may well be off reliving a deposition. Demonstration of empathy and understanding on the part of the practitioner for the patient's ongoing legal difficulties may be helpful to the patient and may also contribute to the therapeutic alliance with regard to compliance with pain management activities.

Situations in which the patient's extent of disability is questioned create potentially very unpleasant experiences for the patient (Merskey, 1986). These instances are the exception rather than the rule; relevant experts agree that most people who claim to be disabled clearly are disabled. In the majority of cases, representatives of the patient and payer negotiate a fair settlement, and the matter is disposed of as regards compensation. It should be added here, however, that settlement of the claim does not eliminate the residual problems such patients face over the course of their lives, and these will be addressed below. For such patients, though, at least the disability itself and its just compensation are agreed to. Trouble arises when the disability is challenged. As described earlier, claims may be denied by SSA or in Workers' Compensation hearings, or the insurer may decline to settle, leading to a tort proceeding. When this happens, the patient's case enters one or more of the procedural systems outlined above and it is thus, for some period, pending.

Questions regarding the degree to which pending litigation affects the pain patient's experience and behavior have been debated for years (Melzack, Katz, and Jeans, 1985), as have questions regarding the role of ongoing compensation in maintaining pain and disability (Strang, 1985). Work by Miller (1961) has been frequently cited in support of the idea that pending litigation limits treatment progress and that resolution of claims leads to improvement, whatever the outcome. Contrary findings with regard to both these issues have been reported (Mendelson, 1984) and, according to Merskey (1986) predominate. A recent study by Dworkin, Handlin, Richlin, Brand, and Vannucci (1985) suggests that employment status is a more important variable than either pending or achieved compensation in predicting response to treatment.

Given the complex and variable nature of the effects of litigation and compensation on patient behavior, it is surprising to note the confidence with which many practitioners characterize litigating patients. Beals (1984), for example, states a series of paradoxes in the compensation laws as follows: "Paradox I, Financial compensation discourages return to work. . . . Paradox II, The appeal process increases disability. . . . Paradox III, An open claim inhibits return to work" (pp. 235–236). One can cite data to support these assertions, and the author does, yet contrary findings also abound. The point I would like to make here is that the widespread expectation that such concepts have relevance in virtually all cases may, itself, color the patient–provider transaction. This may be a problem even when the expectation is correct, that is, when the patient's behavior is being influenced by the financial contingency, but it is especially problematic when the expectation is in error. Thus, pending litigation may or may not materially affect the patient's experience of his pain, his reaction to it, and his relations with providers. To the extent providers expect such effects, however, their relations with the patient may be colored, and this operates both in evaluation and treatment contexts.

With regard to evaluation, in tort proceedings it is characteristic for both plaintiff and defense attorneys to employ experts, usually physicians, but occasionally psychologists, who testify as to the validity and extent of the patient's pain-related disability. In order to do this, the expert must evaluate the patient, usually by examining him and reviewing his medical records. This evaluation process may be experienced by the patient as neutral to friendly in the case of the plaintiff expert, and as neutral to hostile in the case of the defense expert. Given the contest structure of our judicial proceedings, this is true, even assuming both experts approach the evaluation absolutely without prejudice, and it may alter the patient's behavior in a number of ways. For example, his ability to be self-revealing, his confidence in the sympathy of the practitioner, and his comfort in the evaluation setting is likely to be greater in the presence of the plaintiff expert as opposed to the defense. This is important because it suggests that the experts, in fact, see different sides of the patient, that the role of the particular evaluator to some degree alters that which is to be evaluated, namely, the patient and his pain. This bears some similarity to the problem originally noted in physical science; that the process of measurement alters what is being measured, thus throwing into question the possibility of objectivity. In the present situation, furthermore, the particular person making the measurement may *differentially* alter the thing being measured, depending on his role in the litigation scenario.

The treating provider, under these conditions, may be working at cross-purposes with a contingency which operates against minimizing the effects and experience of pain. Clinically, this may express itself in irregular compliance and slow progress as the patient experiences more pain than he might, were he able to focus his attention away from his pain. This need not operate at a conscious level, and the patient does not intend its result, yet it may adversely affect treatment during the period of pending litigation. It should be reiterated here, however, that the provider must not assume that the patient's behavior is so determined since, in the majority of cases, it is not (Mendelson, 1982).

Granting the caveats mentioned above, it must be admitted that there may be cases in which the patient makes a conscious choice to maximize his apparent disability for the sake of compensation, just as there may be cases in which potential payers are aware of the reality of the patient's disability, yet minimize it to avoid making payment. Crass, rather cynical profit motives would seem to animate the latter situation, if it occurs. With regard to the former, however, the patient's behavior raises questions. Profit may be the apparent motive, but we must wonder what sort of circumstances give rise to an adaptation in this person such that being disabled is preferable to recovery and return to work. In the vast majority of these cases, the potential financial gains for pain patients are not great; they are compensatory and limited in magnitude. Thus, if a treating provider becomes convinced that a patient is actually malingering, this observation explains very little. It should lead to an exploration of the patient's life circumstances, which apparently put the patient in such a position that feigning disability is the best adaptation he can make to his life as he sees it (Ludwig, 1980).

As noted, malingering is a rarity in any case, a point emphasized by the Commission on the Evaluation of Pain (1987). From the patient's point of view, therefore, the claim is valid and his or her subjective experience of pain and discomfort confirms this. If there is a legal proceeding, if the claim is denied, or if a suit must be filed, then someone in a position of some power in relation to the patient, the potential payer, is challenging some aspect of the claim. This will be aversive for the patient to varying degrees, dependent upon the basis of the challenge and the specifics of the case. At a minimum, the challenge delays resolution and compensation which, in themselves, are troubling. If the basis of the denial is a disagreement over either liability or the amount of the award, it seems likely that the patient's experience will be less potentially psychologically damaging than if it is alleged that he is faking or exaggerating.

It is worth noting that pain patients are in a particularly vulnerable position in these situations because, to the extent that pain is claimed as a basis for compensation, to that extent the claim rests on a subjective state which is only partially correlated with objective findings (Commission on the Evaluation of Pain, 1987). Examination of subjective states and underlying motives may fall to the psychiatrist or psychologist. The fact is that such assessments are difficult if not impossible to make with surety and experts will often disagree. The patient may thus see his fate resting on the findings of an inexact science whose practitioners probe and opine concerning areas about which he feels, with some justification, that he knows better than they do (i.e., his own subjective state). Popularly held misconceptions that only "crazy people" are seen by psychiatrists or psychologists do not make such examinations any easier for the patient.

For the treating provider, the point made above regarding duration of the proceedings can be reiterated here. These patients may suffer considerable anxiety and distress if they perceive that their honesty or sanity is being questioned. The empathy and support of a provider may be helpful, particularly if he is viewed as expert in the areas under question. To the extent the patient and therapist have established a trusting and open relationship, the therapist can play an especially important and reassuring role, should the patient's case involve allegations of malingering or exaggeration.

Turning last to the issue of the complexity of the systems, the fact is that some patients will experience these systems as procedural labyrinths whose rules are obscure and whose wheels grind slowly. The outlines presented earlier convey a simplicity that may not be reflected in the actual workings of these systems for particular patients. In part because of this complexity, the patient often must rely on the help of an attorney as he pursues his claim. This puts him in a state of relative dependency on his attorney, much as any patient, when ill, is dependent on his doctor. The thinking of Mandler (1972) regarding the relationship between lack of perceived control of events and the experience of anxiety may be relevant here, as may Seligman's (1975) work on feelings of helplessness and consequent depression. For some people, the experience of having to rely so heavily on the advice and judgment of another is difficult, no matter how trustworthy the confidant. Should the case go badly, there are many opportunities for the patient to torment himself (and perhaps his attorney) with second guesses and ruminations. Would a different attorney have been of more help? Should he have accepted an earlier offer from the defense? There is no end to such questions, and often no point, but they may preoccupy the patient and interfere with his ability to pursue the more important tasks of rehabilitation and adaptation. One of the factors that contributes to such questioning is the fact that the patient is a layman and is therefore to some degree subjectively helpless as his case moves through the system. The practitioner working with such a patient may be helpful to him by providing realistic feedback and a context in which the patient can share his doubts and concerns. The purpose here is not to give legal advice, of course, but rather to help the patient sort out realistic from unrealistic questions.

Ongoing Problems of the Disabled Pain Patient

The patients we have been discussing share the fact that they have sustained an injury severe enough to prevent them from working, at least at the level they worked before injury. They have worked their way through one or more of the compensation mechanisms and have come out the other end with some sort of resolution. For many of them, the result is a

monthly disability check which is well below their premorbid
level of income. For others, a lesser level of compensation based
on a judgment of partial disability may have been achieved,
while others will receive only SSA support. Patients involved in
a successful tort proceeding may have received larger sums to
compensate them for lost income commensurate with realistic
expectations, given their earning history. It is important to
remember, however, that, from the patient's point of view, the
optimal outcome he can hope for if the system works as it is
supposed to is a sum zero; he is compensated for his losses,
possibly for his pain and suffering, and, with the rare exception
of punitive damages, that is all. Furthermore, this optimal
outcome is, for most patients, not achieved. In fact, for some no
compensation may be forthcoming.

Given these realities, a provider working with disabled
pain patients after resolution of their cases faces people who
may have a host of difficulties of which pain is only one, and
often not the most disturbing. It may be useful, therefore, to
review some of these areas of potential difficulty, both because
they may impair the patient's ability to pursue pain management strategies and because they deserve attention in their own
right. Other chapters in the present volume discuss specific
pain interventions in detail, so there is no need to review them
again. The purpose here is rather to note that, in working with
patients who are disabled, these interventions may need to be
modified or fine-tuned to account for the special needs of such
patients.

Among the most difficult adjustments patients must make
concerns adaptation to the earlier mentioned role changes
consequent to loss of accustomed employment. There is a
sizable literature on the psychological and medical consequences of unemployment, and it has relevance here (Cobb,
1974). These people suffer an increased incidence of a number
of stress-related medical illnesses, show evidence of depression
and anxiety, and frequently encounter marital difficulties,
including sexual dysfunction, estrangement, and divorce.
These same symptoms may be seen following work loss due to
disability (Heinrich, Cohen, and Nabiloff, 1982). In these
patients, furthermore, there usually is lacking the peer support

which is seen in industrial lay off unemployment where many members of community may be similarly affected (Cobb, 1976), and social support has been reported to ameliorate the negative health consequences of unemployment (Gore, 1978).

These observations suggest several potentially useful avenues of intervention. First, vocational rehabilitation should play a pivotal role in the long-term management of disabled pain patients (Derebery and Tullis, 1986). If the patient is unable ever to return to his accustomed employment, thorough exploration of alternatives is essential, and provision of such vocational services is often part of Workers' Compensation programs. If, for whatever reason, a particular patient has not been offered these services, the provider working with the pain problem may facilitate that contact. In addition, the success of both the vocational and pain management efforts may be increased if the approaches are coordinated. The patient's motivation to pursue often difficult physical therapy exercises may be increased if such activities are articulated in explicit ways to achievement of vocational goals. There is some evidence that pain programs emphasizing return to work as part of treatment do better than similar programs not emphasizing work activities (Catchlove and Cohen, 1982). It is important, therefore, that providers working with patients showing pain related disability be familiar with the laws regarding provision of vocational rehabilitation services applicable to the jurisdictions from which his patients come, and that he have a working relationship with the people who provide those services in both the private and public sectors.

Relevant here also is the distinction noted earlier between charity and entitlement concepts of help for the disabled. Patients who have gone through any of the systems discussed and are receiving support are, by definition, entitled to such support, yet, some patients experience these awards as "welfare," which they equate with "charity," and experience as demeaning. Such individuals thus find themselves in circumstances which effectively force them to accept what they see as charity from the government, a situation which, construed this way, is injurious to the person's sense of pride and self-worth. Some people take as self-evident that one should work for what one gets and that things gotten without work qualify as charity. With patients who feel this way, the provider may be of help in drawing the distinction between insurance-driven compensation, for which the patient, in fact, has paid, and charitable gifts, for which the patient has not paid and which, in most cases, he has not received. In short, insurance programs are in no way at odds with the work ethic, and it should be argued forcefully that this is a matter of fact, not opinion. The laws are clearly intended as entitlements based on medical status. If the patient believes that these entitlements are gifts, he is simply mistaken. Helping the patient to see this may improve his sense of self-worth.

The psychological symptoms of depression and anxiety represent treatable conditions. If pain patients have these problems, they deserve the attention of appropriate professionals (Merskey, 1986). It is necessary, therefore, that providers of pain management services to this group of people be sensitive to the presence of these symptoms and be able either to treat them or to make the appropriate referral. It is wise to be particularly aware of the possibility of masked depression (Aronoff and Evans, 1985). Patients may be reluctant to reveal low mood, feeling that such revelation is an expression of weakness. Vegetative signs may be dismissed by the patient as being irrelevant or somehow due to the pain. It is therefore good practice, especially with patients who tend toward stoicism, to check periodically for vegetative signs. Referral for psychiatric evaluation and possible chemotherapy may spare the patient considerable unnecessary suffering and successful treatment of affective symptoms may translate into improved motivation and progress with pain management strategies.

A final area of potential concern is the family system of the patient with disabling pain (Mohamed, 1982). The role changes inherent in disability status may alter family dynamics in a profound way. Should significant psychological symptoms trouble the patient, they will modify his behavior in relation to family members who, in turn, react differently to him in a reciprocal cycle of maladaptation. The fact of reduced income, which many of these families face, stresses the system as adjustments in living circumstances and life-style are made.

Given these stresses, the possibility that family therapy is indicated should be considered. Treatment issues and goals will differ from case to case, but likely themes include improving and clarifying communication within the family concerning feelings about changing roles, and improving problem solving and negotiating skills as the family copes with its changing economic status.

CONCLUSION

In this chapter, we have looked at the types of legal issues patients with disabling pain and injury may face, and examined some of the potential psychological effects of these procedures and of disability status more generally. Perhaps the most important point to be made is the obvious one that these proceedings are usually not pleasant for any of the parties involved. Even in situations of minimal controversy, for example, when there is no question that the patient is totally disabled and entitled to SSA or Workers' Compensation, the process may be protracted and the patient is subject to the potential indignities of winding his way through a bureaucratic system which he may not understand and which is staffed by persons of varying degrees of refinement and sympathy. When, on the other hand, the patient's claim is questioned, when it is denied at early points in SSA or Workers' Compensation review, or when there is tort liability involved, the proceeding for the plaintiff may be particularly unpleasant. If the issue comes to litigation based on questions regarding the legitimacy of the claim of disability in the view of the potential payor, it is the patient's credibility that is being questioned. As a result, he is called upon to prove that his pain is real and disabling. He may be asked to do this repeatedly, in various forums, under hostile cross-examination, and in the face of experts who say that he is faking or deluded. This sort of procedure may expose many aspects of the patient's and his family's personal and financial circumstances to the scrutiny of disinterested or hostile strangers. For many people, furthermore, issues of health and illness are seen as private or even embarrassing, yet the process requires a glaringly public airing of the patient's bodily defects and behavioral incapacities. Clearly, the circumstances of litigation surrounding pain complaints are rife with possible assaults on the patient's self-esteem. His view of himself as a competent and contributing member of society may be challenged in subtle or obvious ways, and the result may be depression, anxiety, anger, and hostility.

These effects on psychological state may translate into interpersonal problems and conflicts. The disabled person must cope with an altered work role and this often implies ceasing effectively to be the provider in the family. The resulting dependency may be in sharp conflict with strongly held values which equate work with worth, and which may be shared values among the patient, his spouse, his extended family, and his friends. If the patient's disability is challenged, these already troubling adjustments to role change are dramatically worsened. Thus, litigation places an additional strain on an already stressed family and social system, and marital discord or even dissolution is not infrequent among litigating patients. Isolation from friends, particularly from friendships that are work related, may leave the patient estranged from all of his accustomed support persons.

Two main points emerge of relevance for the provider working with patients in these circumstances. First, the provider should have some understanding of the legal realities the patient faces. These may be protracted and difficult and will occupy much of the patient's energy. The therapeutic alliance will be facilitated if the patient senses that the therapist genuinely understands what the patient is experiencing. Second, the disabled pain patient often has many difficulties in addition to the presenting complaint of pain and these will interact with the pain experience in complex ways. Treatment requires a sensitivity to the patient as a whole and a working relationship with other relevant providers.

REFERENCES

Aronoff, G. M., & Evans, W. O. (1985), Evaluation and treatment of chronic pain at the Boston Pain center. In: *Evaluation and Treatment of Chronic Pain*, ed. G. M. Aronoff. Baltimore: Urban & Schwarzenberg, pp. 495–502.

Beals, R. K. (1984), Compensation and recovery from injury. *J. W. Med.*, 140/2:233–237.

Catchlove, R., & Cohen, K. (1982), Effects of a directive return to work approach in the treatment of workmen's compensation patients with chronic pain. *Pain*, 14:181–191.

Cobb, S. (1974), Physiological changes in men whose jobs were abolished. *J. Psychosom. Res.*, 8:245–258.

———(1976), Social support as a moderator of life stress. *Psychosom. Med.*, 38:300–314.

Commission on the Evaluation of Pain (1987), Report of the Commission on the Evaluation of Pain. *Soc. Sec. Bull.*, 50/1:13–44.

Derebery, V. J., & Tullis, W. H. (1986), Low back pain exacerbated by psychosocial factors. *W. J. Med.*, 144:574–579.

Dworkin, R. H., Handlin, D. S., Richlin, D. M., Brand, L. & Vannucci, C. (1985), Unraveling the effects of compensation, litigation and employment on treatment response in chronic pain. *Pain*, 23:49–59.

Fordyce, W. E. (1986), Learning processes in pain. In: *The Psychology of Pain*, 2nd. ed., ed. R. A. Sternbach, New York: Raven Press, pp. 49–66.

Gore, S. (1978), The effect of social support in moderating the health consequences of unemployment. *J. Health & Soc. Behav.*, 19:157–165.

Heinrich, R. L., Cohen, M. J. & Nabiloff, B. D. (1982), Rehabilitation of pain patients: Coping in interpersonal contexts. In: *Psychological Approaches to the Management of Pain*, eds. J. Barber & C. Adrian. New York: Brunner/Mazel, pp. 118–136.

Kentucky Workers' Compensation Law, Kentucky Revised Statute Chapter 342 (1982).

Ludwig, A. M. (1980), *Principles of Clinical Psychiatry*. New York: Free Press.

Mandler, G. (1972), Helplessness: Theory and research in anxiety. In: *Anxiety: Current Trends in Theory and Research*, Vol. 2, ed. C. D. Spielberg. New York: Academic Press, pp. 363–374.

Melzack, R., Katz, J., & Jeans, M. E. (1985), The role of compensation in chronic pain: Analysis using a new method of scoring the McGill pain questionnaire. *Pain*, 23:101–112.

Mendelson, G. (1982), "Not cured by a verdict." Effect of legal settlement on compensation claimants. *Med. J. Austral.*, 2:132–134.

———(1984), Compensation, pain complaints, and psychological disturbance. *Pain*, 20:169–177.

Merskey, H. (1986), Psychiatry and pain. In: *The Psychology of Pain*, 2nd ed., ed. R. A. Sternbach. New York: Raven Press, pp. 97–120.

Miller, H. G. (1961), Accident neurosis. *Brit. Med. J.* (Clin. Res.), i:919–925; 992–998.

Miller, I. W., & Norman, W. H. (1979), Learned helplessness in humans: A review and attribution theory model *Psycholog. Bull.*, 86:93–118.

Mohamed, S. (1982), The patient and his family. In: *Psychosocial Factors in Rehabilitation* ed. R. Roy & E. Tunks. Baltimore: Williams & Wilkins, pp. 145–150.

Price, D. N. (1984), Workers' Compensation: 1976–1980 benchmark revisions. *Soc. Sec. Bull.*, 477: 3–23.

Seligman, M. E. (1975), *Helplessness*. San Francisco: W. H. Freeman.

Social Security Disability Benefit Reform Act of 1984.

Strang, J. P. (1985), The chronic disability syndrome. In: *Evaluation and Treatment of Chronic Pain* ed. G. M. Aronoff. Baltimore: Urban & Schwarzenberg, pp. 603–624.

Trout, J., & Mattson, D. R. (1984), A 10-year review of the supplemental security income program. *Soc. Sec. Bull.*, 47 1:3–24.

Part II

DIAGNOSTIC ISSUES IN CHRONIC PAIN

In the consideration of diagnostic issues in chronic pain, Drs. Randal France and Ranga Rama Krishnan of Duke University Medical Center present a systems approach to the assessment and management of chronic pain. Their systems' model includes the role of multiple factors in the development and maintenance of chronic pain states, the sequelae to chronic pain, the factors that interact in the development of these sequelae, and the progression and effect of the sequelae on chronic pain syndrome. Considered are both organic and functional factors of pain and the evaluation of personality traits consistent in chronic pain.

There is no other measure that has been used more extensively than the Minnesota Multiphasic Personality Inventory (MMPI). Dr. Douglas K. Snyder addresses the assessment of chronic pain with the MMPI, including the specific scales and profile configurations playing a prominent role in the evaluation of psychological factors contributing to chronic pain, as well as other physical disorders. In addition, a review of the most current empirical studies relating to the MMPI diagnosis and the treatment of chronic pain are discussed. Efforts to delineate distinguishing psychological features of specific pain subgroups are also explored, and the chapter concludes with specific guidelines for incorporating the MMPI in the assessment of chronic pain syndromes.

Drs. Brena and Sanders, of the Pain Control and Rehabilitation Institute of Georgia and Emory University, discuss special features in the diagnosis and management of pain in cancer patients. Reviewed are common physical factors in cancer pain, as are psychological factors in cancer pain. A comprehensive summary of clinical research data in this area, together with multiple approaches to cancer pain management, are explored. Drs. Weisberg and Page address diagnostic issues and personality variables in coping with treatment for life-threatening illness. Key psychological variables related to attribution theory, learned helplessness theory, and theories of learning and reinforcement are explored. Special attention is paid to the personality characteristics of dialysis patients and the use of Millon Behavioral Health Inventory as a unique instrument developed with a nonpsychiatric medical population that has strong application to understanding a multiplicity of factors unique to the chronic pain patient.

Dr. Dan Blazer of the Department of Psychiatry, Duke University Medical Center, addresses a multiaxial approach to the psychosocial assessment and intervention of chronic pain. Considerable attention is addressed toward operational assessment of chronic pain, which is an attempt to reliably describe aspects of the pain experience itself. A conceptual framework for assessing chronic pain is introduced, which incorporates the principles of operational assessment into a comprehensive assessment procedure and presents techniques of psychosocial management of chronic pain that can be helpful in chronic pain assessment.

Dr. Craig D. Waggoner, Director of the Behavioral Rehabilitation Pain Management Program at the Thoms Rehabilitation Hospital and Dr. Frank Andrasik, Professor, Department of Psychology, University of West Florida address in this concluding chapter the behavioral assessment and treatment of recurrent headache pain. Recognizing that headache is among the most commonly presented symptoms in outpatient clinics, Drs. Waggoner and Andrasik thoroughly review the biological bases of both migraine and tension headaches. This is followed by psychological aspects of headache pain, including personality characteristics which are often found in chronic headache patients. Also addressed is the spectrum of behavioral methodologies applied to both the diagnosis and treatment of headache pain. The chapter concludes with consideration of the emerging trends in treatment and appropriately brings to a close this section and volume on chronic pain.

6

The Systems Approach to the Assessment and Management of Chronic Pain

RANDAL D. FRANCE, M.D. AND
KAY RANGA RAMA KRISHNAN, M.D.

Pain is one of the most feared and least understood sensory experiences. It is one of the major biological signals which warns a person that a disease process or injury is occurring and prepares the person for the course of the illness (Sternbach, 1968; Bonica, 1977). Pain is the most common symptom of a disease or injury to motivate a person to seek medical care (Merskey and Spear, 1967). The lessening of the pain symptom often heralds recovery. Szasz (1957) states that pain falls into the category of private data that cannot be simultaneously shared or reported by anyone other than the person experiencing the pain. To obtain information concerning the pain experience, clinicians are totally dependent upon the report of the patient. Engel (1958) stated the capacity to experience pain develops initially from stimulation of the peripheral sensory system but thereafter pain experiences, like visual and auditory experiences, may occur without the corresponding stimulation of the end organs. Merskey (1980) has defined pain as an

K.R.R. Krishnan, R.D. France, & B.J. Urban (1987), Systems approach to chronic pain syndromes, In: *Chronic Pain*, eds. R.D. France, & K.R.R. Krishnan. Washington, DC. American Psychiatric Press. Reprinted by permission.

"unpleasant experience which we primarily associate with tissue damage or describe in terms of tissue damage or both." Expanding on Merskey's definition, the International Association for the Study of Pain (IASP) (1986) defined pain as an "unpleasant sensory and emotional experience we associate with tissue damage or describe in terms of tissue damage" (p. 26).

For unknown reasons, pain persists in some patients despite resolution of the acute illness. In this situation, pain no longer serves as a warning signal but becomes an illness unto itself with enormous impact on the patient and his or her environment.

The chronic pain syndrome is an ancient and puzzling phenomenon (Melzack, 1973; Bonica, 1977). A review of early writings on pain explain chronic pain in mystical, spiritual, and religious terms. A religious explanation for chronic pain dominated Western thinking. Pain was viewed as a punishment inflicted by God for sins committed by the sufferer. The word *pain*, in fact, is derived from the Latin word *poena* meaning penalty or punishment. Aristole's view on pain also had a profound influence in Western thinking. He maintained that the heart was the center of sensation and pain was the result of increase in the sensitivity of touch that was carried by the blood to the heart.

Modern concepts of pain can be traced back to Descartes in the seventeenth century who held that the brain was the center of sensation. He further believed pain was transmitted to the brain by means of small threads running from the skin to the brain. Following his work, major advances in anatomy and physiology led to the localization of specific pain receptors in the periphery and pain pathways from the periphery to the brain. At the end of the nineteenth century, two opposing views of pain were maintained: pain as a biological phenomenon, and, as traditionally believed, pain as a purely emotional experience. In 1895, Strong suggested pain consisted of two elements: the original sensation as initiated by the pain receptor and the message carried to the brain by the pain pathways, and the psychic reaction or processing caused by the sensation (Bonica, 1977). Hardy, Wolff, and Goodell (1952) expanded this theory to include the belief that cutaneous pain experience is similar for all individuals, whereas the reaction to pain is a complex physiological process involving cognitive functioning of the individual, and is influenced by past experiences, psychological factors, and social environment.

Melzack and Wall (1965) have incorporated the early and recent observations on the pain phenomenon and developed a theory on the perception of acute pain termed the *gate control theory*. The acute pain experience is the net effect of the incoming pain sensation to the transmission cell in the spinal cord balanced against the excitory and inhibitory mechanisms in the central nervous system (CNS) which are, in turn, influenced by biochemical, physiological, and psychological mechanisms in the CNS.

Indeed, our knowledge of pain has increased greatly in the twentieth century. The neurophysiology of pain is better understood at present and considerable advances have been made in diagnostic methods and medical and surgical treatments of pain. While we are better able to treat and diagnose acute pain, chronic pain remains an enigma.

The scope of the chronic pain problem is enormous. Chronic pain is one of the most significant health problems in clinical practice. Chronic pain is the most frequent cause of disability in the United States (NIH, 1979), while low back pain is the most common cause of compensation payments (Rowe, 1969). The economic effects of chronic pain have been estimated to cost the U.S. economy $40 to 50 billion annually (NIH Publication, 1979). The cost includes medical services, loss of work productivity, and compensation payments. After an extensive review of health related behaviors, Houpt, Orleans, George, and Brodie (1979) concluded that despite the differences in sample populations, lack of control groups, and varying definitions of clinical problems, chronic back pain is among the most expensive and costly of disabilities. A National Institute of Health (NIH) panel (NIH, 1979) concluded that the four most frequent causes of chronic pain are: chronic recurrent headaches, low back pain, arthritis, and cancer pain. It is estimated that at least one-third of Americans suffer from persistent or recurrent pain requiring medical treatment (Bonica, 1980).

Chronic pain is defined as the persistence of daily occurring pain for more than six months (Sternbach, 1974; Mc-Creary and Jamison, 1975; Black, 1975). Nociception is present despite the lack of an explanatory anatomical or physiological basis. Unlike the defined and predictable course of acute pain generated by an underlying disease, patients and clinicians are often unable to ascribe meaning to the persistence of pain. This is often the case where etiological evaluation and treatment provides little understanding and relief of the continual pain. One does not have to work long with chronic pain patients to see the multiplicity of causative factors and resulting affective and behavioral reactions that in themselves may lead to an illness. Hence, the presence of the pain complaint may communicate nociception alone and/or develop from the suffering of nociception over an extended period of time. At times, it might be a behavior designed to obtain socioeconomic or interpersonal gains, a maladaptive coping style, or a symbol of distress. Similarly, the chronic pain may represent an affective state such as depression or anxiety. Often the complaint of persistent pain and the associated emotions and behaviors is multidetermined from the above described factors. The importance of the behavioral and psychological factors in the assessment and management of chronic pain syndromes is increasingly recognized.

The question remains as to how to integrate the diverse facets of the clinical picture presented by a chronic pain patient. To understand the chronic pain syndrome, the clinician must take into account both the anatomical and physiological basis of the illness as well as the psychological and behavioral aspects. The purpose of this chapter is to provide a knowledge base and framework which clinicians can use to assess and better manage patients with chronic pain.

A systems approach offers the clinician a framework to include and integrate diverse causative factors in the pathogenesis of chronic pain, and a flexibility to understand the impact of these factors over the course of the chronic pain syndrome. The systems approach provides structure, mutability, and integration at different conceptual levels. The system, as described in Figure 6.1, can be focused on the individual patient with chronic pain or generalized to understand a particular chronic pain syndrome. Further, this approach provides a framework for understanding and assessing chronic pain syndromes as well as a framework for the development and examination of hypothesis.

Systems Model for Chronic Pain

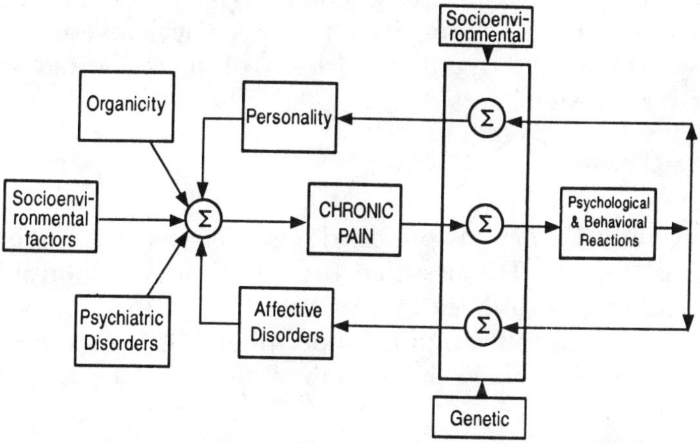

Figure 6.1. Systems model for chronic pain. K.R.R. Krishnan, R.D. France, & B. J. Urban (1987), Systems approach to chronic pain syndromes, In: *Chronic Pain*, eds. R. D. France, & K.R.R. Krishnan. Washington, DC. American Psychiatric Press. Reprinted by permission.

SYSTEMS MODEL

A basic systems model for chronic pain syndromes is presented in Figure 6.1. This figure illustrates: (1) the role of multiple factors in the development and maintenance of chronic pain states; (2) the sequelae to chronic pain; (3) the factors that interact in the development of these sequelae; (4) the progression of the sequelae; and (5) the effect of the sequelae on the chronic pain syndrome. Although the basic model as illustrated appears static, the dynamic nature of the process described must be kept in mind. The symbol Σ refers to sum of the various factors which interact at a particular point or node. There are at least five possible factors that intersect at the node leading to the pathogenesis of a particular chronic pain syndrome. They are: (1) organic factors; (2) personality; (3) socioenvironmental factors; (4) affective disorders; and (5) psychiatric disorders other than affective disorders. The separation of affective disorders from other psychiatric disorders is primarily based upon the close link between pain and depression, and the attention given to the clinical investigation of these two related syndromes. Each of these factors will be briefly discussed.

Organic Factors

Bonica (1977) has provided a guideline for clarifying the organic factors. He classified organic factors responsible for chronic pain into three groups based upon the origin of the apparent nociceptive input: (1) peripheral; (2) central; and (3) peripheral-central. Each of these factors will be briefly discussed.

Peripheral Origin. Any biochemical, mechanical, or thermal stimuli continually acting on pain receptors can generate a chronic pain state. In addition, a change in the sensitization may be caused by some of the pain-producing substances or by psychological or environmental factors. This mechanism may be responsible for the persistant pain of arthritis, some types of cancer, myocardial ischemia, peptic ulcer, peripheral nerve injury, perhipheral neuropathy, and pain of herniated disc. As there is a progression in the severity in any of these illnesses, the reactive psychological and behavioral reactions to the chronic pain and resulting disability may progress to the point of an illness in themselves.

Central Origin. Lesions that occur in the CNS can produce a chronic pain syndrome know as central pain. The exact mechanism of this disorder is unknown but evidence suggests a loss of descending inhibitory influences or loss of sensory inputs (Melzack and Loeser, 1978). Examples of central pain include: injury to the spinal cord (pain in paraplegics); cardiovascular accident in the thalamus (thalamic syndrome); and cortical areas (traumas). Many of these patients complain of spontaneous aching, burning, or shooting pain and have dysesthesias, hyperalgesias, formications, and other unusual sensations. In many cases the pain is poorly localized. Nonpainful stimuli can give rise to pain. Psychological factors clearly contribute to the pain. Anxiety and depressed states increase the level of central pain. However, there is little evidence to support a psychological cause for the central pain syndrome, but rather, the emotional disturbances exaggerate the chronic pain syndrome.

Peripheral-Central Origin. Abnormalities of both the peripheral and central portions of the somatosensory nervous system can generate a chronic pain state. The pathophysiology of these abnormalities is not well understood and it is possible that several mechanisms are involved. An initial injury produces a reflex response that in turn may cause abnormal changes in tissue. Examples of this mechanism are: reflex sympathetic dystrophy that develops following an injury to an extremity producing muscle spasm, vasospasticity, liberation of pain producing substances, and sensitization of nociceptors to nonnoxious stimuli. Psychological distress may contribute substantially to the exaggeration of this type of pain.

Chronic pain may also be due to a decrease in the number of large fibers in peripheral nerves that are known to exert an inhibitory influence on the activity of nociceptive transmission. This is the likely mechanism responsible for pain in neuralgia, diabetic neuropathy, toxic neuropathy, herniated disc, and trigeminal neuralgia. In addition, a decrease in inhibitory influences originating in the reticular formation of the brain stem, which is dependent on normal sensory input, may lead to a chronic pain syndrome. Examples of this disorder are phantom limb pain and causalgia.

The role of organic factors in the pathogenesis of pain disorders where the primary cause is not organic (i.e., in psychiatric disorders) is not well understood and further investigation is necessary.

Personality traits and/or disorders are separated from psychiatric disorders to clarify the role of each in the chronic pain syndrome. Personality traits are defined as enduring patterns of perceiving, relating to, and thinking about the environment in one's self, and exhibit in a wide range of important social and personal contacts (APA, 1980). Only when these traits become inflexible, maladaptive, and cause significant impairment in social and occupational functioning, or cause subjective distress are they considered as personality disorders (APA, 1980). For the purpose of understanding the term *personality*, Figure 6.1 refers not only to the core personality of the patient but also to the effects of the superimposed illness behavior and psychological function.

The importance of relationships between personality traits and chronic pain has long been recognized, but the exact nature has been the subject of disagreement. However, the variations in response to pain from one patient to another fuels the interest. Brown, Nemiah, Barr, and Barry (1954) describe the importance of personality factors in the chronic pain syndrome. They described these patients as having the following: (1) a vague history of present illness with confusing chronology; (2) expressions of either open or veiled resentment toward medical personnel for supposed neglect; (3) dramatic descriptions of reactions and of symptoms; (4) difficulty in localization and description of pain; (5) accompanying anxiety and depression; and (6) failure of usual forms of treatment indicating the presence of complicating psychological factors.

In evaluating personality traits using the Minnesota Multiphasic Personality Inventory (MMPI), Hanvik (1951) reported acute and chronic low back patients without physical findings could be differentiated from low back pain patients with organic findings. Patients without physical findings showed elevations on MMPI scales of hypochondriasis and

hysteria and scale of depression relatively low. This configuration is called the conversion V. In this study, patients with
physical findings showed normal personality profiles on the
MMPI. In a similar study, Sternbach, Murphy, Akeson, and
Wolf (1973a) were unable to find a difference in the conversion
V scale scores between patients with and without physical
findings. Lynn and Eysenck (1961) utilized the Eysenck Personality Inventory (EPI) to describe the personality traits in
chronic pain patients. They showed the experience of pain to
be associated with extroversion and the inhibition to pain with
introversion. Similarly, Woodforde and Merskey (1961) showed
that patients with pain of physical origin were actually more
anxious, depressed, and subject to signs of neuroticism as
compared to a group of patients with psychogenic pain. Kissen
(1964) showed relief of pain is associated with a fall in the level
of neuroticism and anxiety on the EPI. This may suggest the
elevated scores on the neuroticism scale (measure of the
likelihood of an emotional breakdown) is, at least in part, a
result of the pain.

Using the MMPI to evaluate the effects of personality on
duration of pain, Philip (1974) showed female patients with low
back pain had significantly elevated scores of hysteria, depression, and hypochondriasis, whereas females with acute pain
from fractures had only slightly elevated scores. Sternbach,
Wolf, Murphy, Akeson (1973b) found similar findings in that
patients with chronic forms of pain had increased scores on the
MMPI scales of hypochondriasis and hysteria, and patients with
acute pain seldom had these elevations. From these studies it
appears personality traits are altered in chronic pain patients as
compared to patients with acute pain, but the question remains
whether certain personality traits predispose an individual to
the maintenance of a chronic pain state whereas other patients
with the same physical diagnosis do not develop chronic pain.

The effects of personality traits on the outcome of pain
treatment have likewise been evaluated using the MMPI.
Wilfling, Klonoff, and Kokan (1973) showed patients scoring
significantly lower on the hysteria, hypochondriasis, and depression scales had greater success from spinal fusion than the
group with elevated scales. Another study (Beals and Hickman,

1972) reported patients with multiple surgeries scored higher on hysteria and hypochondriasis scales than patients with one surgery, acute pain, extremity injury, or than normals. Sternbach et al. (1973b) has suggested that specific profiles on the MMPI are important in predicting outcome. Patients with low back pain who have an elevated depressive subscale can be expected to have a favorable response to treatment whereas those with a dominant hysterical component respond poorly to surgery and psychological treatment. He stated that patients with the classic conversion V profile may or may not respond favorably.

Psychodynamic theory has been applied to the understanding of the relationship between pain and personality. Freud (1895) defined pain as an affective response to actual loss or injury, and Rangell (1953) described pain as a psychological defense against a core conflict or psychotic process. Szasz (1957) has described pain as arising from the threated loss of, or damage to, the body, either real or imagined.

Eisenbud (1937) and Weiss (1947) both emphasized the role of repressed hostility in pain patients. Similarly, Engel (1951) in a study of atypical facial pain, showed pain was associated with the experience of guilt from overt hostility. Engel (1959) has stated that certain patients are likely to develop a pain syndrome because of their psychodynamics, and has named patients in this group "pain-prone." These patients are described as having excessive guilt feelings where the experience of pain serves as a punishment to relieve the guilt feelings. Life histories of these patients reveal poor tolerance to success and repeated episodes of suffering and defeat. Further, they are unable to express anger directly and usually turn anger on themselves. They often have a history of physical abuse as a child and during rearing, pain had been used to promote discipline. Parents of these patients were only attentive when the child was either sick or hurt. Engel stated these psychodynamics can be found in various psychiatric disorders including depression, conversion disorder, neurotic, and personality disorders. In follow-up studies on the psychodynamic nature of pain, Tingling and Klein (1966) report on fourteen men with psychogenic pain. They discern conflicts over aggression and dependency as well as behavioral characteristics such as solitary hunting, reckless driving, and depression. Walters (1961) studied a group of patients with chronic pain without organic findings, and suggested that the injury is personalized with the most common sites being the neck and head, chest, and lower back.

Blumer and Heilbronn (1982) have furthered these concepts and have melded a profile consisting of Axis I and Axis II (DSM-III) disorders as well as psychodynamic considerations. He described these pain patients as being moralistic, having difficulty acknowledging negative affects, and so instead, displacing them onto somatic concerns. These patients have typical histories marked by personal and family histories of depression and alcoholism, physical abuse, and models of invalidism or pain. They tend to be workaholics and are "solid citizens" in their premorbid state and become depressed and somatically preoccupied.

Despite all of these attempts at validating the notion of a relationship between personality and depression, there have been few systematic studies aimed at clarifying a relationship between premorbid personality and pain and clarifying the relationship between pain, premorbid personality, and the alterations of personalities subsequent to pain.

To summarize, little is known about the influence of premorbid personality on chronic pain. There has been a tendency to confuse personality traits seen at the time of evaluation of chronic pain patients with premorbid personality. Such a tendency does not take into account the fact that chronic pain can itself induce changes in intrapsychic and interpersonal function and behavioral patterns which may become enduring patterns of perceiving, relating to, and thinking about the environment in one's self. These included changes can be exhibited in a wide range of important social and personal contexts. This is represented in the systems model.

The model generates the following questions about pain and personality: (1) Do certain premorbid personality factors influence pain and the pain experience? (2) Are these personality changes secondary to the pain experience? (3) What variables influence personality adaptation to the chronic pain experience? The systems model, as described, postulates the following: (1) Personality influences the development of chronic pain. (2) Chronic pain produces psychological and behavioral changes which, in turn, in the presence of certain genetic and socio-environmental factors can alter personality factors; that is, enduring patterns of perceiving, thinking, and relating to an environment in one's self.

AFFECTIVE DISORDER

Depression is often found in chronic pain patients (Romano and Turner, 1985; Fishbain, Goldberg, Meagher, Steele and Rosomoff, 1986). In many patients, the depression follows the onset of pain, whereas in others the pain is part of the symptom complex of depression (Krishnan, France, Pelton, McCann, Davidson and Urban, 1985a). Pain is one of the major psychopathological disorders found in chronic pain patients (Romano et al., 1985; Fishbain et al., 1986; France, Krishnan, Houpt, and Urban, in press; Kramlinger, Swanson, and Maruta, 1983). The presence of depression in chronic pain patients significantly elevates general levels of psychological distress, as compared to chronic pain patients without the presence of major depression (France et al., in press). Some authors have postulated that chronic pain is a variant of the depressive disease spectrum (Blumer et al., 1982) a form of masked depression (Lesse, 1968; Lopez-Ibor, 1972), or that depression is inevitable in chronic pain patients (Hendler 1984; Wilson, Blaser, Nashold, 1986). On the other hand, other authors have failed to document the presence of depression in all chronic pain patients and relate the occurrence of depression (Pilowsky, Chapman, Bonica, 1977; France et al. 1986a) with the development of chronic pain (France et al., in press; France, Houpt, Skott, Krishnan, and Varia, 1986). It is clear that clinicians and investigators have noted the close association between chronic pain and depression, but despite continual efforts to clarify the relationship, many questions remain. The separation of affective disorders from other psychiatric disorders (Figure 6.1) is primary for clarification of the clinical presentation of both syndromes in the chronic pain patient, for an understanding of the literature concerning chronic pain and depression, and for the generation of hypotheses to elucidate the relationship between the two syndromes. The model as presented posits that chronic pain may lead to the development of various affective disorders, and depression as a specific psychiatric disorder can lead to a chronic pain syndrome. We will discuss the former relationship initially. In evaluating the depressive disorder that develops in chronic pain patients, at least four possible relationships exist: (1) pain may be a symptom of depression; (2) depression may be a complication of chronic pain; (3) pain and depression are linked inextricably; and (4) pain and depression coexist but are not related.

Hendler (1983) considers depression to be a normal illness behavior in patients with chronic pain. He states that almost all chronic pain patients will pass through a period of depression. He has conceptualized four stages of response to pain akin to the stages of dying. It should be noted that the stages should not be considered rigidly but rather taken as a useful method of understanding the way in which patients cope with pain. In addition, it should be noted these stages are based on clinical experience which has not yet been studied or validated. The relationship between depression as an illness behavior and depression as a psychopathological disorder is unclear, as is the difference between the two. Just as grief following a loss can precipitate depression as a psychopathological disorder, so too can loss secondary to chronic pain precipitate depression.

Despite several studies of depression and chronic pain syndromes, the data concerning its prevalence can best be described as unreliable (Romano et al., 1985). Depression and chronic pain syndromes have been reported to vary from less than 10 percent all the way to 100 percent (Romano et al., 1985). The wide variation in the prevalence of depression is probably related to one of several factors: (1) lack of a uniform definition of depression (i.e., symptom, mood, or syndrome); (2) nature of the chronic pain; (3) setting where the study was carried out; and (4) variability in the assessment method. Only four studies have utilized Research Diagnostic Criteria (RDC) for the assessment of depression. Kramlinger et al. (1983)

noted 25 percent of chronic pain patients satisfied RDC for major depression. Lindsay and Wyckoff (1981) reported 31 percent of 300 patients were depressed by RDC. Krishnan et al. (1985a) studied the incidence of major depression using RDC in an inpatient setting, and found 40 percent of patients presenting with major depression. In a similar study, France et al. found a 20 percent incidence of major depression as defined by RDC to occur in chronic pain patients presenting to a pain clinic. It also should be noted that approximately 20 percent of patients in each study showed no evidence of depression. In addition, France et al. (in press) showed the occurrence of depression in chronic pain patients was not related to the duration of the chronic pain when examining major depression. However, when evaluating the occurrence of chronic forms of depression, it appears there is a strong correlation between the onset of chronic depression and onset of chronic pain. This finding may be explained by the close similarity of diagnoses between the two disorders and difficulty in separating out the two syndromes.

France, Houpt, Skott, Krishnan, and Varia (1986) failed to show a relationship between the occurrence of depression is chronic low back pain patients in certain clinical and demographic features such as age, gender, race, marital status, educational level, employment status, presence or absence of litigation, and number of operations for pain.

In an attempt to clarify the relationship between chronic pain and depression, a number of authors studied the plasma cortisol response to dexamethasone (Atkinson, Kremer, and Risch, 1983; France, Krishnan, Houpt, and Maltbie, 1984a; France and Krishnan 1985; Syvalakti, Hyyppa, and Salminen, 1985). In these reports, approximately 40 percent of chronic pain patients with major depression had nonsuppression of cortisol following dexamethasone administration. It appeared the rate of nonsuppression was not related to the presence or absence of organic findings in the chronic pain patients (Engel, 1958). France et al. studied the thyrotropin-releasing hormone stimulating test in a group of chronic pain patients with and without the presence of major depression. This test is a measure in the change of serum thyroid stimulating hormone levels following the administration of a standard amount of thyroid releasing hormone. Unlike the dexamethasone suppression test, the thyrotropin-releasing hormone stimulation test for depression is reported to be both a trait and state marker (Loosen and Prange, 1982). Approximately 30 percent of chronic pain patients showed a blunted thyroid stimulating hormone response to thyroid releasing hormone. There was no statistical difference between chronic pain patients with or without the presence of major depression. From a review of the present studies on the dexamethasone suppression test and the thyrotropin-releasing hormone stimulating test, it appears that the dexamethasone suppression test is a state marker for the presence or absence of major depression in chronic pain and the thyrotropin-releasing hormone stimulating test may be a trait marker common to both syndromes.

At the current time we cannot predict which chronic pain patients will develop major depression. Some preliminary studies indicate genetic factors may play a role. Schaffer, Donlan, and Bittle (1980), in a study of twenty chronic pain patients, reported patients with chronic pain had a high familial incidence of depression. Seventy-three percent of chronic pain patients with depression and 40 percent of those without depression had a family history of depressive spectrum disorder. Blumer et al. (1982) reported a high incidence of mental disorders such as depression in families of chronic pain patients. They reported 42 percent of these patients had first-degree relatives with a mental disorder. France, Krishnan, and Trainor (1986) examined the incidence of depression and alcoholism in first-degree relatives of 100 chronic pain patients with and without depression. A higher incidence of major depression was found in first-degree relatives of those patients with depression than those without depression. The familial incidence of alcohol dependency was similar in both groups of patients. These studies confirm the possibility that the occurrence of major depression in chronic pain may be related to genetic vulnerability to depression in these patients.

Depression is frequently seen as a complication of chronic pain. Depressed mood may be part of the normal illness behavior or may be part of a psychopathological disorder. The incidence of depression as a psychopathological disorder varies considerably across different studies. This discrepancy may be due to the clinical setting and different criteria used to define depression. Different subtypes of depression such as major depression, reactive depression, and chronic depression (dysthymic disorder) may be clearly identified in chronic pain patients. Symptoms of depression, especially neurovegetative symptoms and symptoms of anxiety, serve as useful discriminators of these subtypes (Kramlinger et al., 1983; Davidson, Krishnan, France, and Pelton, 1985; Krishnan et al., 1985b). Assessing depression amongst chronic pain patients is important because of the therapeutic implications as to the presence of depression in these patients.

Pain complaints are commonly seen in depressive disorders (Spear, 1967; Gallemore and Wilson, 1969; von Knorring 1975; Delaplaine, Ifabumuyi, Merskey, and Zarfas, 1978; Mathew, Weinman, and Misales 1981; Lindsay and Wuckoff, 1981; von Knorring, Perris, Eisemann et al., 1983a). The incidence of pain complaints in depressed patients ranges from 30 to 84 percent. Many of the above studies did not use operationally defined diagnoses or a structured interview to make the diagnosis of depression. The occurrence of pain complaints in different subtypes of depression is not well understood. Von Knorring et al. (1983a) have shown that 50 percent of patients with unipolar depression have pain complaints. Forty-four percent of bipolar patients in the depressed phase have pain complaints. Sixty-nine percent of patients with reactive depression were observed to have pain complaints in another study (Perris, 1966). Lesse (1968) reported pain is characteristic of patients with agitated depression. Others have reported pain complaints are more common in neurotic depression than in endogenous depression (Bond, 1967; Delaplaine et al., 1978).

As stated earlier, pain may serve to solve unconscious conflicts (Breuer and Freud, 1895). Several authors have noted a relationship between pain, aggression, hostility, and guilt (Walters 1961; Merskey, 1965a; Tingling et al., 1966; Blumer et al., 1982). Von Knorring, Perris, Eisemann, Eriksson, and Perris (1983b) showed interjected aggression in depressed patients with pain complaints. However, they did not find an association between guilt and the occurrence of pain in depressed patients. It is reported that elements of depression precede the physical complaints in patients using pain as a defense (Freud, 1895; Engel, 1959).

Since pain is a common complaint in depression, the question arises whether this is a change in the sensitivity to pain in depressed patients with pain complaints. Earlier studies have shown depressed patients have a higher pain threshold (Hall and Stride, 1954; Hemphill, Hall, and Crookes, 1962; Merskey 1965a). It has been shown that pain threshold increased in depressed patients with and without pain complaints (von Knorring, 1975). Davis, Buschbaum, and Bunney (1979) reported an increase in pain threshold in bipolar patients as well as unipolar patients, and the increase is seen in both the depressed and manic phase. From these studies and the reported incidence of pain complaints in depressed patients, it appears the occurrence of pain complaints in patients with depression is related to factors other than changes in the pain threshold of depressed patients.

In summary, it is well documented that depressed patients often present with pain complaints, and chronic pain patients often develop a depressive illness. Establishing the exact nature of the pain and depression in a patient has enormous clinical implications. Bradley (1963) had demonstrated that in patients where pain and depression occur simultaneously, effective treatment results in resolution of both symptoms, and in patients where pain precedes the occurrence of depression, successful treatment of the depression results in resolution of the depressive symptomatology but not in pain. Despite the close association between pain and depression and previously described investigational studies, many questions remain.

PSYCHIATRIC DISORDERS

Pain may also be part of a symptom complex of various psychiatric disorders including somatization disorder, conversion disorder, psychogenic pain disorder, generalized anxiety disorder, dementia, schizophrenia, malingering, and factitious

disorders. The model proposed suggests chronic pain may be:
(1) part of the symptom complex of these disorders; (2) organic
pathology and personality variables can influence the development of chronic pain in these disorders; and (3) chronic pain
resulting from these disorders can lead to both the development of depression and/or changes in personality, just as in the
case of the other primary causes for the development of
chronic pain.

When pain occurs in patients with schizophrenia and is not
related to organic conditions, pain may be part of a delusional
or somatizing process. If the pain is based upon a delusional
process, the pain is unusual and bizzare in description and
ill-defined. The pain behavior is not appropriate to the pain
complaint. Delusional pain is relatively uncommon in schizophrenic patients (Merskey, 1965b). Pain as part of a somatizing
process is more commonly seen in these patients than delusional pain. It should also be noted that there is a relative pain
insensitivity in schizophrenic patients as compared to non-
schizophrenic patients and controls (Davis, Buschbaum, van
Kammen, and Bunney, 1979; Stengel, Oldham, and Ehrenberg, 1955). Pain complaints are commonly seen among patients with anxiety disorders (Spear, 1967). Patients suffering
from anxiety have low pain thresholds compared to patients
with major depression and other neurotic conditions (Hemphill
et al., 1952). Pain is commonly seen in the somatization
disorder as one of the multiple somatic complaints characteristic of this syndrome. Pain can also be an associated symptom
in conversion disorders. In the psychogenic pain disorder
(DSM-III), pain is the predominant symptom. In DSM-III-R,
this classification will be changed to idiopathic pain disorder.
Characteristics of this syndrome are as follows: (1) severe and
prolonged pain; (2) pain present as a symptom is inconsistent
with any pathophysiological mechanism; (3) psychological factors are judged to be etiologically involved in the pain; and (4)
the pain is not due to other mental disorders. In addition,
persistent pain complaints can occur in hypochondriasis, malingering, substance abuse disorders, and personality disorders.

The occurrence of persistent pain in patients with various
psychiatric disorders must be closely evaluated due to the

implications this occurrence has in each of the neuropsychiatric syndrome. In addition, the occurrence of new pain complaint in patients with various psychiatric disorders must be assessed in terms of various etiological causes or combinations as presented in the systems model. Thorough formulation of these etiological causes will direct management of the pain complaint in patients with psychiatric disorders.

SOCIOECONOMIC FACTORS

It has been reported that patients with manual labor jobs, limited education, and a personal style which involves denial of emotional distress more commonly develop chronic pain following injury (Gentry, Shows, and Thomas, 1974). In certain pain patients, chronic pain and pain behaviors are strongly influenced by socioenvironmental factors. The behavior of these patients is usually inconsistent with the voiced pain complaints. For example, they may appear to be in severe pain while in a physical examination setting, but appear quite calm and relaxed moments after in the waiting room. Although this behavior can be viewed from several perspectives including psychodynamics, an operant approach is found to be useful in understanding this behavior. For example, in back pain patients during the acute stage, patients learn to assume stiff posture to reduce the pain, learn inactivity, and increase the intake of pain medication, and may also find they can avoid unwanted work, home responsibilities, and family and mental conflicts (Keefe, Block, Williams, and Surwit, 1981). Then, when the pain becomes chronic, the pain complaints may become controlled primarily by their positive social and environmental consequences.

Like those patients with "learned pain disease," as described by Fordyce, Fowler, and Lehmann (1968), Sternbach (1968), Fordyce (1976), and Brena (1978), patients with organic disease for pain can also suffer prolonged disability, social disorder, and illness behavior patterns (Pilowsky et al. 1977). This paradigm causes these patients to resemble patients whose pain behavior is adequately accounted for by the behavior model. In evaluating chronic pain patients, therefore, it is necessary to exercise caution in trying to fit patients completely into either a behavioral or medical construct.

Compensation is a factor which has to be considered in the development of chronic pain (Ross, 1977). The pain in these cases may be a symbol not only of pain but also of other emotions (Porkorny and Moore, 1953). Thus, the main hypotheses from the model are: (1) social and environment factors may initiate chronic pain complaints, and (2) they may play a role in sustaining pain complaints and behaviors. The systems model as presented takes into account the possibility that depending upon the patient and the particular pain disorder, the significance of each of these factors may vary. In some chronic pain patients, the major initiator for the chronic pain may be primarily organic (e.g., rheumatoid arthritis) or psychiatric (e.g., conversion disorder or psychogenic pain disorder), or socioenvironmental. In others, the development of the chronic pain syndrome may depend upon the complex interplay of all these factors (e.g., as in many patients with chronic low back pain).

EFFECTS OF CHRONIC PAIN

Chronic pain has effects on (1) intrapsychic functioning of the individual where pain, with the attendant limitations of work and pleasure, engenders feelings of helplessness and hopelessness followed by despair, lowered self-esteem, and depression; and (2) interpersonal functioning at a level of the family, work, and society where often either the helplessness gets reinforced with reinforcement of the pain behavior or the patient gets rejected by the consequent despair and depression. The occurrence of maladaptive styles of functioning and behavior patterns are often secondary to social and environmental factors. The reinforcement by family and society of behaviors which increase pain complaints and pain behaviors play a roll in the continuation of the chronic pain (see Figure 6.1). As already noted, various subtypes of depression are common sequelae of chronic pain. These in turn exacerbate chronic pain and the associated distress.

The occurrence of major depression and other psychiatric sequelae may be due to a complex interplay of familial, genetic, intrapsychic, social, and environmental factors. An increased familial incidence of depression in chronic pain patients who become depressed indicates that genetic factors play a role in the development of depression in these patients.

Further, the changes in intrapsychic and interpersonal functioning in the model are postulated to change the personality as described earlier. Evidence for this is suggested by a recent study by Bond showing personality, as measured by the Eysenck Personality Inventory is related to both the severity of pain and variations in complaint behavior (Bond, 1976). Similar observations have been made by Kissen (1964) and Timmenmans and Sternbach (1976). Sternbach and Timmenmans have suggested that changes in personality scores secondary to chronic pain may be reversible. These changes may be secondary to, or influenced by, genetic and socioenvironmental factors.

The main concepts postulated by the systems model are: (1) personality, organic pathology, socioenvironmental factors, and personality disorders may lead to, or interact with, each other in the development of the chronic pain syndrome; (2) the importance of each of these factors varies with each individual patient and type of pain problem; (3) the development of the chronic pain syndrome can initiate psychological and behavioral changes which in themselves may lead to an illness; (4) socioenvironmental and genetic factors influence changes that can occur in chronic pain patients; (5) psychological and behavioral changes may in turn lead to alterations in personality; (6) alterations in personality depend upon genetic and socioenvironmental factors; (7) psychological and behavioral changes secondary to chronic pain may lead to the development of various types of depressive disorders; and (8) personality changes may in turn affect the course of chronic pain. In reviewing Figure 6.1, it should be noted that at each node any of the given factors may be absent or present to varying degrees. The utility of the model provides a basis for treatment (i.e., treating the condition and its sequelae); for assessment (i.e., assessing the significance of each of the factors for a given patient); and for research (i.e., testing the above hypothesis for particular pain disorders).

ASSESSMENT

The systems approach as outlined in Figure 6.1 gives a rational and systematic approach for assessing chronic pain patients. The presence of organic factors, personality issues, psychiatric disorders, and socioenvironmental factors has to be evaluated in each patient. Thus, careful clinical, psychological, and behavioral examinations along with ancillary laboratory and radiographic evaluations have to be done. History and the evaluation of family interactional patterns by interviewing the family also should be done when possible. A thorough physical examination needs to be performed to assess the presence of other physical illnesses or physical changes that may have resulted from the chronic pain syndrome itself or past treatments. For the assessment of the pain complaint, several instruments are commonly used. They are the McGill Pain Questionnaire (Melzack 1975), Hendler Pain Inventory (Hendler, Viernstein, Gucev, and Long 1979), Visual Analog Scale (Huskisson 1983), and numerical scaling of pain intensity. These scales are not diagnostic instruments by themselves but serve to supplement clinical and diagnostic assessments by rating the intensity or quality of the pain complaint. It is also necessary to assess the effects of chronic pain on the life-style of the patient and his or her family, occupation, leisure activity, and economic status. Direct observation (Keefe, Crisson, and Trainor, 1987) and video recording (Keefe and Block, 1982a) of body movements and pain behavior, as well as a review of the patient's activity record (Fordyce, 1976), serve to identify styles of function. In addition, a psychophysiological assessment can occur with the use of surface electromyography (Keefe, Brown, Scott, and Ziesat, 1982). Electrodes are placed over muscles believed to be involved in the patient's pain problem. This technique is particularly useful in muscular-based pain problems.

Typically, the assessment of personality traits in the chronic pain patient is made by use of the Minnesota Multiphasic Inventory (MMPI) (Sternbach et al., 1973). Levels of psychological distress can be quantified by the use of the Symptom Checklist-90-R (Derogotis, 1977). This is a ninety-item self-reported inventory that measures nine primary symptom dimensions as well as three global indices of distress. The Beck Depression Inventory provides a good index of a general level of depressive symptomatology (Beck and Beamesderfer, 1974). This is a twenty-one item self-rating questionnaire which is convenient and readily adaptable to a general pain patient population (France, Houpt, Skott, Krishnan, and Varia, 1986a). The Montgomery–Asberg Depression Rating Scale (France, Houpt, Skott, Krishnan, and Varia, 1986a; von Knorring, 1975) and the Hamilton Depression Rating Scale (Krishnan et al., 1985a) are two observer rating scales of depressive symptomatology that have successfully and reliably been used in the assessment of chronic pain patients.

An intelligence test and neuropsychological test are often useful in the evaluation of chronic pain syndromes. Patients with chronic pain can present with significant intellectual and cognitive deficiencies that must be considered in treatment planning.

Behavioral assessment protocols and measures of coping strategies provide an understanding of operant mechanisms (Keefe, Brown, Scott, and Ziesat, 1982). Ideally, the interview should be conducted with the spouse and other family members regarding activities and changes in family interactions. Standardized behavioral assessment of pain behavior can also provide information regarding the role of environmental factors and day-to-day behavioral patterns in relationship to pain. The presence of psychiatric disorders secondary to chronic pain need to be assessed in a systematic and clinical interview and operationally defined diagnostic criteria applied. The dexamethasone suppression test may have some utility in identifying major depression in some chronic pain patients. However, the utility of this test is yet to be established.

MANAGEMENT

The management of the chronic pain patient should be individually tailored following careful assessment. If treatable organic factors are found, then the treatment should be first directed toward it (i.e., the treatment of ulcer, trigeminal neuralgia, herniated nucleus pulposus, etc.), and the rest of the treatment should be based upon the assessment of the various components of the system.

If maladaptive patterns of behavior are clearly identified, then a program designed to reduce and eliminate the behavioral pattern is instituted. The operant mechanisms which reinforce pain behaviors are commonly seen in chronic low back pain patients. The working hypothesis supporting the operant conditioning approach is that the patient's pain behavior is maintained by social consequences (e.g., attention from spouse or family, avoidance of unwanted responsibilities). Operant conditioning methods are used for patients who: (1) have minimal or no physical findings to account for their pain; (2) show a disproportionally high level of pain behaviors; (3) demonstrate dramatic variability in behavior from one time to another; (4) are extremely inactive; and (5) are dependent on pain medications. The operant conditioning programs are focused on two goals—increasing activity and decreasing narcotic intake. Patients are placed on a structured activity program in which they are required to be up and out of bed during a scheduled number of minutes per hour. The uptime goals are increased gradually. By avoiding high levels of activity, the likelihood that patients will exhibit excessive pain behaviors is reduced. If pain behaviors do occur, they are given minimal attention. Medications are also given in a "pain cocktail" administered on a time contigent basis rather than linked to a pain complaint. The use of a pain cocktail becomes particularly important in patients with drug dependency problems. A time contigent administration is also useful in patients who overuse pain medications following overactivity. After the baseline analgesic requirement is determined, it is then incorporated into a liquid base and decreased slowly over time. Withdrawal of addictive medications is done at a slower rate than physiologically required. Pain cocktails are also often used as the prescribed means of getting a steady blood level of analgesic even when narcotic abuse is not the problem. Some patients show considerable improvement by simply offering a steady analgesic blood level.

This type of operant conditioning programs is best implemented on inpatient units (Houpt, Keefe, and Snipes, 1984). However, these can also be done on an outpatient basis with support from the family. Self-control methods which teach patients to exert control over their own behavioral affective and physiological reactions to pain are also useful when pain behavior is more than is expected.

Self-management techniques are again indicated in cases when: (1) there is no evidence of ongoing tissue pathology and when medical and surgical treatment is not possible; (2) pain behaviors are not that strongly entrenched; and (3) there is little evidence that positive reinforcement or secondary gains are maintained by pain behavior. A variety of self-management techniques are currently used either alone or in combination in treatment programs. These include biofeedback, cognitive behavior therapy, and multimodal approaches.

Biofeedback is used to help patients control muscle activity. Self electrodes are placed over target muscles and feedback from electromyographic activity by either audio or visual display is used to teach patients to control activity (Keefe 1982; Keefe, 1987). Biofeedback is often combined with progressive relaxation techniques to enhance benefits (Wolfe, Nacht, and Kelly 1982). These approaches have been used for headache, phantom limb pain (Sherman, Gall, and Gormly, 1979), and low back pain (Wolfe et al., 1982).

Training chronic pain patients in cognitive behavioral methods designed to reduce pain is often useful (Rybstein-Blinchick, 1979; Turner, 1979). Effective pain management programs often use a wide variety of techniques, including biofeedback, relaxation training, medication reduction, and self-directed physical exercise (Tan, 1982). Appropriate physical therapy designed to promote strength and mobilization of muscles is especially useful in chronic low back pain patients.

Sometimes when the pain is due to organic factors but the

organic factors are not readily treatable, then methods of altering nociception either by blocking or by augmenting nerve impulses are useful (Urban, 1984; Urban, 1987). Nerve blocks are useful only when a clearly identifiable nerve is involved. Blocks can either be temporary or permanent. Permanent blocks are rarely applied to chronic pain of nonmalignant origin (Katz, 1979). Similarly, neurodestructive surgery is also used very rarely (Loeser, 1977). Specialized destructive techniques for individual pain syndromes are occasionally indicated. Temporary nerve blocks often enhanced by corticosteriods are sometimes useful in alleviating chronic pain (Urban, in press).

Psychiatric disorders, especially depression, either major or chronic depression, can often accompany chronic pain. Appropriate treatment is that for depression in general, namely, tricyclic antidepressants, ECT, and so on. Serotonic reuptake blocking tricyclics are often preferred as it is felt that serotonin reuptake blocking drugs are useful in reducing pain (France et al., 1984b) When psychiatric disorders are the primary problem and pain is secondary, specific treatment has to be directed toward the psychiatric disorder (e.g., therapy for conversion disorders, hysteria, etc., and neuroleptics for psychosis).

Psychotropic drugs, especially antidepressants, are also used in the treatment of chronic pain with and without depression. The use of these drugs depend upon specific pain syndromes.

Headaches

Antidepressant medications are reported to be effective in the treatment of migraine (Mahloudji, 1969; France and Krishnan, 1987). Couch, Ziegler, and Hassanien (1976) showed that amitriptyline reduces the frequency of headaches by 50 percent. There was little relationship between depression and improvement in migraine headaches. Noone (1977) showed desipramine reduced frequency and duration of migraine headaches. Sherwin (1979) showed that amitriptyline reduced tension headaches in patients with depression. Okasha, Ghaleb, and Sadek (1973) showed that both doxepin and amitriptyline in low doses (50 mg day) were effective in reducing tension headaches in patients with and without depression.

Facial Pain

Lascelles (1966) showed phenelzine was useful in alleviating facial pain. Gessell (1973) showed amitriptyline also had therapeutic benefit in this syndrome.

Postherpetic Neuralgia

Taub (1973) showed amitriptyline was effective in the treatment of postherpetic neuralgia in patients with and without depression. Watson, Evans, Reed, Merskey, and Goldsmith (1982) showed amitriptyline was better than placebo and that there was no correlation between relief of depression and relief of pain.

Diabetic Neuropathy

Turkington (1980) showed that both imipramine and amitriptyline were effective in the treatment of chronic pain associated with diabetic neuropathy.

Low Back Pain

Imipramine was found to be no better than placebo in the treatment of low back pain without depression (Jenkins, Ebbutt, and Evans, 1976). Amitriptyline was also not effective in a double-blind study (Pilowsky, Hallett, Bassett, Thomas, and Penhall, 1982), but open-label studies suggest the opposite (Szasz, 1957).

Despite the frequent use of antidepressants in the treatment of chronic pain, their mechanism of action remains unknown. However, based on clinical experience, it appears low doses of antidepressants (50–75 mg/day) are effective in treating chronic pain without depression. Furthermore, it has been reported that the onset of pain relief is quicker than the relief of depression. Thus, it is important to use these medications depending upon the type and nature of pain and any associated neuropsychiatric disorder.

Besides antidepressants, neuroleptics such as haloperidol and fluphenazine are used for treating chronic refractory pain (Merskey and Hester, 1972; Maltbie, Cavenar, Sullivan, Hammett, and Zung, 1979). However, in view of side effects such as tardive dyskinesia, it is best to restrict their use to cancer and pain related to terminal illness.

Other psychotropic medications have been periodically recommended. Again, caution is indicated when using benzodiazepines and/or stimulants because of the addictive potential. Further, benzodiazepines have not been particularly effective in the treatment of chronic pain. Stimulants such as metamphetamines have been useful, primarily for increasing the analgesic effect of opioid drugs. Nonsteroidal analgesic drugs are useful primarily in the treatment of pain associated with chronic inflammatory diseases such as arthritis.

Individual counseling to help patients adjust to the loss associated with the chronic pain is often indicated. Marital and family counseling to help the patient and his family accept and cope with the illness play a major role in reducing the reactive distress associated with chronic pain and disability. Reconstructive psychotherapy for chronic pain patients whose pain arises from personality disorders, somatizing disorder, hypochondriasis, and malingering have limited benefit and are often contraindicated since this type of therapy promotes regression and disorganization of adaptive mechanisms.

Given the complexity of chronic pain syndromes, the best treatment can be given only in multidisciplinary settings. This can be accomplished both in an inpatient and outpatient setting. Psychiatrists, psychologists, orthopedists, neurologists, neurosurgeons, anesthesiologists, nurses, physical therapists, and psychiatrists constitute part of these multidisciplinary teams.

Pain patients are very accepting of the concept of pain clinics and the multidisciplinary approach offered by these programs. Within the context of pain clinics, they are willing to accept psychological intervention, especially when such recommendations are reinforced by their personal physicians. Since the time Bonica (1974) and Hudson and Pratt (1979) started the pain clinic concept, the number of pain clinics has rapidly grown.

The systems approach which we have outlined here, when used in such a setting, can be a very effective tool in the assessment and management of chronic pain patients.

SUMMARY

A systems approach to the assessment and management of chronic pain is presented. The approach allows for an understanding of chronic pain syndromes in the individual patient who presents with persistent pain. It also provides a framework for assessing the various aspects of chronic pain and assisting and tailoring individual programs for the treatment of chronic pain syndromes.

REFERENCES

American Psychiatric Association (1980), *Diagnostic and Statistical Manual of Mental Disorders*, 3rd ed. Washington, DC: American Psychiatric Press.

Atkinson, E., Kremer, E.F., & Risch, S.C. (1983), Neuroendocrine function and endogenous opioid peptide systems in chronic pain. *Psychosom.*, 24:899–913.

Beals, R.K., & Hickman, N.W. (1972), Industrial injuries of the back and extremities. *J. Bone & Jnt. Surg.*, 34:1593–1611.

Beck, A.T., & Beamesderfer, A. (1974), Assessment of depression: The depression inventory. In: *Psychological Measurements in Psychopharmacology, Modern Problems in Pharmacopsychiatry*, Vol. 7, ed. P. Pichot. Basel, Switzerland: Karger, pp. 151–169.

Black, R.G. (1975), The chronic pain syndrome. *Surg. Clin. N. Amer.*, 55:999–1011.

Blumer, D., & Heilbronn, M. (1982), Chronic pain as a variant of depressive disease: the pain-prone disorder. *J. Nerv. Ment. Dis.*, 170:381–406.

Bond, M.R. (1967), *Pain: Its Nature, Analgesics, and Treatment*. New York: Churchill Livingstone.

———— (1976), Pain and personality in cancer patients. In: *Advances in Pain Research and Therapy*, Vol. 1, eds. J.J. Bonica & D. Albe-Fessard. New York: Raven Press.

Bonica, J.J. (1974), Organization and function of a pain clinic. *Adv. Neurol.*, 4:433–443.

———— (1977), Neurophysiological and pathologic aspects of acute and chronic pain. *Arch. Surg.*, 112:750–761.

———— (1980), Pain research and therapy; past and current status and future needs. In: *Pain Discomfort and Humanitarian Care*, eds. L.K.Y. Ng & J.J. Bonica. New York: Elseyier North Holland.

Bradley, J.J. (1963), Severe localized pain associated with the depressive syndrome. *Brit. J. Psychiatry*, 109:741–745.

Breuer, J., & Freud, S. (1895), Studies on Hysteria. *Standard Edition*, 2. London: Hogarth Press, 1955.

Brena, S.F. (1978), *Chronic Pain. America's Hidden Epidemic.* New York: Atheneum.

Brown, T., Nemiah, J.C., Barr, J.S., & Barry, H. (1954), Psychological factors in low back pain. *New Eng. J. Med.*, 251:123–128.

Couch, J.R., Ziegler, D.K., & Hassanien, R. (1976), Amitriptyline in the prophylaxis of migraine. *Neurol.*, 26:121–127.

Davidson, J.R.T., Krishnan, K.R.R., France, R.D., & Pelton, S. (1985), Neurovegetative symptoms in chronic pain and depression. *J. Affect. Disord.*, 9:213–218.

Davis, G.G., Buschbaum, M.S. & Bunney, W.E. (1979), Analgesia to painful stimuli in affective illness. *Amer. J. Psychiat.*, 136:1148–1151.

———— Buschbaum, M.S., van Kammen, D.P. & Bunney, W.E. (1979), Analgesia to pain stimuli in schizophrenia and its reversal by naltrexone. *Psychiat. Res.*, 1:61–69.

Delaplaine, R., Ifabumuyi, O.I., Merskey, H., & Zarfas, J. (1978), Significance of pain in psychiatric hospital patients. *Pain*, 4:361–366.

Derogotis, L. (1977), Symptom Check List-90-R (SCL-90-R), Manual I, Derogatis: Baltimore. Unpublished manuscript, April.

Eisenbud, J. (1937), The psychology of headache. *Psychiat. Quart.*, 2:592–619.

Engel, G.L. (1951), Primary atypical facial neuralgia. A hysterical conversion symptom. *Psychosom. Med.*, 15:375–379.

———— (1958), Psychogenic pain. *Med. Clin. N. Amer.*, 42:1481–1496.

———— (1959), 'Psychogenic' pain and the pain-prone patient. *Amer. J. Med.*, 26:899–918.

Fishbain, D.A., Goldberg, M., Meagher, B.R., Steele, R., & Rosomoff, H. (1986), Male and female chronic pain patients categorized by DSM-III Psychiatric Diagnostic Criteria. *Pain*, 26:181–197.

Fordyce, W.E., Fowler, R.S., & Lehmann, J.F. (1968), Some implications of learning in problems of chronic pain. *J. Chron. Dis.*, 21:105–107.

———— (1976), *Behavioral Methods for Chronic Pain and Illness.* St. Louis, MO: C.V. Mosby.

France, R.D., Krishnan, K.R.R., Houpt, J.L., & Maltbie, A.A. (1984a), Differentiation of depression from chronic pain using a comparison of DST and diagnostic criteria. *Amer. J. Psychiat.*, 141:1577–1579.

———— Houpt, J.L., & Ellinwood, E.H. (1984b), Therapeutic effects of antidepressants in chronic pain. *Gen. Hosp. Psychiat.*, 6:55–63.

———— Krishnan, K.R.R. (1985), The dexamethasone suppression test as a biological marker of depression in chronic pain. *Pain*, 21:49–55.

———— Houpt, J.L., Skott, A., Krishnan, K.R.R., & Varia, I.M. (1986), Depression as a psychopathological disorder in chronic low back pain patients. *J. Psychosom. Res.*, 30:127–133.

———— Krishnan, K.R.R., & Trainor, M. (1986), Chronic pain and depression. III. Family history study of depression and alcoholism in chronic low back pain patients. *Pain*, 24:185–190.

———— ———— (1987), Psychotropic drugs in chronic pain. In: *Chronic Pain*, eds. R.D. France & K.R.R. Krishnan. Washington, DC: American Psychiatric Press.

———— ———— Houpt, J.L., & Urban, B.J. (1987), Clinical characteristics of depression subtypes in chronic pain patients. *South. Med. J.*, 28:188–191.

Freud, S. (1895), Inhibitions, symptoms and anxiety. *Standard Edition*, 20:169–172. London: Hogarth Press, 1955.

Gallemore, J.L., & Wilson, W.D. (1969), The complaint of pain in the clinical setting of affective disorders. *S. Med. J.*, 62:551–555.

Gentry, W.D., Shows, W.D., & Thomas, M. (1974), Chronic low back pain. A psychological profile. *Psychosom.*, 15:174–177.

Gessel, A.H. (1973), Electromyographic biofeedback and tricyclic antidepressants in myofascial pain-dysfunction syndrome: Psychological prediction of outcome. *J. Amer. Den. Assn.*, 91:1048–1052.

Hall, K.R.L., & Stride, E. (1954), The varying response to pain in psychiatric disorders: A study in abnormal psychology. *Brit. J. Med. Psychol.*, 27:48–60.

Hanvik, L.J. (1951), MMPI profiles in patients with low back pain. *J. Consult. Psychol.*, 15:350–353.

Hardy, J.D., Wolff, H.D., & Goodell, H. (1952), *Pain, Sensations and Reactions*, Baltimore: Williams & Wilkins.

Hemphill, R.E., Hall, K.R.L., & Crookes, T.G. (1952), A preliminary report on fatigue and pain tolerance in depressive and psychoneurotic patients. *J. Ment. Sci.*, 98:433–440.

Hendler, N.A., Viernstein, M., Gucer, P., & Long, D. (1979), A preoperative screening test for chronic back pain patients. *Psychosomat.*, 20:801–805.

—— (1983), The four stages of pain. In: *Diagnosis and Treatment of Chronic Pain*, eds. N. Hendler, D. Long, & T.N. Wise. Littleton, MA: John Wright PSG.

—— (1984), Depression caused by chronic pain. *J. Clin. Psychiat.*, 45:30–36.

Houpt, J.L., Orleans, C.S., George, L.K., & Brodie, H.K.H. (1979), *The Importance of Mental Health Services to General Health Care*. Cambridge, MA: Ballinger Publishing.

—— Keefe, F.J., & Snipes, M. (1984), The clinical specialty unit: the use of the psychiatry inpatient unit to treat chronic pain syndrome. *Gen. Hosp. Psychiat.*, 6:65–70.

Hudson, J.S., & Pratt, T.H. (1979), Pain clinics: Their value to the general practitioner. *South. Med. J.*, 72:845–847.

Huskisson, E.C. (1983), Visual analogue scales. In: *Pain Measurement and Assessment.* New York: Raven Press, pp. 33–37.

IASP Subcommittee on Taxonomy (1986), Classification of chronic pain: Description of chronic pain syndromes and definitions of pain terms. *Pain Supplement 3.*

Jenkins, D.G., Ebbutt, A.F., & Evans, C.D. (1976), Tofranil in the treatment of low back pain. *J. Int. Med. Res.*, 4:28–40.

Katz, J. (1979), Current role of neurolytic agents. In: *Advances in Neurology*, Vol. 4, New York: Raven Press, pp. 47–476.

Keefe, F.J. (1982), Behavioral assessment and treatment of chronic pain. Current status and future directions. *J. Consult. Clin. Psychiat.*, 50:896–899.

—— Block, A. R. (1982), Development of an observational method for assessing pain behavior in chronic low back pain. *Behav. Ther.*, 13:363–375.

—— —— Williams, R.B., & Surwit, R.S. (1981), Behavioral treatment of chronic pain; Clinical outcome and individual differences in pain relief. *Pain*, 11:221–231.

—— Brown, C., Scott, D.S., & Ziesat, H. (1982), Psychological assessment of chronic pain. In: *Assessment Strategies in Behavioral Medicine*, eds. F.J. Keefe & J.A. Blumenthal. New York: Grune & Stratton.

—— Crisson, J.E., & Trainor, T. (1987), Observational methods for assessing pain: A practical guide. In: *Applications in Behavioral Medicine and Health Psychology: A Clinician's Sourcebook*, eds. J.A. Blumenthal & D.C. McKee. Sarasota, FL: Professional Resource Exchange.

—————— (1987), Behavioral assessment methods for chronic pain. In: *Chronic Pain*, eds. R.D. France & K.R.R. Krishnan. Washington, DC: American Psychiatric Press.

Kissen, D.M. (1964), The influence of some environmental factors on personality inventory scores in psychosomatic research. *J. Psychosom, Res.*, 8:145–152.

Kramlinger, K.G., Swanson, D.W., & Maruta, T. (1983), Are patients with chronic pain depressed? *Amer. J. Psychiat.*, 140:747–749.

Krishnan, K.R.R., France, R.D., Pelton, S., McCann, U.D., Davidson, J., & Urban, B.J. (1985a), Chronic pain and depression. I. Classification of depression in chronic low back pain patients. *Pain*, 22:279–287.

—————— —————— —————— —————— —————— (1985b), Chronic pain and depression. II. Symptoms of anxiety in chronic low back pain patients and their relationship to subtypes of depression. *Pain*, 22:289–294.

Lascelles, R.G. (1966), Atypical facial pain and depression. *Brit. J. Psychiat.*, 112:651–659.

Lesse, S. (1968), Masked depression: Diagnostic and therapeutic problems. *Dis. Nerv. Syst.*, 29:169–173.

Lindsay, P.G., & Wyckoff, M. (1981), The depression-pain syndrome and its response to antidepressants. *Psychosomat.*, 22:571–577.

Loeser, J.D. (1977), Neurosurgical control of chronic pain. *Arch. Surg.*, 112:880–883.

Loosen, P.T., & Prange, A.J. (1982), Serum thyrotropin response to thyrotropin-releasing hormone in psychiatric patients: A review. *Amer. J. Psychiat.*, 139:405–416.

Lopez-Ibor, T.J. (1972), Masked depression. *Brit. J. Psychiat.*, 120:245–258.

Lynn, A., Eysenck, H.L. (1961), Tolerance for pain, extraversion and neuroticism. *Percept. Mot. Skills*, 12:161–162.

McCreary, C., & Jamison, K. (1975), The chronic pain patient. In: *Consultation-Liaison Psychiatry*, ed. R.O. Pasnau. New York: Grune & Stratton, pp. 205–217.

Mahloudji, M. (1969), The migraine syndrome. *Brit. Med. J.*, 1:182–183.

Maltbie, A.A., Cavenar, J.O., Sullivan, J.L., Hammett, E.B., & Zung, W.W.K. (1979), Analgesia and haloperidol: A hypothesis. *J. Clin. Psychiat.*, 40:323–326.

Mathew, R., Weinman, M., & Misales, M. (1981), Physical symptoms of depression. *Brit. J. Psychiat.*, 139:293–296.

Melzack, R., & Wall, P.D. (1965), Pain mechanisms: A new theory. *Sci.*, 150:971–979.

—————— (1973), *The Puzzle of Pain*. New York: Basic Books.

—————— (1975), The McGill Pain Questionnaire: Major properties and scoring methods. *Pain*, 1:277–299.

—————— Loeser, J.D. (1978), Phantom body pain in paraplegics: Evidence for a central "pattern generating mechanism" for pain. *Pain*, 4:195–210.

Merskey, H. (1965a), The effects of chronic pain upon the response to noxious stimulus by psychiatric patients. *J. Psychiat. Res.*, 8:405–419.

—————— (1965b), The characteristics of persistent pain in psychological illness. *J. Psychosom. Res.*, 9:291–298.

—————— Spear, F.G. (1967), *Pain, Psychological and Psychiatric Aspects*, London: Balliere, Tindall & Cox.

—————— Hester, R.A. (1972), The treatment of chronic pain with psychotropic drugs. *Postgrad. Med. J.*, 48:594–598.

—————— (1980), The role of the psychiatrist in the investigation and treatment of pain. In: *Pain*, ed. J.J. Bonica. New York: Raven Press, pp. 249–260.

NIH (1979), Report on the panel on pain to the National Advisory Neurological and

Communicative Disorder and Stroke Council. Washington DC: NIH Publication No. 81:1912.

Noone, J.F. (1977), Psychotropic drugs and migraine. *J. Intern. Med. Res.*, 5:66–71.

Okasha, A., Ghaleb, H.A., & Sadek A. (1973), A double-blind trial for the clinical management of psychogenic headache. *Brit. J. Psychiat.*, 122:181–183.

Perris, C. (1966), A study of bipolar (manic-depressive) and unipolar recurrent depressive psychoses. *Acta Psychiat. Scand. Suppl.* 194.

Philip, E.L. (1974), Some psychological characteristics associated with orthopedic complaints. *Curr. Pract. in Orthoped. Surg.*, 2:165–176.

Pilowsky, I., Chapman, C.R., & Bonica, J.J. (1977), Pain, depression and illness behavior in a pain clinic population. *Pain*, 4:183–192.

————— Hallett, E.C., Bassett, D.L., Thomas, P.G., & Penhall, R.K. (1982), A controlled study of amitriptyline in the treatment of chronic pain. *Pain*, 14:169–179.

Porkorny, A.D., & Moore, F.J. (1953), Neuroses and compensation: Psychiatric disorders following injury in compensable situations. *Arch. Indus. Hyg. & Occup. Med.*, 8:547–563.

Rangell, L. (1953), Psychiatric aspects of pain. *Psychosom. Med.*, 15:22–37.

Romano, J.M., & Turner, J.A. (1985), Chronic pain and depression: does the evidence support a relationship? *Psychol. Bull.*, 97:18–34.

Ross, W.D. (1977), How to get a neurotic worker back on the job successfully. *Occup. Health & Safety*, 46:20–23.

Rowe, M.L. (1969), Low back pain in industry: A position paper. *J. Occup. Med.*, 11:161–169.

Rybstein-Blinchick, E. (1979), Effects of different cognitive strategies in the chronic pain experience. *J. Behav. Med.*, 2:93–102.

Schaffer, C.B., Donlan, P.T., & Bittle, R.M. (1980), Chronic pain and depression: A clinical and family history survey. *Amer. J. Psychiat.*, 137:118–120.

Sherman, R.A., Gall, T.V., & Gormly, J. (1979), Treatment of phantom limb pain with muscular relaxation training to disrupt the pain anxiety-tension cycle. *Pain*, 6:47–56.

Sherwin, D. (1979), New method for treating headaches. *Amer. J. Psychiat.*, 136:1181–1183.

Spear, F.G. (1967), Pain in psychiatric patients. *J. Psychosom. Res.*, 11:187–193.

Stengel, E., Oldham, A.J., & Ehrenberg, A.S.C. (1955), Reactions to pain in various abnormal states. *J. Mental Sci.*, 101:52–69.

Sternbach, R.A. (1968), *Pain: A Psychophysiological Analysis.* New York, Academic Press.

————— Murphy, R.W., Akeson, W.H., & Wolf, S.R. (1973), Chronic low-back pain: The low-back "loser." *Postgrad. Med.*, 53:135–138.

————— Wolf, S.R., Murphy, R.W., & Akeson, W.H. (1973b), Aspects of chronic low back pain. *Psychosomatics*, 14:52–56.

————— (1974), *Pain Patients: Traits and Treatment.* New York, Academic Press.

Syvalakti, E., Hyyppa, M.T., & Salminen, J.K. (1985), Depression and the dexamethasone test (DST) in patients with non-specific somatic complaints. *Ann. Clin. Res.*, 17:148–151.

Szasz, T.S. (1957), *Pain and Pleasure: A Study of Bodily Feeling.* London: Tavistock Publications.

Tan S-Y. (1982), Cognitive and cognitive-behavioral methods for pain control: A selective review. *Pain*, 12:201–228.

Taub, A. (1973), Relief of postherpetic neuralgia and psychotropic drugs. *J. Neurosurg.*, 39:235–239.

Timmenmans, G., & Sternbach, R.A. (1976), Human chronic pain and personality: A canonical correlation analysis. In: *Advances in Pain Research and Therapy*, Vol. 1, eds. J.J. Bonica & D. Albe-Fessard. New York: Raven Press.

Tingling, D.C. & Klein, R.F. (1966), Psychogenic pain and aggression: The syndrome of the solitary hunter. *Psychosom. Med.*, 28:738–748.

Turkington, R.W. (1980), Depression masquerading as diabetic neuropathy. *JAMA*, 243:1147–1150.

Turner, J.A. (1979), A comparison of progressive relaxation training and cognitive behavioral therapy for chronic low back pain. Paper presented at the American Pain Society Meeting, San Diego, CA.

Urban, B.J. (1984), Treatment of chronic pain with nerve blocks and stimulation, *Gen. Hosp. Psychiat.*, 6:43–47.

———— (1987), Treatment of chronic pain by local modulation of nociception. In: *Chronic Pain*, eds. R.D. France & K.R.R. Krishnan. Washington, DC: American Psychiatric Press.

von Knorring, L. (1975), The experience of pain in depressed patient. *Neuropsychobiol.*, 1:155–165.

———— (1975), *The Experience of Pain in Patients with Depressive Disorders: Clinical and Experimental Study*. Doctoral dissertation, Umea University Medical Dissertations, Umea, Sweden.

———— Perris, C., Eisemann, M., Eriksson, U., & Perris, H. (1983a), Pain as a symptom in depressive disorders. II. Relationship to personality traits as assessed by means of KSP. *Pain*, 17:377–384.

———— ———— ———— ———— ———— (1983b), Pain as a symptom in depressive disorders. I. Relationship to diagnostic subgroup and depressive symptomatology, *Pain*, 15:19–26.

Walters, A. (1961), Psychogenic regional pain alias hysterical pain. *Brain*, 84:1–18.

Watson, C.P., Evans, R.J., Reed, K., Merskey, H., & Goldsmith, L. (1982), Amitriptyline versus placebo in postherpetic neuralgia. *Neurol.*, 32:671–673.

Weiss, E. (1947), Psychogenic rheumatism. *Ann. Inter. Med.*, 26:890–900.

Wilfling, F.J., Klonoff, H., & Kokan, P. (1973), Psychological, demographic and orthopedic factors associated with prediction of outcome of spinal fusion. *Clin. Orthoped. & Rel. Res.*, 90:153–160.

Wilson, W.P., Blazer, D.G., & Nashold, B.S. (1986), Observations on pain and suffering. *Psychosom.*, 17:73–76.

Wolfe, S.L., Nacht, M., & Kelly, J.L. (1982), EMG feedback training during dynamic movement for low back patients. *Behav. Ther.*, 13:395–406.

Woodforde, J., & Merskey, H. (1961), Personality traits of patients with chronic pain. *J. Psychosom. Res.*, 16:167–172.

7

Assessing Chronic Pain with the Minnesota Multiphasic Personality Inventory (MMPI)

DOUGLAS K. SNYDER, PH.D.

No other instrument has been as widely or intensively examined for its utility in evaluating the psychological components of chronic pain as has the Minnesota Multiphasic Personality Inventory (MMPI). The reasons for this arise both from the nature of chronic pain in general, and the psychometric properties of this instrument in particular. As Keefe (1982) noted in his review of behavioral assessment and treatment of chronic pain, behavioral and psychological dimensions have received increasing recognition for their critical role in the development and maintenance of pain syndromes. Keefe argued that conventional treatments for acute pain are usually ineffective for chronic pain, and that medications are limited by their temporary effectiveness and potential side effects; in addition, surgical alternatives to eliminate underlying tissue damage may be exhausted by the time the chronic pain patient presents for treatment. Pheasant, Gilbert, Goldfarb, and Herron (1979) determined that the number or duration of preoperative symptoms and extent of objective physical findings were unrelated to surgical outcome. Fordyce, Brena, Holcomb, deLateur, and Loeser (1978) concluded that "physician diagnostic judgments about chronic pain are themselves burdened with the hazard of limited reliability. . . . When dealing with chronic pain, medical analysis of the significant parameters involved is not yet precise" (p. 302).

Butcher and Finn (1983) noted several reasons for incorporating objective personality measures into clinical assessment procedures. Among other advantages, objective measures are: (1) less vulnerable than interview and other subjective approaches to nonsystematic sources of error; (2) more cost-efficient means of screening for psychopathology; (3) useful for identifying reliable subgroups within clinical populations covarying with treatment response; and (4) valuable for generating clinical hypotheses derived from normative findings and applying these idiographically to individual cases.

The MMPI has a long tradition of empirical research spanning nearly forty years relating individual scales and profile configurations to individual differences within medical and psychiatric populations, identifying emotional factors contributing to patients' somatic complaints, and predicting patients' response to surgery and other medical and psychiatric treatments. As Sternbach (1982) noted, "Only the Minnesota Multiphasic Personality Inventory (MMPI) has a clinically useful profile with sizeable medical and psychiatric patient norms" (p. 14).

OVERVIEW OF THE MMPI

The Minnesota Multiphasic Personality Inventory comprises 566 statements which the patient indicates as being either "true" or "false" as applied to him or herself. These statements cover a wide range of attitudes, affect, cognitions, and behaviors including a broad range of neurologic, cardiorespiratory, gastrointestinal, and psychiatric symptoms. The MMPI can be administered individually or in groups, after which respondents' answer sheets can be scored either manually or through one of many commercially available computerized scoring and test-interpretation services. Standard scoring procedures provide scores on four validity and ten clinical scales. Raw scores on each are transformed to T-scores having a mean of 50 and a standard deviation of 10; consequently, on any given scale approximately two-thirds of individuals from the general population would be expected to have scores from 40 to 60T, with 95 percent expected to fall between 30 to 70T. Separate norms are employed for men and women, with T-scores plotted on a standard profile form.

The MMPI was developed by Hathaway and McKinley at the University of Minnesota, and was first published in 1943. For the most part, scales were developed employing an empirical criterion-keying approach in which test items for a given scale were determined by identifying those items that discriminated between patients comprising a specific diagnostic group and nonpsychiatric controls, consisting primarily of relatives and visitors of patients in the University of Minnesota Hospitals. Specific diagnostic groups used in the development of eight of the ten clinical scales included those with primary diagnoses of hypochondriasis, depression, hysteria, psychopathic deviate, paranoia, psychasthenia, schizophrenia, and hypomania. By the early 1950s, it became widely recognized that MMPI scales reflected constellations of personality and behavioral attributes extending well beyond those implied by specific diagnostic labels; consequently, scales were assigned consecutive numbers and decreasing emphasis was placed on original scale names. Interpretive guidelines for individual scales and scale combinations have been developed on the basis of scales' relationships to independent relevant criteria identified on an empirical basis.

A brief description of the four validity and ten clinical scales is offered below. More extensive descriptions of these scales and profile configurations can be found in any number of comprehensive textbooks on the MMPI, including Dahlstrom, Welsh, and Dahlstrom (1972, 1975), Graham (1977), and Lachar (1974).

Validity Scales

?–(Cannot Say)—Total number of items omitted or double-marked; scores over 30 may invalidate a profile. Invalid responses can be reduced considerably by emphasizing instructions to answer every item.

L–(Lie)—Reflects a general, deliberate evasive response set through items expressing valued behaviors which, in fact, are rarely characteristic of even highly conscientious individuals.

F–(Frequency)—Comprises items answered infrequently ($\leq$ 10%) by normals. Reflects an atypical response set characterizing severe psychopathology or an attempt to "fake bad."

K–(Correction)—Empirically derived to improve the predictive accuracy of five clinical scales by reducing their number of false negative decisions ("test misses"); fractions of K are added to the Hs, Pd, Pt, Sc, and Ma scales. Elevations on K reflect patients' subtle defensiveness and guardedness.

Clinical Scales

1–(Hs—Hypochondriasis)—A stable "trait" scale reflecting undue concern about health and a seeking of sympathy through exaggeration of vague somatic complaints. Because of the heterogeneous nature of item content, high scores on this scale (above 65T) are unlikely to result exclusively from bona fide physical disorders.

2–(D—Depression)—A sensitive index of current affect reflecting poor morale, moodiness, and feelings of hopelessness. Assesses general dissatisfaction and discomfort in living, and is the most frequent high-point scale in profiles of psychiatric patients.

3–(Hy—Hysteria)—Originally developed to identify patients with conversion symptoms; item content reflects (a) general denial of good physical health, and (b) denial of psychological or emotional problems or interpersonal discomfort.

4–(pd—Psychopathic deviate)—Fairly stable measure reflecting tendencies toward impulsivity, low frustration tolerance, and poor social adjustment.

5–(Mf—Masculinity/Femininity)—Among males, high scores reflect a nontraditional sex-typed orientation including creativity, sensitivity, and passivity; low scores indicate emphasis on traditional male interests and attitudes. Among females, high scores suggest assertiveness, self-confidence, and high activity; low scores reflect passivity and sensitivity.

6–(Pa—Paranoia)—Assesses tendencies toward hypersensitivity, rigidity, suspiciousness and, at higher levels, paranoid ideation including delusions of persecution or grandeur.

7–(Pt—Psychasthenia)—Reflects generalized anxiety, excessive doubt and indecision, difficulties in concentration, unreasonable fears, compulsions, and obsessions.

8–(Sc—Schizophrenia)—Assesses tendencies toward unusual thought processes, lack of deep interests and apathy, social alienation, and peculiarities of perception and cognition.

9–(Ma—Hypomania)—Indicates tendencies toward elevated mood, high activity, excitability and irritability, and social gregariousness.

0–(Si—Social introversion)—High scores reflect lack of confidence and discomfort in social situations, and tendencies toward social withdrawal.

Scales 1, 2, and 3 (Hs, D, and Hy) have been designated as a "neurotic triad" and are those scales most frequently cited as characterizing chronic pain patients and predicting a broad range of independent pain-related criteria. A variety of profile patterns or "codetypes" involving significant elevations on these scales (above 70T) or relatively high scores (below 70T but higher than other profile scales) have been identified as moderating patients' affective and behavioral response to physical difficulties. Five of these codetypes warrant particular attention.

The 1-3/3-1 codetype (Hs and Hy ≥ 70T and higher than remaining scales) comprises the most frequent profile configuration observed among chronic pain patients (with an incidence of 35–60%), although this pattern is found among only

5 to 15 % of general medical patients and 3 to 5% of psychiatric outpatient samples (Webb, 1970; Schwartz and Krupp, 1971; Louks, Freeman, and Calsyn, 1978). This codetype reflects tendencies toward somatic preoccupation and exaggeration of physical complaints, often with conspicuous absence of sustained symptomatic depression or anxiety. This pattern results from a selective endorsement of somatic items and denial of social anxiety (Hs and Hy) without endorsement of depressive and anxiety items (D and Pt). Even when the patient reports depressive symptoms, this affect typically is focused exclusively on physical complaints with denial of any other emotional stressors. Characteristic defenses include repression and denial; common psychiatric diagnoses include one of the psychophysiologic or somatoform disorders (somatization, conversion, psychogenic pain, or hypochondriacal disorder). When elevations on Hs and Hy also exceed scale 2 (D) by 10 or more T-points, the 1-3/3-1 codetype is described as a "conversion-V" reflecting immaturity, dependency, reliance on somatic expression of underlying emotional conflict, and resistance to psychological interpretations.

By comparison, the 1-2/2-1 profile (Hs and D $\geq$ 70T and higher than remaining scales) characterizes patients who also exhibit excessive preoccupation with somatic complaints, but without the same conspicuous absence of subjective emotional distress; the most prominent features include somatic discomfort and pain. When Hs comprises the higher of these scales, a somatization or hypochondriacal syndrome is likely to predominate with recurrent, multiple somatic complaints unsubstantiated by objective physical findings. Unlike conversion disorders, various symptoms of depression, anxiety, fatigability, and irritability may prevail—particularly if the elevation on D exceeds that on Hs. This pattern appears relatively stable and unresponsive on a long-term basis to either medical or psychological interventions.

The 1-8/8-1 codetype is relatively infrequent among chronic pain patients, but characterizes individuals with a history of vague physical complaints that may seem particularly peculiar or bordering on somatic delusions. This pattern reflects the hypochondriacal emphasis of scale 1 and the schizoid mentation and bizarre sensory experiences reflected in item content of scale 8. Patients exhibiting this profile configuration typically exhibit interpersonal anxiety and social withdrawal.

The 2-3/3-2 profile type suggests mixed symptomatology involving at least moderate distress (depression, tension, nervousness, and anxiety) coupled with multiple somatic complaints. Although many patients with this codetype are diagnosed as suffering depressive reactions, those with physical complaints often fail to respond to traditional medical interventions. Defense mechanisms of repression and denial predominate. Depressed affect is often displayed only fleetingly; physical complaints and emotional distress may be employed to gain the support and nurturance of others, and response to psychotherapy is typically poor.

In contrast to the codetypes described above, the 2-7/7-2 profile reflects a predominance of emotional distress with less involvement of somatic complaints other than those symptoms typically associated with depression (fatigability, sleep disturbance, decreased appetite) and autonomic responses to anxiety. Depressed mood, nervousness, lack of self-confidence, and a ruminative style prevail. Patients obtaining this codetype are likely to be pessimistic worriers, intropunitive, and preoccupied with their personal deficiencies. Psychotropic medications and/or psychotherapy often afford considerable symptomatic relief.

In the review that follows, empirical findings consistently demonstrate the disproportionate incidence of significant elevations on these scales among MMPI profiles of chronic pain patients, and indicate their association with independent criteria, including degree of functional incapacitation and response to treatment. However, studies vary in their emphasis on individual scales versus configural analyses and in their interpretation of these findings.

EMPIRICAL INVESTIGATIONS OF CHRONIC PAIN

Prototypic Profiles of Combined Pain Groups

Swanson, Swenson, Maruta, and McPhee (1976) described the MMPIs of twenty-two men and twenty-six women admitted to a pain-management program on the basis of chronic pain of several years' duration, multiple operations, treatment failures, prolonged disability, and dependency on medication; the majority of patients suffered from neurologic (50%) and/or orthopedic (76%) difficulties, with many exhibiting unrelated but complicating medical (28%) difficulties, or psychiatric (32%) conditions. Group mean profiles for pain patients were significantly higher than the mean profiles for 50,500 general medical patients on MMPI scales comprising the neurotic triad (Hs, D, and Hy) in addition to Sc and Ma. Mean scores on the neurotic triad ranged from 65 to 75T for women and 70 to 80T for men in the pain-management program, and were consistently 10 to 20 T-score points higher than those for the general medical sample.

Pilling, Brannick, and Swenson (1967) examined the MMPI profiles of 221 male and 341 female medical and surgical patients referred for psychiatric evaluation on the basis of minimal physiologic or anatomic findings. These patients produced significant elevations across several scales (mean scores on Hs, D, and Hy from 70 to 75T, and on Pt and Sc from 65 to 70T). The most frequent two-point codes, accounting for 42 percent of the patients, were of the following type: 1-3/3-1, (18%), 2-7/7-2 (10%), 1-2/2-1 (8%), and 2-3/3-2 (6%). However, group mean profiles within this sample were distinctly different for those patients having significant pain complaints (*n* = 182) and those without pain (*n*=380). Both sexes in the former group had distinctly higher scores on Hs and Hy than their counterparts without pain, with female pain patients producing a mean profile characterized by a 3-1 codetype and male pain patients a 1-2-3 codetype; by contrast, patients referred for psychiatric evaluation without pain showed an inverted-V pattern on the neurotic triad.

In presenting the mean MMPI profile for a diverse sample

of 100 chronic pain patients referred to a university pain clinic for evaluation, Fordyce et al. (1978) showed these patients to obtain significant elevations on all three scales of the neurotic triad (69 to 72T) relative to other scales (at or below 61T); scores on obvious subscales of D and Hy were substantially higher than patients' scores on subtle components of these measures, whereas scores on obvious components of Pd and Pa were significantly lower. In addition, patients reporting less walking activity during the two weeks prior to examination scored significantly higher on Hs and D (72 to 73T) compared to subjects describing greater walking activity.

Finally, Naliboff, Cohen, and Yellen (1982) correlated self-ratings of functional limitation with MMPI scores for four chronic illness groups characterized by low-back pain, migraine headaches, hypertension, or diabetes. Functional limitation ratings received validational support from spouse and physical-therapist ratings and observed performance during a maximum speed walk (r's ranging from 0.34 to 0.53 in absolute value). Self-ratings of functional limitation correlated substantially with neurotic triad scales of the MMPI ($r=0.56$, 0.45, and 0.55 for Hs, D, and Hy respectively). However, measures of illness type, age, and chronicity added little or no predictive power above that of functional limitation alone for these three scales, suggesting that there was no unique relationship between illness type and MMPI elevations over and above what could be accounted for by functional limitation differences among these groups.

Although composite MMPI profiles of mixed chronic pain samples typically exhibit significant elevations on scales comprising the neurotic triad, these studies have been criticized for their implication that personality factors relate to various pain syndromes in a consistent manner without respect to the locus or nature of the underlying physical disorder. Consequently, numerous investigations have been conducted of more specific groups classified by pain descriptors and, in some cases, by presumed etiology of the pain complaints. A review of such studies follows.

STUDIES OF SPECIFIC PAIN GROUPS

Arthritis

In a review of psychological dimensions of arthritis, Achterberg-Lawlis (1982) notes both the prevalence of the disease (50 million Americans suffering from the condition with 600,000 new cases annually) and its heterogeneity. Citing the differences across studies in research methods, clinical samples, and comparison groups, Hoffman (1974) concludes that the integration and interpretation of psychological studies of patients suffering from arthritis are rendered virtually impossible. Nevertheless, these difficulties notwithstanding, results of MMPI studies of arthritic samples over the past thirty years yield surprisingly consistent results and provide a psychometric standard against which to compare individual profiles.

Moos and Solomon (1964) contrasted the group mean MMPI profile from forty-nine female rheumatoid arthritic medical center patients with the mean profile generated by fifty-three of their healthy female family members (some of whom possibly had incipient or latent rheumatoid disease). The arthritic sample produced a profile with moderate elevations between 65 and 68T on Hs, D, and Hy with scores on remaining profile scales below 58T; by comparison, the nonarthritic family controls produced mean profile scale scores all less than 55T. Moos and Solomon cite the striking similarity between profiles of their clinical group and the arthritic samples of seventy-five male VA patients of Cohen (1949) and fifty male VA arthritics of Wiener (1952). Similar group mean profiles were reported for thirty-five female and ten male rheumatoid arthritic outpatients by Nalven and O'Brien (1964), and for twenty-four and twenty-two female arthritic patients by Spergel, Ehrlich, and Glass (1978), with mean scores on the neurotic triad (Hs, D, and Hy) all at 67 to 69T and scores on remaining scales between 50 and 60T. Bourestom and Howard (1965) reported similar findings for seventy-seven female patients with rheumatoid arthritis, but obtained a more pathological profile for a smaller sample of seventeen male arthritics with six of ten clinical profile scales at or above 65T.

Polley, Swenson, and Steinhilber (1970) compared MMPIs from 726 rheumatoid arthritis outpatients with 50,000 general medical patients and 1576 "normal healthy controls" undergoing examination but without complaints or medical findings. The arthritic sample produced scores on the neurotic triad from 63 to 64T with remaining scales below 55T, in contrast to scores on the neurotic triad averaging 60 to 61T for the general medical sample and 58 to 60T for the "healthy" controls. However, Polley et al. also determined that arthritic patients differed from general medical patients at $p < 0.01$ on ten individual items, most reflecting specific somatic concerns or conditions attributable to rheumatoid arthritis. The authors concluded that "the predominant or statistically significant differences in responses to the MMPI test in patients with rheumatoid arthritis are most readily explained on the basis of the symptoms and effects of a disease that is chronic, painful, and potentially disabling to various degrees" (p. 48).

As Hoffman (1974) notes in her review, these studies fail to address issues of intra- and intersubject variability in profiles, seriously compromising predictive utility when group results are applied idiographically. For example, potential distinct subgroups characterized by "conversion-V" configurations on the neurotic triad in contrast to patients obtaining peak scores on scale 2 would remain unidentified in these studies and could be expected to generate the "flattened" scores on the neurotic triad averaging 67 to 70T. However, the consistency in MMPI profiles for arthritic patients across seven studies and nearly 1,000 subjects suggests that individual profiles showing clinical elevations significantly above 70T on Hs, D, or Hy or above 60T on remaining profile scales lend themselves increasingly to interpretation of psychological components contributing to the individual's pain complaints.

Chronic Low Back Pain

MMPI studies of chronic low back pain (CLBP) patients outnumber by far those of any other pain group. Many of these reflect efforts to delineate homogeneous subgroups within the back pain population, or to distinguish between "organic" and "functional" groups for whom objective physical findings may or may not be sufficient to account for the patient's various complaints; others reflect attempts to identify aspects of MMPI profiles predictive of patients' response to medical and psychological interventions. Studies of CLBP patients falling in either of these categories are described later in this chapter. However, the literature also contains more circumscribed MMPI studies of low back pain patients describing typical profile characteristics, relating these to independent criteria, and elaborating on general interpretive issues.

Gentry, Shows, and Thomas (1974) presented a psychological profile including both biographical as well as psychometric features for fifty-six inpatients with low back pain referred for evaluation by orthopedic surgeons. All patients had sustained one or more prior spinal operations with limited improvement. Both male and female patients produced conversion-V configurations (Hs and Hy above 70T and 5 to 10 points higher than D), with remaining scales at or below 60T. The authors suggested that patients' profiles reflected "a tendency to manifest marked somatic concern (complaints), to use denial and repression as major psychological defense mechanisms, to interpret problems in living in rational and socially acceptable terms, as well as a poor prognosis for remotivation and a contrasting appearance of being externally extroverted and sociable and internally self-centered, demanding, and dependent" (p. 175).

However, the extent to which low back pain patients uniformly exhibit conversion-V configurations has been challenged by numerous investigations. Donovan, Dwyer, White, Batalin, Skerritt, and Bedbrook (1981) presented findings from fifty chronic low back pain patients, all of whom were functionally impaired, but only eighteen of whom had undergone prior surgery. Of forty MMPIs obtained for this sample, thirty-six were abnormal with twenty-seven involving significant elevations on the neurotic triad (Hs, D, and Hy); however, of these, only eleven involved conversion-V configurations while sixteen reflected inverted-V (depressed) patterns. Similarly, Naliboff, Cohen, and Yellen (1983) noted that although the mean profile for seventy-two CLBP patients in their study reflected a conversion-V configuration, this pattern was *not* the most frequent codetype in their sample and in fact was "an artifact of averaging several clinically distinct profiles of equal frequency" (p. 846).

Several explanations have been posited for elevations on the neurotic triad among CLBP patients. Kinder, Curtiss, and Kalichman (1986) found a measure of trait anxiety (Spielberger et al., 1983) to correlate significantly ($p < 0.05$) with Hs, D, and Hy for forty-two male and thirty-five female patients with chronic back pain of musculoskeletal origin (r's ranging from 0.34 to 0.44 for males and 0.54 to 0.66 for females); they concluded that results "confirm the need for treatment modalities aimed at decreasing anxiety that are commonly used in the treatment of chronic pain patients" (p. 660). Using a measure of general and low back pain cognitive distortion with 138 CLBP patients, Smith, Aberger, Follick, and Ahern (1986) determined that cognitive distortion was related to general distress on the MMPI (D, Pt, and Sc) but not somatization (Hs and Hy), and that these findings were not moderated by extent of physical disability or severity or duration of pain.

McCreary, Turner, and Dawson (1981) factor-analyzed the responses of 102 chronic low back pain patients to the McGill Pain Questionnaire (Melzack, 1975) and related these dimensions to subjects' scores on the MMPI; they concluded that patients with higher scores on the neurotic triad (Hs, D, and Hy) had a tendency to describe their pain as more intense, frightening, unbearable, and burdensome. Using a Rorschach measure (F%) of rigidity and constriction in a sample of 148 low back pain patients, Leavitt and Garron (1982) found that increasing elevations on Hs, D, and Hy were associated with *lower* levels of self-dramatization and lability; they suggested that "the tense, constrained and emotionally inexpressive patient whose complaints may well be psychogenic may well be underdiagnosed as suffering from a psychological disturbance marked by conversion" (p. 24).

Diagnostic issues related to "conversion" and hysterical processes as they relate to the Hy scale have been discussed at length by Caldwell and Chase (1977), Watson (1982), and Prokop (1986). Caldwell and Chase asserted that elevations on

Hy reflect hysteroid mechanisms of repression involving primary (rather than secondary) gain and reduction of pain–fear acquired through conditioning. The authors proposed that "the reduction of pain-fear reinforces a wide range of behaviors including both (1) a high level of body-pain protection and (2) interpersonal behaviors that avoid emotional upset and its intensification of subjective pain" (p. 146); these behaviors are hypothesized to account for higher scores of chronic low back pain patients on the Hy scale. However, in an analysis of MMPI item endorsement in a sample of 144 pain patients compared to general medical and nonpatient control groups, Watson (1982) determined that pain patients' elevations on Hy reflected *greater* admission of somatic problems and *lesser* denial of psychological difficulties, arguing against Caldwell and Chase's model of hysteroid dynamics being reflected on this scale.

In a study comprising three independent samples of psychiatric, general medical, and chronic pain patients, Mc-Grath and O'Malley (1986) also found consistent negative correlations between Hy subscales assessing admission of physical difficulties and denial of psychological problems, although the smallest correlation (− 0.28) was obtained in the chronic pain sample. Based on correlations with remaining MMPI profile scales, the authors concluded that simultaneous elevations on K, Hs, and Hy provided the best indicator of the denial of psychological factors associated with a physiological disorder.

Similarly, Prokop (1986) challenged the inference of hysterical personality dynamics in CLBP patients with MMPI profiles of the conversion-V type, based on item overlap between Hs and Hy and scores on Hy subscales for fifty-three female and forty male CLBP patients. Prokop's conclusions regarding the interpretation of conversion-V configurations for this population warrant inclusion:

> The presence of an unusual focus on physical symptomatology may thus be inferred to exist in the low back pain patient presenting a Conversion V profile, but the inference that these symptoms indicate conversion dynamics may not be justified without additional evidence,

whether from subscale analysis, analysis of the balance of the MMPI profile, or history. Instead, the Hy elevation may reflect a need to call attention to confusing or frightening physical symptoms, or it may suggest another somatoform disorder, such as hypochondriasis, and thus may not be indicative of hysterical personality functioning. Alternatively, the Hy elevation may reflect an operantly developed and controlled focus on physical symptoms, with little or no suggestion of other psychopathology. [p. 561].

Headaches

Blanchard, Andrasik, Neff, Arena, Ahles, Jurish, Pallmeyer, Saunders, Teders, Barron, and Rodichok (1982) have noted that chronic recurring headaches afflict up to 40 percent of the adult population. In a review of early MMPI studies of headache sufferers, Harrison (1975) concluded that headache samples of diverse types typically exhibited conversion-V patterns on the neurotic triad. More recent studies have contrasted MMPI profiles differentiated by specific headache subgroups. Kudrow and Sutkus (1979) compared MMPIs of 113 male and 145 female headache patients grouped into six categories: (1) migraine; (2) contraction; (3) mixed migraine/contraction; (4) cluster; (5) posttraumatic cephalgia; and (6) conversion cephalgia. For both males and females, MMPI profiles of migraine and cluster headache patients were indistinguishable and least deviant with scores on Hs, D, and Hy between 60 and 65T, but significantly higher than controls' scores on these scales (50 to 55T). Contraction and mixed headache types were also indistinguishable for both sexes, with scores on the neurotic triad ranging from 70 to 75T for males and 65 to 70T for females. Posttraumatic and conversion cephalgia (constant or near constant headache of moderate to severe intensity and duration of at least one year) produced the most deviant mean profiles, with scores on Hs, D, and Hy for conversion and male posttraumatic headaches from 75 to 80T and for female posttraumatic headaches from 65 to 75T.

These results were generally confirmed by Sternbach, Dalessio, Kunzel, and Bowman (1980) in a study of forty-six male and 136 female headache patients grouped into vascular (migraine), muscle contraction (tension), and mixed categories. For both sexes, MMPI profiles of muscle contraction and mixed headache sufferers were higher than those from vascular sufferers, which were higher than the MMPI profile for 50,000 general medical patients (Swenson, Pearson, and Osborne, 1973). Sternbach et al. argued that the lower scores on neurotic scales obtained by the vascular group were likely due to pain-free intervals between attacks.

Andrasik, Blanchard, Arena, Teders, Teevan, and Rodi-chok (1982) divided twenty male and seventy-nine female headache patients into four categories of migraine, muscle contraction, mixed migraine–contraction, and cluster subtypes. Headache groups fell along a continuum of psychological disturbance, beginning with cluster patients showing minimal distress, continuing through migraine and mixed types, and ending with muscle contraction patients revealing the greatest amount of disturbance. However, contraction headache patients obtained only moderate mean scores on the neurotic triad (64 to 66T), although one-third had scores on Hs and/or Hy exceeding 70T. The authors emphasized the extent of overlap of MMPI score values among the four headache subtypes, despite statistically significant differences in group means.

Several MMPI studies have suggested a possible role of personality factors in either the etiology or treatment of headache disorders. Sovak, Kunzel, Sternbach, and Dalessio (1981) determined that migraine sufferers successfully treated with a standard drug regimen revealed only minimal changes on the MMPI, suggesting the chronicity of personality dynamics associated with this condition. Werder, Sargent, and Coyne (1981) and Blanchard et al. (1982) found the MMPI to predict treatment response of chronic headache patients administered a relaxation–training and/or biofeedback regimen.

Menstrual Distress and Gynecologic Pain

Relatively few studies have examined the relationship of MMPI scores to women's complaints of menstrual and premenstrual distress or chronic pelvic pain, despite the prevalence of the former and the recent inclusion of a periluteal phase (premenstrual) dysphoric disorder in a draft of DSM-III-R (American Psychiatric Association, 1986). Investigations in this area have been limited in scope and divergent in findings, precluding reliable conclusions or interpretive guidelines. Hain, Linton, Eber, and Chapman (1970) administered the MMPI and a menstrual history questionnaire to seventy-one first-year nursing students and determined that women reporting irregularity of menstrual cycle and symptoms (abnormal flow and abdominal swelling, premenstrual depression, and irritability) were characterized by significantly lower scores on the K scale and higher scores on Pd, Pt, Sc, and Ma. Gruba and Rohrbaugh (1975) found for a nonspecific sample of sixty undergraduate women that both menstrual and premenstrual symptoms of pain, functional restriction, autonomic reactions, and dysphoria were consistently and significantly correlated with Hs, Hy, Pt, and Sc, and that these correlations were only marginally reduced when controlling for intermenstrual (baseline) symptoms and an MMPI dissimulation (F-K) response set. Correlations between the MMPI and both pain and affect ratings were consistently higher premenstrually than menstrually, but yielded no differential association of specific symptom patterns and MMPI scales.

Castelnuovo-Tedesco and Krout (1970) identified elevated scores on Hs, D, and Hy (from 67 to 70T) for a sample of forty women complaining of chronic pelvic pain, although no comparisons were conducted of women with and without clear physical pathology; a comparison group of twenty-five women with pelvic pain sampled from a different setting produced a similar but lower mean profile. Similar MMPI findings for thirty-seven women with chronic pelvic pain were obtained by Renaer, Vertommen, Nijs, Wagemans, and Van Hemelrijck (1979), with scores on the neurotic triad from 60 to 70T and remaining scales below 55T; mean scores on Hs and Hy for 15 of the women without a clear organic basis to their pelvic pain were 5 to 8 T-points higher than those for twenty-two women whose pain resulted from endometriosis, although these differences were not statistically significant.

Other Specific Groups

Other relatively isolated MMPI studies of specific pain groups have been conducted. Small (1976) reported on the MMPIs of twenty-four male and twenty-six female patients presenting with temporomandibular joint (TMJ) dysfunction treated with conservative (nonsurgical and psychological) measures; forty of these patients' profiles were classified as "abnormal," with twenty-eight exhibiting a conversion-V configuration on scales Hs, D, and Hy. Mean MMPI scale scores and specific criteria for classifying profiles were not reported. The author interpreted the favorable response of these forty patients to conservative treatment (in contrast to only three of ten patients with "normal" profiles) as supporting the role of psychological factors in the pain syndromes of the former group.

Finally, in a study of 144 patients with arteriosclerotic heart disease, Bakker and Levenson (1967) compared the profiles of seventy-five patients complaining of angina pectoris and sixty-nine without angina at their initial visit; both groups produced elevations on the neurotic triad (Hs, D, and Hy from 65 to 70T and remaining scales below 60T), with the angina group being significantly higher ($p < 0.05$) on Hs and Hy. Of greater interest, however, were differences between patients without angina at the initial visit who did ($n = 6$) or did not ($n = 43$) report angina at six-month follow-up; the small group of patients who subsequently developed angina initially produced more deviant MMPIs (scores on the neurotic triad from 70 to 78T) with significantly higher scores on Hs and Hy than patients remaining pain-free.

THE ROLE OF DEPRESSION IN CHRONIC PAIN

Considerable disagreement can be found in the clinical and research literature regarding the relationship of depression to chronic pain. In a recent review, Beutler, Engle, Oro'-Beutler, Daldrup, and Meredith (1986) noted that 50 percent of medical patients exhibit significant depressive features and over 20 percent warrant diagnoses within the depressive spectrum; major depressive syndromes have been found to characterize at least 30 percent of patients experiencing chronic pain (Turner and Romano, 1984; Love, 1987). Beutler et al. concluded that prolonged inhibition of intense interpersonal anger or other emotional experience coinciding with prolonged stress may be a common correlate or precursor of depression, chronic pain, and disease susceptibility. In noting the frequently observed pain–depression linkage, arguments have been proffered citing each as a cause and/or result of the other. It could be expected, then, that elevations on scale 2 (depression) of the MMPI among chronic pain patients would receive particular attention.

Sternbach (1976) argued that in acute pain states the predominant affect is anxiety but that, in chronic pain states, the severity and duration of pain are more strongly associated with depression which may or may not be "masked" by somatic features. He suggested that relieving chronic pain alleviates depression and, similarly, that treating the depression (with antidepressants or other nonpharmacologic interventions) "either reduces the pain or makes it more bearable" (p. 294). Sternbach (1977) also argued that continuing antianxiety agents past the acute pain stage tends to potentiate depression.

Parker, Doerfler, Tatten, and Hewett (1983) administered the MMPI to thirty male VA patients with chronic pain of at least three months' duration, along with the Beck Depression Inventory (BDI) (Beck, Ward, Mendelson, Mock, and Erbaugh, 1961) and the McGill Pain Questionnaire. Neither the BDI nor the MMPI depression (D) scale correlated above chance with any of the McGill pain measures; by contrast, the MMPI psychasthenia (Pt) and hypochondriasis (Hs) scales predicted patients' tendencies to describe their pain in emotional terms (e.g., exhausting or terrifying) and to report higher pain intensities, respectively.

In a study of sixty-two male and eighty-six female chronic pain patients, Garron and Leavitt (1983) administered the MMPI and other affect and pain measures to three groups of patients with recent (0–6 months, $n = 39$), relatively longstanding (6 to 24 months, $n = 35$), and chronic (more than 24 months, $n = 74$) low back pain. Although findings were limited by the cross-sectional nature of their design, the authors concluded that chronic low back pain results in increased somatic preoccupation, passive dependence, and vegetative aspects of depression (overconcern with physical functioning and disturbances of sleep, appetite, and libido), but does not result in increases in psychopathological mood states or in the pain itself. They added that, "These increases in apparent psychopathology seem to affect aspects of the self that might result in a less productive life style" (p. 492).

Maruta, Swanson, and Swenson (1976) compared the group mean MMPI profiles of twenty-six low back pain patients with twenty-six depressed patients matched for age and sex; all patients had been admitted to the psychiatric service of a general hospital. Both groups exhibited elevated scores on all three scales comprising the neurotic triad; however, the low back pain group obtained higher scores on Hs and Hy (with greater differences on these scales among men) and lower scores on D (with greater mean differences for women).

At least two methodological issues contribute to inconsistencies in the literature relating pain to depression on the MMPI. The first involves the inconsistent criteria used to define "chronic" pain, ranging from three months (Parker et al.) to twenty-four months (Garron and Leavitt). More critical has been the failure to control for the configural relationship of the depression (D) scale to the Hs and Hy scales; the behavioral and affective expressions of a given elevation on scale 2 vary markedly depending on whether the D score reflects the high-point scale in an inverted-V pattern or a score relatively lower than Hs and Hy in a conversion-V configuration. For example, results presented earlier for Pilling et al. (1967) indicated that among medical and surgical patients with minimal physical findings referred for psychiatric evaluation, mean profiles for patients without pain showed distinctly *lower* scores on Hs and Hy than patients with pain, although both groups had comparable scores on the depression (D) scale.

EMPIRICALLY DERIVED CHRONIC PAIN MMPI
SUBGROUPS

Studies of the sort described above have been criticized widely over the past ten years for their frequent failure to differentiate among homogeneous subgroups of patients within specific pain populations. Presumably one could identify subgroups on the basis of presenting symptoms (beyond general locus of pain as reflected above), pain descriptors, response to treatment, psychological measures, or presumed etiology as evaluated by physical findings. Studies of the latter type abound, and typically use physicians' judgments for classifying patients into "functional," "organic," and "mixed" groups. Investigations of this type are reviewed later, but have been criticized for their unreliable grouping of patients by presumed etiology on the basis of highly fallible indicators (Bradley, Prieto, Hopson, and Prokop, 1978).

Furthermore, classifying patients on the basis of physical findings or other pain-related criteria and then evaluating group differences on various psychological measures restricts one to delineating the probability of obtaining some particular pattern of test responses given independent external criteria (i.e., $P(R_i|C_j)$), rather than the conceptually more appealing and predictively more useful probability of observing relevant external criteria (pain characteristics, physical findings, or treatment response) given some particular pattern of psychometric indicators ($P(C_i|R_j)$) (Wiggins, 1973). Consequently, the advantages of the MMPI as a multidimensional measure of personality functioning and the availability of multivariate taxonomic clustering algorithms have led to numerous studies aimed at identifying homogeneous MMPI subgroups of pain patients on an empirical basis and evaluating subgroup differences across independent behavioral criteria.

Sternbach (1974) laid the conceptual foundations for research in this area in presenting four theoretically derived prototypic profiles labeled (a) "hypochondriasis" (scores on Hs, D, and Hy from 75 to 85T with Hs highest, Pt and Sc 70 to 75T, and remaining scales below 65T); (b) "reactive depression" (scores on Hs, D, and Hy from 70 to 75T with D highest, and remaining scales below 65T); (c) "somatization reaction" (conversion-V pattern with Hs and Hy from 70 to 75T and remaining scales below 60T); and (d) "manipulative reaction" (Hs, D, Hy, and Pd from 70 to 75T with remaining scales below 67T). Sternbach suggested that only patients with MMPI profiles reflecting reactive depressions or somatization reactions are likely to exhibit a favorable response to treatment.

In the first empirical study of this nature, Bradley, Prokop, Margolis, and Gentry (1978) derived homogeneous MMPI subgroups for 548 low back pain patients and replicated profile types across sex and across three cohorts within sex. Three of four profile types derived for women generally confirmed Sternbach's theoretically derived hypochrondriasis, depression, and somatization types; a fourth group was characterized by a mild conversion-V pattern within normal limits on the MMPI (55 to 70T). Mean profiles for male subgroups replicated three of the types derived for women, with the absence of a clear somatization type (Hs and Hy above 70T and remaining scales below 60T).

Hart (1984) replicated the four profile types identified by Bradley et al. in a sample of seventy male chronic pain patients with heterogeneous complaints. In a follow-up to their own study, Prokop, Bradley, Margolis, and Gentry (1980) applied cluster analysis to 123 male and 221 female patients with multiple pain complaints excluding low back pain. Results across sex were less consistent than for the Bradley et al. (1978) study. Elevated and subclinical (below 70T) hypochondriacal patterns were derived for both sexes; an additional somatization (conversion-V) type was identified for women with multiple pain complaints, in contrast to a reactive depression type for men. Adams, Heilbronn, and Blumer (1986) identified just two subgroups in a cluster analysis of MMPIs from seventy-two chronic pain patients; one group exhibited a conversion-V pattern within normal limits, while the other group obtained elevated scores on all three scales of the neurotic triad ranging from 70 to 72T.

Armentrout, Moore, Parker, Hewett, and Feltz (1982) derived MMPI subgroups for 240 male VA chronic pain patients and subsequently examined subgroup differences across ratings on the McGill Pain Questionnaire and related measures. Three cluster profiles were derived, including two highly elevated hypochondriasis and depressive reaction groups (scores on relevant scales from 80 to 100T), and one subclinical (below 70T) hypochondriacal group. Patients in the two groups comprising the highly elevated profiles reported significantly greater pain severity and accompanying symptoms (including impaired self-esteem, sleep difficulties, and decreased sexual frequency) than patients in the subclinical group, but did not differ from each other on these dimensions. McCreary (1985) reported similar findings for replicated MMPI subgroups of 401 chronic low back pain patients treated nonsurgically and followed up six to twelve months posttreatment. He noted that patients comprising two groups with unelevated MMPIs (scores below 70T) generally reported better outcome (greatest decrease in pain intensity from pretreatment to follow-up) than patients comprising three elevated MMPI subgroups.

Bernstein and Garbin (1983) subjected the MMPI profiles of seventy-seven female pain patients to a clustering algorithm and derived five profile types including one normal profile (comprising 16 percent of the sample) and four profiles remarkably consistent with the theoretically derived profile types of Sternbach (1974). McGill et al. (1983) applied cluster analysis to forty-six male and forty-six female low back pain patients and related four resultant profile types to subjects' reported pain history and physical therapists' ratings of improvement. MMPI mean profiles for the four groups reflected somatization (conversion-V), reactive depression, and elevated and subclinical hypochondriacal configurations. Patients comprising the subclinical group (all scales below 65T) were distinguished by a shorter duration of pain, fewer prior hospitalizations or back surgeries, and lower estimated pretreatment pain than the other three groups; subjects in the somatization (conversion-V) group were less likely to report a clear precipitant to their pain. Following treatment, patients comprising the subclinical group reported less overall pain but did not differ from subjects in the other three groups in amount of analgesics used, amount of daily activity, or range of motion.

However, the importance of elevations on the neurotic triad (Hs, D, and Hy) to the relative exclusion of elevations on remaining scales—even when scores on the neurotic scales are below 70T—was highlighted by Bradley and Van der Heide (1984) in a study of ninety-six male and 218 female back pain patients. Although disruption of daily activities was generally correlated with overall profile elevation, profile subgroups with elevations primarily on Hs, D, and Hy reported greater affective disturbance and disruption of activities than did subgroups with elevations on *both* the neurotic triad and additional scales (especially Pd and Sc). In addition, profile subgroups with subclinical elevations on the neurotic triad (60 to 69T) exhibited poorer adjustment than did subgroups having all clinical scales below 60T.

Similar findings were obtained by Snyder and Power (1981) in a cluster analysis of 141 chronic pain patients referred for psychiatric evaluation whose MMPI profiles fell entirely within normal limits (below 70T). Snyder and Power delineated five profile types among these unelevated MMPIs, including four characterized by scores on the neurotic triad ranging from 60 to 65T. Patients comprising the fifth profile type (all clinical scales below 55T) reported the shortest duration of pain; were least likely to report multiple pain complaints, impaired work ability, or previous surgery or psychiatric treatment; and were least likely to describe family members with similar or identical pain complaints.

COMPARISONS OF PATIENTS WITH "FUNCTIONAL" VERSUS "ORGANIC" PAIN

MMPI studies aimed at identifying patients whose pain syndrome comprises a substantial psychological component abound, evolving in part from the high cost to both the individual and the health care system in undertaking extensive medical interventions unlikely to elicit subjective pain relief. Typically such studies attempt to delineate characteristics of the MMPI profile discriminating between patients with clear physical findings accounting for their pain complaints and either those pain patients without physical 'findings or those whose physical findings are insufficient to account for the severity of their pain or extent of their functional limitations. These investigations have been criticized on numerous grounds, including (1) their reliance on subjective and unreliable judgments of physicians; (2) artificial bifurcation of "organic" versus "functional" classifications; (3) frequent failure to employ appropriate multivariate or configural analyses; and (4) conceptual deficiencies in viewing the relationship between psychological factors and subjective pain as linear rather than reciprocal (Bradley et al., 1978; Elkins and Barrett, 1984).

The merit of these criticisms notwithstanding, MMPI studies of this genre yield a pattern of consistent findings across numerous independent investigations. To the extent that replicable profile differences emerge between groups of pain patients classified on the basis of objective physical findings and physicians' judgments—regardless of the deficiencies of such criteria—these findings demand closer examination for their diagnostic and treatment implications. Issues warranting consideration include the extent to which MMPI profile characteristics can be employed either to confirm or rule out psychological or physical components to the patient's pain syndrome, the relative utility of scale-by-scale versus configural profile analyses, and the likelihood of classification error in different patient populations.

In the original prototypic study in this area, Hanvik (1951) compared the mean MMPI profiles for thirty "proved" organic low back pain patients with thirty cases without clear physical findings, matched on age, SES, marital status, IQ, and race. Mean scores for the organic group were all below 60T; by contrast, the mean profile for patients in the functional group exhibited a classic conversion-V pattern (Hs = 73, D = 63, Hy = 69 and remaining scales below 60T). Differences in mean MMPI profiles between pain patients with and without physical findings have been found repeatedly since Hanvik's study, typically identifying significant differences on the neurotic triad (Hs, D, Hy) and, less consistently, on Pd and Pt. McCreary, Turner, and Dawson (1977) compared group mean profiles for forty-seven female and thirty-two male low back pain patients divided into organic (n = 42) and functional (n = 37) groups. The mean profile for the functional group was significantly higher ($p < 0.01$) on Pd and, to a lesser extent ($p < 0.05$), higher on Hs, Hy, Sc, Ma, and Si and lower on K; the functional group had mean scores on the neurotic triad ranging from 73 to 77T, in contrast to scores on these scales from 63 to 67T for the organic group. Similarly, Turner and McCreary (1978) compared mean MMPI profiles for thirty-nine low back pain patients judged by physicians to have a substantial psychological component to their pain with twenty-five patients not judged to have a functional component; scores for the functional group were significantly higher on Hs, Hy, Sc, and Si scales.

Shaw and Matthews (1965) compared thirty-two patients with a wide range of neurologic symptoms suggestive of central nervous system (CNS) dysfunction but without physical findings (X-ray, EEG, brain scan, or spinal fluid analysis) to thirty-two patients with symptoms "unequivocally referrable" to organic brain damage; the pseudoneurologic mean profile reflected a prototypic conversion-V pattern (Hs = 72, D = 63, Hy = 73 with remaining scales below 65T) in comparison to scale scores consistently below 65T for the neurologic group. In a study noted earlier, Renaer et al. (1979) determined that the mean scores on Hs and Hy for fifteen women complaining of chronic pelvic pain without a clear organic basis were 5 to 8 T-points higher than scores for a comparison group of women whose pelvic pain could be attributed to identifiable organic pathology.

By contrast, some studies have failed to find differences in MMPI profiles for patients dichotomized into functional versus organic groups. Sternbach et al. (1973) reported no significant differences in the MMPIs of low back pain patients with (n = 81) and without (n = 36) positive physical findings; both groups produced mean elevations on the neurotic triad ranging from 67 to 72T. Similarly, Cox, Chapman, and Black (1978) could find no significant differences in the mean MMPI profiles of patients with chronic pain of unknown etiology and those whose pain onset could be linked to a surgical event; both groups obtained scores on Hs, D, and Hy ranging from 70 to

75T, with scores on remaining scales below 62T. Based on such negative findings, Rosen, Frymoyer, and Clements (1980) suggested that the MMPI should be used *not* to predict the presence or absence of physical findings, but rather the appropriateness of the pain disability. In a follow-up study, Rosen, Johnson, and Frymoyer (1983) employed K-corrected T-scores on Hs and Hy to predict the classification of forty-nine pain patients judged to exhibit an inappropriate degree of incapacitation relative to their physical findings versus seventy-four patients judged to exhibit appropriate pain-related limitations; reclassification of patients based on a score on either scale $\geq$ 70T resulted in 82 percent overall accuracy and 79 percent correct identification of the "inappropriately disabled" group.

Other investigators have argued for expanded classification of patients into functional, organic and "mixed groups," the latter comprising patients whose pain syndromes are judged to evolve from an exacerbation of physical pathology on a psychological basis. Freeman, Calsyn, and Louks (1976) examined the mean MMPI profiles of thirty-six male VA low back pain patients classified into functional, organic, and mixed groups on the basis of physical findings and extent of pain complaints. Both the functional and mixed groups produced highly elevated scores on the neurotic triad (ranging from 73 to 87T) but did not differ from each other; however, both groups were significantly higher on these scales than the organic group (Hs, D, and Hy from 63 to 67T and remaining scales below 60T). The authors concluded that elevations on Hs and Hy are likely to confirm a psychological component to patients' pain complaints, but do not rule out organic factors. Calsyn, Louks, and Freeman (1976) extended these findings to sixty-two patients with chronic low back pain divided evenly into organic and mixed groups, and found patients with exacerbating psychological factors to have significantly higher scores on the neurotic triad (from 75 to 85T) compared to scores on these scales for the organic group (from 63 to 67T with remaining scales below 65T).

Although analyses of group mean profiles tend to reveal higher scores for functional and mixed groups on Hs and Hy, these studies do not address the relative incidence of 1-3/3-1 codetypes in patients judged to have a significant psychological component to their pain syndrome. Chaney, Williams, Cohn, and Vincent (1984) compared the MMPIs of twenty-six trauma patients evaluated at least six months postaccident with twenty-six patients who were judged to have an organically based illness and twenty-six judged to have a psychological basis to their pain syndrome; 42 percent of patients in the functional group obtained a 1-3/3-1 profile, in contrast to only 15 percent of the trauma patients and 8 percent of the organic group. Louks et al. (1978) sorted MMPI profiles of seventy-four low back pain patients previously classified as functional, organic, or mixed into six profile types based on criteria of Pichot, Perse, Lekeoux, Dureau, Perez, and Rychewaert (1972); the authors determined that conversion-V patterns accounted for 58 percent of the functional patients, in contrast to 45 percent of mixed and 35 percent of organic patients. However, Schwartz, Osborne, and Krupp (1972) showed that a representative sample of 178 medical patients obtaining conversion-V patterns were somewhat more likely to be judged as having a significant psychological component to their physical complaints if they were younger (below forty years in age) and female.

The disproportionate incidence of 1-3/3-1 profiles among various pain samples has been compared to the incidence of such profiles in general medical samples. Gilberstadt and Jancis (1967) observed 1-3/3-1 codetypes in just 14 percent of eighty-eight male veterans seeking admission to a VA general hospital. In an extensive study of 50,000 general medical patients, Schwartz and Krupp (1971) identified 4,051 patients where Hs and Hy were the highest scales and at least one of these was $\geq$ 70T. However, when more restrictive criteria were imposed requiring that Hy exceed D by 10 T-points and remaining scales be $\leq$ 70T, the incidence dropped to 1,398; additional criteria that Hs exceed D by 10 T-points and Hy exceed Pd by 10 T-points further reduced the incidence to 820, or less than 2 percent of the total sample. This stands in sharp contrast to the much higher incidence of 1-3/3-1 codetypes among chronic pain patients and, particularly, among patients judged independently to have a substantial psychological basis to their pain.

Overall, findings from these studies suggest that high scores on the MMPI, and particularly on those scales comprising the neurotic triad, confirm a significant psychological component to the patient's pain complaints and functional limitations, but do not rule out underlying physical pathology. The higher the profile, the more likely that psychological factors play a significant and disproportionately greater role in the patient's pain syndrome. However, as Meehl and Rosen (1955) noted in their classic discussion of base rates and the efficiency of psychometric indicators, in a setting where the only patients referred for psychological evaluation are those pain patients for whom physical findings are absent, it would be unwise to rule out psychological factors *solely* on the basis of a low MMPI.

PREDICTING RESPONSE TO TREATMENT

While studies described above have attempted to identify etiologic and presumed prognostic differences among patients' pain syndromes, others have examined more directly the ability of the MMPI to predict treatment response. These vary considerably in the type and chronicity of pain evaluated, method of treatment, length of time between initial testing and assessment of outcome, and analysis of individual scales versus profile configurations. As in the previous areas reviewed, however, the extant literature presents significant findings replicated across diverse investigations offering strong diagnostic and treatment implications.

In an early study of 151 industrially injured patients six months following discharge from a disability prevention program, Beals and Hickman (1972) identified a positive correlation between patients' "total adjustment score" derived from the MMPI and the number of back operations. Their findings also suggested that increased duration of unemployment resulted in individuals' profiles changing from an inverted-V on the neurotic triad to a conversion-V reflecting both relative increases in the elaboration and exaggeration of symptoms (Hs and Hy) and a decrease in subjective depression (D). In another early study limited by its retrospective nature, Wilfling, Klonoff, and Kokan (1973) related current MMPIs of twenty-six male VA patients to their response to spinal fusion for low back pain two to nine years earlier; patients with good outcome had a mean profile with all scores below 60T, in contrast to elevated scores on the neurotic triad (Hs, D, and Hy) for patients exhibiting either fair or poor response. In addition, singly operated patients (n = 15) had lower mean MMPIs (neurotic triad 61 to 65T) than multiply operated subjects (n = 11, neurotic triad 72 to 78T in a hypochondriacal pattern).

Wiltse and Rocchio (1975) examined the ability of preoperative MMPIs to predict treatment response of sixty-eight men and sixty-two women to chymopapain injection therapy who otherwise would have undergone laminectomy for relief of low back pain. Overall, 48 percent of patients showed functional recovery one year postoperatively. However, for patients with Hs and Hy below 65T, favorable response climbed to 87 percent; in contrast, only 25 percent of individuals having scores on Hs and Hy above 74T exhibited successful outcome. Similarly, Blumetti and Modesti (1976) found that for forty-two patients treated surgically for intractable back pain, individuals in the unimproved group (n = 23) at six-month follow-up scored significantly higher preoperatively on scales Hs and Hy of the MMPI; they suggested a cutoff score of 75T on Hs and 70T on Hy for predicting poor outcome.

Waring, Weisz, and Bailey (1976) failed to find individual MMPI scales predictive of treatment response in twenty men and fourteen women evaluated for low back pain; however, the small group of unfavorable responders (n = 5) were distinguished by a mild conversion-V pattern within normal limits (all scores below 70T). Jamison, Ferrer-Brechner, Brechner, and McCreary (1976) identified a nonsignificant trend toward lower Hs and Hy scores for sixteen treatment-success cases in a heterogeneous chronic pain sample relative to twenty-one poor responders; the authors attributed their nonsignificant findings to the restricted range in their sample since their facility served as a "last-resort" clinic.

The problem of restricted range presents itself in other studies as well. Pheasant et al. (1979) examined preoperative

MMPIs for fifty-four men and forty-nine women undergoing surgery for low back pain; mean MMPI profiles for patients divided into poor, fair, or good response groups were all significantly elevated, with scores on the neurotic triad above 70T. However, the poor outcome group had mean Hs and Hy scores at 78 to 79T, compared to $\leq$ 73T for fair and good outcome patients; in addition, a conversion-V pattern was associated with relatively poor outcome, especially for multiply operated cases. Cummings, Evanski, Debenedetti, Anderson, and Waugh (1979) found that pretreatment MMPIs did not discriminate between "improved" and "unimproved" male VA chronic pain patients following a six-week inpatient psychiatric treatment program; both groups (n = 37 each) produced nearly identical profiles characterized by high scores on Hs (79 to 82T), D and Hy (72 to 76T), with remaining scores at or below 65T.

Trief and Yuan (1983) followed up the work status of seventy-nine subjects participating in a six-week rehabilitation program for whom further medical–surgical treatment had been deemed inappropriate; of thirty-one persons with "poor risk" codetypes (those involving elevations on one or more scales of the neurotic triad) only seven (23%) had returned to work, compared to forty-three of forty-eight individuals (90%) not exhibiting these codetypes. At the other end of the distress spectrum, Zaretsky, Lee, and Rubin (1976) examined the ability of the MMPI to differentiate among relatively normal subjects responding or not to acupuncture for induction of oral analgesia; no significant group differences were found.

In contrast, Smith and Duerksen (1980) found strong, positive correlations (from 0.59 to 0.73) between Hs, D, and Hy and postsurgical ratings of pain alleviation for a heterogeneous sample of thirty-one chronic pain patients; a Pain Assessment Index (PAI) derived from a combination of five MMPI scales (Hs, D, Hy, Pt, and Ma) accurately classified twenty-nine of thirty-one cases (94%) as surgical "successes" or "failures." In a follow-up study, Turner et al. (1986) found the PAI to have 79 percent accuracy in classifying surgical outcome for 106 low back pain patients undergoing lumbar laminectomy and discectomy, with 87 percent accuracy in predicting work status at least one year later; however, prediction from either Hs or Hy alone or in combination afforded comparable overall accuracy, with higher sensitivity but lower specificity rates.

Shipman, Greene, and Laskin (1974) examined the MMPIs of 120 patients with myofascial pain dysfunction (MPD) syndrome subjected to three different placebo conditions. They found that patients having their highest score on either Hs or D responded most favorably to "ordinary" placebo (drug-placebo or dental splint without occlusal platform); by comparison, the "strong" placebo (enthusiastic dispensing of placebo drug) prompted the most improvement in persons having their highest score on Hy. Gentry, Newman, Goldner, and von Baeyer (1977) compared the MMPIs of fifty-five chronic low back pain patients with their response to a graduated spinal block (GSB); the two diagnostic approaches agreed in their classification of "organic" and "functional" cases only 55 percent of the time. Patients diagnosed as "functional" by the GSB had slightly higher scores on Hs; however, both groups showed conversion-V configurations on the neurotic triad.

Maruta et al. (1979) contrasted the MMPIs of thirty-four patients who responded favorably to a nonsurgical pain-management program with the profiles of thirty-five who did not; outcome criteria included acceptance of the need to live with pain, reduction of pain-related medication, and motivation to remain off medication. Patients exhibiting successful outcome scored lower on Hs, D, and Hy although these differences did not reach statistical significance; the authors subsequently adopted a cutting score of 80T on Hs and Hy in a seven-item prognosis scale. McCreary and Colman (1984) also found the MMPI to predict medication usage among 100 chronic low back pain patients; individuals using narcotics combined with other drugs (mild analgesics, antidepressants, or sedatives) scored significantly higher on the Hs and Hy scales than subjects using either no medications or else mild analgesics or single narcotics not in combination.

Blanchard, Andrasik, Neff, Arena, Ahels, Jurish, Pallmeyer, Saunders, Teders, Barron, and Rodichok (1982) examined the MMPIs of seventeen men and seventy-four women with chronic headache of diverse types treated with relaxation training or, when this failed, with additional biofeedback. For twenty-seven migraine patients treated with relaxation alone, positive outcome was strongly related to *higher* scores on Hy (r = 0.46), consistent with placebo effects identified by Shipman et al. (1974). By contrast, in a study of 112 chronic pain patients treated either surgically or psychiatrically, Strassberg, Reimherr, Ward, Russell, and Cole (1981) found that better outcome on both medical and subjective measures twenty months post-treatment was associated with MMPI scores suggesting lower defensiveness (lower K) and less of a psychological overlay to the pain complaints (lower Hs and Hy); however, the MMPI's ability to predict long-term success varied as a function of the nature of the outcome measures and the type of treatment received.

Finally, predictive studies employing configural analyses have found a consistent association between poor treatment response and MMPI codetypes involving high elevations on either Hs or Hy. Herron and Pheasant (1982) studied preoperative and follow-up MMPIs of sixty-nine patients who had undergone low back surgery for discogenic disease from one to eleven years previously. Preoperative Hs and Hy scales were only modestly associated with treatment response; however, patients comprising the "poor" outcome group (n = 20) produced a mean profile distinguished by a mild conversion-V pattern, in contrast to lower Hs and Hy and higher D scores for patients exhibiting "fair" response and consistently lower scores on all scales for patients comprising the "good" outcome group. Similarly, Long (1981) related preoperative MMPIs to surgical outcome assessed six to eighteen months later for forty-four patients treated for low back pain; only Hs discriminated between mean profiles characterizing treatment successes and failures. However, patients with elevations on Hs and Hy characterized by a conversion-V, or with less of an elevation on these scales in conjunction with an elevation on Pd, were characteristically surgery failures; all patients with substantial elevations on the Pd scale alone also exhibited poor treatment outcome.

Additional support for configural analyses was presented by McCreary, Turner, and Dawson (1979) in a study of seventy-nine patients treated for chronic low back pain of at least six months' duration; overall, treatment was successful in 50 percent of these cases. However, among patients exhibiting codetypes involving elevations on both Hs and Hy (1-3/3-1, 1-2-3), only 39 percent experienced significant pain relief and only 25 percent returned to normal activities; in contrast, among patients exhibiting neurotic codetypes excluding Hs (2-3/3-2), 88 percent reported significant reduction in pain and 67 percent described functional recovery. The authors concluded that, "Based upon the present results, it seems preferable to use codetypes rather than single scales on the MMPI-derived predictors of outcome" (p. 284).

Conclusions

The collective findings of empirical studies described above lend strong support to inclusion of the MMPI in the assessment of patients being treated for chronic pain. Notable strengths of the MMPI include: (1) its broad empirical foundations underlying interpretive guidelines with medical, psychiatric, and normal populations; (2) research spanning forty years aimed specifically at distinguishing features of chronic pain syndromes; (3) the ability to identify homogeneous subgroups within chronic pain samples; and (4) the degree to which the MMPI can predict even long-term success to medical and psychological treatment programs. However, none of these factors should be viewed as a basis for "blind interpretation" of patients' MMPI profiles with disregard for data accrued from physical examination, laboratory findings, or clinical interview; rather, the MMPI provides a psychometric standard and background against which other findings may be more objectively scrutinized.

Fordyce (1976) presented a conceptual model for integrating MMPI data with other clinical findings in assessment of the chronic pain patient; he proposed that the MMPI provides strong indications of the patient's preparedness to signal pain, the subjective cost of pain behaviors, other personal difficulties for which the chronic pain syndrome may provide subjective relief, susceptibility to addiction, responsiveness to suggestion or placebo, and reinforcement potential of increased activity. In these and other domains, research findings from more than 100 studies across diverse samples and settings yield the following conclusions and interpretive guidelines:

1. Patients with chronic pain can be expected to obtain significant elevations on scales comprising the neurotic triad (Hs, D, and Hy), with scores on these measures typically ranging from 65 to 75T and exceeding scores on other scales. Significant elevations on these scales are disproportionately prevalent among chronic pain samples compared to general medical and psychiatric control groups.

2. The similarity of group mean profiles across samples differing in the nature or locus of pain (e.g., arthritis, low back pain, headache, or pelvic pain) suggests that differences in such pain disorders are unlikely to result from individual differences in personality functioning; rather, mean profile differences among specific pain groups on the MMPI appear more closely related to degree of functional impairment.

3. Within chronic pain samples there exist considerable individual differences both in profile shape and overall elevation. A growing body of research literature confirms the ability to identify homogeneous subgroups of chronic pain patients, replicable across settings, gender, and diverse pain populations. Moreover, these subgroups vary along pain-related dimensions including degree of subjective distress, functional impairment, and treatment response.

4. High scores on the Hs (hypochondriasis) and Hy (hysteria) scales have consistently been related to increased chronicity and intensity of pain, decreased activity levels, general functional limitations, excessive reliance on medications, and poor response to medical and psychological treatment.

5. Scores on Hs and Hy demonstrate greater utility in evaluating the appropriateness of a patient's disability

than in predicting the presence or absence of physical findings. Significant elevations on these scales provide substantial evidence of a psychological component to the patient's pain syndrome, but do not rule out contributing physical factors.

6. Elevations on D (depression) appear related to factors other than chronicity of the pain syndrome, including degree of functional impairment and general activity level.

7. In a heterogeneous sample of chronic pain patients with minimal physical findings, referred for evaluation of potential response to surgery, elevations on Hs (above 75T) appear particularly effective in predicting poor outcome. By comparison, elevations on Hy (above 70T) are somewhat less predictive of treatment failure, particularly if accompanied by only moderate or low scores on Hs; individuals with 2-3/3-2 codetypes may have an increased potential for favorable response to placebo effects, although this appears to vary with type of pain and intervention modality.

8. The majority of research findings indicate the superiority of predicting treatment response from codetypes rather than on the basis of individual scales. In particular, the behavioral and affective attributes associated with given elevations on D or Hy are strongly moderated by scores on Hs and, to a lesser extent, by scores on K (correction) and Pt (psychasthenia).

9. The most frequently observed profile configurations among chronic pain patients include the 1-3/3-1, 1-2/2-1, 2-3/3-2, and 2-7/7-2 codetypes. Evidence indicates that these codetypes offer stronger prediction of treatment response than psychiatric diagnosis. For example, individuals with either the 2-3 or 2-7 profile may receive a diagnosis of reactive depression on the basis of clinical interview; however, research findings suggest a more guarded prognosis for persons obtaining the former (2-3) code. Patients with codetypes reflecting peak elevations on the Hs (hypochondriasis) scale appear to have the least favorable prognosis.

10. Interpretive decision rules should be adjusted across settings to reflect differences in base rates for such factors as type of pain, nature of treatment alternatives, and preselection of patients on the basis of minimal physical findings or their limited response to previous interventions. For example, in a setting where patients typically have undergone multiple operations and for whom further surgical interventions appear questionable, cutoff scores on Hs and Hy may be set substantially lower with decision alternatives based on profile configurations within normal limits.

The psychological assessment of chronic pain extends well beyond evaluating the degree of "functional involvement" in the patient's pain syndrome. As Sternbach (1976) noted, "Far more important than the question of whether pain is psychological or physical in origin is the issue of whether there are treatable psychological or physical findings" (p. 297). There exists a broad consensus that if the patient has objective findings which justify surgery, then such an intervention should be undertaken regardless of the psychological findings. However, where a strong psychological component has been identified as contributing to the patient's pain syndrome—even in the presence of clear organic pathology—prudence dictates psychological consultation and use of nonmedical interventions aimed at improving the emotional context in which surgery occurs.

The research literature demonstrates impressive gains over the past decade in the breadth and sophistication of empirical investigations employing the MMPI in chronic pain populations. Prominent among these have been efforts to identify homogeneous subgroups covarying with pain-related descriptors and treatment response. Research objectives should continue to emphasize delineation of those dimensions moderating prediction of relevant criteria from the MMPI, including biographic, physiologic, and treatment factors.

REFERENCES

Achterberg-Lawlis, J. (1982), The psychological dimensions of arthritis. *J. Consult. & Clin. Psychol.*, 50:984–992.

Adams, K. M., Heilbronn, M., & Blumer, D. P. (1986), A multimethod evaluation of the MMPI in a chronic pain patient sample. *J. Clin. Psychol.*, 42:878–886.

American Psychiatric Association. (1986), *DSM-III-R in Development: Second draft*. Washington, DC: American Psychiatric Association.

Andrasik, F., Blanchard, E.B., Arena, J. G., Teders, S. J., Teevan, R. C., & Rodichok, L. D. (1982), Psychological functioning in headache sufferers. *Psychosom. Med.*, 44:171–182.

Armentrout, D. P., Moore, J. E., Parker, J. C., Hewett, J. E., & Feltz, C. (1982), Pain-patient MMPI subgroups: The psychological dimensions of pain. *J. Behav. Med.*, 5:201–211.

Bakker, C. B., & Levenson, R. M. (1967), Determinants of angina pectoris. *Psychosom. Med.*, 29:621–633.

Beals, R. K., & Hickman, N. W. (1972), Industrial injuries of the back and extremities. *J. Bone & J. Surg.*, 54A:1593–1611.

Beck, A. T., Ward, C. H., Mendelson, M. M., Mock, J., & Erbaugh. J. (1961), An inventory for measuring depression. *Arch. Gen. Psychiat.*, 4:561–571.

Bernstein, I. H., & Garbin, C. P. (1983), Hierarchical clustering of pain patients' MMPI profiles: A replication note. *J. Pers. Assess.*, 47:171–172.

Beutler, L. E., Engle, D., Oro'-Beutler, M. E., Daldrup, R., & Meredith, K. (1986), Inability to express intense affect: A common link between depression and pain? *J. Consult. & Clin. Psychol.*, 54:752–759.

Blanchard, E. B., Andrasik, F., Neff, D. F., Arena, J. G., Ahles, T. A., Jurish, S. E., Pallmeyer, T. P., Saunders, N. L., Teders, S. J., Barron, K. D., & Rodichok, L. D. (1982), Biofeedback and relaxation training with three kinds of headache: Treatment effects and their prediction. *J. Consult. & Clin. Psychol.*, 50:562–575.

Blumetti, A. E., & Modesti, L. M. (1976), Psychological predictors of success or failure of surgical intervention for intractable back pain. In: *Advances in Pain Research and Therapy*, Vol. 1, eds. J. J. Bonica & D. Albe-Fessard, New York: Raven Press, pp. 323–325.

Bourestom, N.C., & Howard, M.T. (1965), Personality characteristics of three disability groups. *Arch. Phys. Med. & Rehab.*, 46:626–632.

Bradley, L. A., Prieto, E. J., Hopson, L., & Prokop, C. K. (1978), Comment on "Personality organization as an aspect of back pain in a medical setting." *J. Pers. Assess.*, 42:573–578.

———Prokop, C. K., Margolis, R., & Gentry, W. D. (1978), Multivariate analyses of the MMPI profiles of low back pain patients. *J. Behav. Med.*, 1:253–272.

———Van der Heide, L. H. (1984), Pain-related correlates of MMPI profile subgroups among back pain patients. *Health Psychol.*, 3:157–174.

Butcher, J. N., & Finn, S. (1983), Objective personality assessment in clinical settings. In: *Clinical Psychology Handbook* eds. M. Hersen, A.E. Kazdin, & A.S. Bellack. New York: Pergamon, pp. 329–344.

Caldwell, A. B., & Chase, C. (1977), Diagnosis and treatment of personality factors in chronic low back pain. *Clin. Orthopaed. & Rel. Res.*, 129:141–149.

Calsyn, D. A., Louks, J., & Freeman, C. W. (1976), The use of the MMPI with chronic low back pain patients with a mixed diagnosis. *J. Clin. Psychol.*, 32:532–536.

Castelnuovo-Tedesco, P., & Krout, B. M. (1970), Psychosomatic aspects of chronic pelvic pain. *Psychiat. in Med.*, 1:109–126.

Chaney, H. S., Williams, S. G., Cohn, C. K., & Vincent, K. R. (1984), MMPI results: A comparison of trauma victims, psychogenic pain, and patients with organic disease. *J. Clin. Psychol.*, 40:1450–1454.

Cohen, D. (1949), *Psychological Concomitants of Chronic Illness: A Study of Emotional Correlates of Pulmonary Tuberculosis, Peptic Ulcer, the Arthritides, and Cardiac Disease*. Doctoral dissertation, University of Pittsburgh, Pennsylvania.

Cox, G. B., Chapman, C. R., & Black, R. G. (1978), The MMPI and chronic pain: The diagnosis of psychogenic pain. *J. Behav. Med.*, 1:437–443.

Cummings, C., Evanski, P. M., Debenedetti, M. J., Anderson, E. E., & Waugh, T. R. (1979), Use of the MMPI to predict outcome of treatment for chronic pain. In: *Advance in Pain Research and Therapy* Vol. 3, eds. J. J. Bonica, J. C. Liebeskind, & D. G. Albe-Fessard. New York: Raven Press, pp. 667–670.

Dahlstrom, W. G., Welsh, G. S., & Dahlstrom, L. E. (1972), *An MMPI Handbook:* Vol. 1. *Clinical Interpretation*, rev. ed. Minneapolis: University of Minnesota Press.

————— —————(1975), *An MMPI Handbook:* Vol. 2 *Research Applications*, rev. ed. Minneapolis: University of Minnesota Press.

Donovan, W. H., Dwyer, A. P., White, B. W. S., Batalin, N. J., Skerritt, P. W., & Bedbrook, G. M. (1981), A multidisciplinary approach to chronic low-back pain in Western Australia. *Spine*, 6:591–597.

Elkins, G. R., & Barrett, E. T (1984), The MMPI in evaluation of functional versus organic low back pain. *J. Pers. Assess.*, 48:259–264.

Fordyce, W. E. (1976), *Behavioral Methods For Chronic Pain and Illness*. St. Louis: C. V. Mosby.

————Brena, S. F., Holcomb, R. J., deLateur, B. J., & Loeser, J. D. (1978), Relationship of patient semantic pain descriptions to physician diagnostic judgments, activity level measures and MMPI. *Pain* 5:293–303.

Freeman, C., Calsyn, D., & Louks, J. (1976), The use of the Minnesota Multiphasic Personality Inventory with low back pain patients. *J. Clin. Psychol.*, 32:294–298.

Garron, D. C., & Leavitt, F. (1983), Chronic low back pain and depression. *J. Clin. Psychol.*, 39:486–493.

Gentry, W. D., Newman, M. C., Goldner, J. L., & von Baeyer, C. (1977), Relation between graduated spinal block technique and MMPI for diagnosis and prognosis of chronic low-back pain. *Spine*, 2:210–213.

————Shows, W. D., & Thomas, M. (1974), Chronic low back pain: A psychological profile. *Psychosom.*, 15:174–177.

Gilberstadt, H., & Jancis, M. (1967), "Organic" versus "functional" diagnoses from 1-3 MMPI profiles. *J. Clin. Psychol.*, 23:480–483.

Graham, J. R. (1977), *The MMPI: A Practical Guide*. New York: Oxford University Press.

Gruba, G. H., & Rohrbaugh, M. (1975), MMPI correlates of menstrual distress. *Psychosom. Med.*, 37:265–273.

Hain, J. D., Linton, P. H., Eber, H. W., & Chapman, M. M. (1970), Menstrual irregularity, symptoms and personality. *J. Psychosom. Res.*, 14:81–87.

Hanvik, L. J. (1951), MMPI profiles in patients with low back pain. *J. Consult. Psychol.*, 15:350–353.

Harrison, R. H. (1975), Psychological testing in headache: A review. *Headache*, 13:177–185.

Hart, R. R. (1984), Chronic pain: Replicated multivariate clustering of personality profiles. *J. Clin. Psychol.*, 40:129–133.

Hathaway, S.R., & McKinley, J. C. (1943), *The Minnesota Multiphasic Personality Schedule.* Minneapolis: University of Minnesota Press.

Herron, L. D., & Pheasant, H. C. (1982), Changes in MMPI profiles after low-back surgery. *Spine,* 7:591–597.

Hoffman, A. L. (1974), Psychological factors associated with rheumatoid arthritis: Review of the literature. *Nursing Res.,* 23:218–234.

Jamison, K., Ferrer-Brechner, M. A., Brechner, V. L., & McCreary, C. P. (1976), Correlation of personality profile with pain syndrome. In: *Advances in Pain Research and Therapy,* Vol. 1. eds. J. J. Bonica, & D. Albe-Fessard. New York: Raven Press, pp. 317–321.

Keefe, F. J. (1982), Behavioral assessment and treatment of chronic pain: Current status and future directions. *J. Consult. & Clin. Psychol.,* 50:896–911.

Kinder, B. N., Curtiss, G., & Kalichman, S. (1986), Anxiety and anger as predictors of MMPI elevations in chronic pain patients. *J. Pers. Assess.,* 50:651–661.

Kudrow, L., & Sutkus, B. J. (1979), MMPI pattern specificity in primary headache disorders. *Headache,* 19:18–24.

Lachar, D. (1974), *The MMPI: Clinical Assessment and Automated Interpretation.* Los Angeles: Western Psychological Services.

Leavitt, F., & Garron, D. C. (1982), Rorschach and pain characteristics of patients with low back pain and "conversion V" MMPI profiles. *J. Pers. Assess.,* 46:18–25.

Long, C. J. (1981), The relationship between surgical outcome and MMPI profiles in chronic pain patients. *J. Clin. Psychol.,* 37:744–749.

Louks, J. L., Freeman, C. W., & Calsyn, D. A. (1978), Personality organization as an aspect of back pain in a medical setting. *J. Pers. Assess.,* 42:152–158.

Love, A. W. (1987), Depression in chronic low back pain patients: Diagnostic efficiency of three self-report questionnaires. *J. Clin. Psychol.,* 43:84–89.

Maruta, T., Swanson, D. W., & Swenson, W. M. (1976), Pain as a psychiatric symptom: Comparison between low back pain and depression. *Psychosom.,* 17:123–127.

—— —— ——(1979), Chronic pain: Which patients may a pain management program help? *Pain,* 7:321–329.

McCreary, C. (1985), Empirically derived MMPI profile clusters and characteristics of low back pain patients. *J. Consult. & Clin. Psychol.,* 53:558–560.

——Colman, A. (1984), Medication usage, emotional disturbance, and pain behavior in chronic low back pain patients. *J. Clin. Psychol.,* 40:15–19.

——Turner, J., Dawson, E. (1977), Differences between functional versus organic low back pain patients. *Pain,* 4:73–78.

—— —— ——(1979), The MMPI as a predictor of response to conservative treatment for low back pain. *J. Clin. Psychol.,* 35:278–284.

—— —— ——(1981), Principal dimensions of the pain experience and psychological disturbance in chronic low back pain patients. *Pain,* 11:85–92.

McGill, J.C., Lawlis, G.F., Selby, D., Mooney,V., & McCoy, C.E. (1983), The relationship of Minnesota Multiphasic Personality Inventory (MMPI) profile clusters to pain behaviors. *J. Behav. Med.,* 6:77–92.

McGrath, R. E., & O'Malley, W. B. (1986), The assessment of denial and physical complaints: The validity of the Hy scale and associated MMPI signs. *J. Clin. Psychol.,* 42:754–760.

Meehl, P. E., & Rosen, A. (1955), Antecedent probability and the efficiency of psychometric signs, patterns, or cutting scores. *Psycholog. Bull.,* 52:194–216.

Melzack, R. (1975), The McGill Pain Questionnaire: Major properties and scoring methods. *Pain,* 1:277–299.

Moos, R. H., & Solomon, G. F. (1964), Minnesota Multiphasic Personality Inventory response patterns in patients with rheumhatoid arthritis. *J. Psychosom. Res.*, 8:17–28.

Naliboff, B. D., Cohen, M J., & Yellen, A. N. (1982), Does the MMPI differentiate chronic illness from chronic pain? *Pain*, 13:333–341.

———— ———— ————(1983), Frequency of MMPI profile types in three chronic illness populations. *J. Clin. Psychol.*, 39:843–847.

Nalven, F. B., O'Brien, J. F. (1964). Personality patterns of rheumatoid arthritic patients. *Arthrit. & Rheum.*, 7:18–28.

Parker, J. C., Doerfler, L. A., Tatten, H. A., & Hewett, J. E. (1983), Psychological factors that influence self-reported pain. *J. Clin. Psychol.*, 39:22–25.

Pheasant, H. C., Gilbert, D., Goldfarb, J., & Herron, L. (1979), The MMPI as a predictor of outcome in low-back surgery. *Spine*, 4:78–84.

Pichot, P., Perse, J., Lekeoux, M. O., Dureau, J. L., Perez, C. I., & Rychewaert, A. (1972), La Personnalité des Sujets Presentant des Douleurs Dorsales Fonchonnelles Valeur De L'Invenlaire Multiphasique De Personnalité Du Minnesota. *Revue de Psychologie Appliqué*, 22:145–172.

Pilling, L. F., Brannick, T. L., & Swenson, W. M. (1967), Psychologic characteristics of psychiatric patients having pain as a presenting symptom. *Can. Med. Assn. J.*, 97:387–394.

Polley, H. F., Swenson, W. M., & Steinhilber, R. M. (1970), Personality characteristics of patients with rheumatoid arthritis. *Psychosom.*, 11:45–49.

Prokop, C. K. (1986), Hysteria scale elevations in low back pain patients: A risk factor for misdiagnosis? *J. Consult. & Clin. Psychol.*, 54:558–562.

————Bradley, L. A., Margolis, R., & Gentry, W. D. (1980), Multivariate analyses of the MMPI profiles of patients with multiple pain complaints. *J. Pers. Assess.*, 44:246–252.

Renaer, M., Vertommen, H., Nijs, P., Wagemans, L., & Van Hemelrijck, T. (1979), Psychological aspects of chronic pelvic pain in women. *Amer. J. Obstet. & Gynecol.*, 134:75–80.

Rosen, J. C., Frymoyer, J. W., & Clements, J. H. (1980), A further look at validity of the MMPI with low back patients. *J. Clin. Psychol.*, 36:994–1000.

————Johnson, C., & Frymoyer, J. W. (1983), Identification of excessive back disability with the Fashingbauer abbreviated MMPI. *J. Clin. Psychol.*, 39:71–74.

Schwartz, M. S., & Krupp, N. E. (1971), The MMPI "conversion V" among 50,000 medical patients: A study of incidence, criteria, and profile elevation. *J. Clin. Psychol.*, 27:89–95.

————Osborne, D., & Krupp, N. E. (1972), Moderating effects of age and sex on the association of medical diagnoses and 1-3/3-1 MMPI profiles. *J. Clin. Psychol.*, 28:502–505.

Shaw, D. J., & Matthews, C. G. (1965), Differential MMPI performance of brain-damaged versus pseudo-neurologic groups. *J. Clin. Psychol.*, 21:405–408.

Shipman, W. G., Greene, C. S., & Laskin, D. M. (1974), Correlation of placebo responses and personality characteristics in myofascial pain-dysfunction (MPD) patients. *J. Psychosom. Res.*, 18:475–483.

Small, E. W. (1976), An investigation into the psychogenic bases of the temporomandibular joint myofascial pain dysfunction syndrome. In: *Advances in Pain Research and Therapy*, Vol. 1, eds, J. J. Bonica & D. G. Albe-Fessard. New York: Raven Press, pp. 889–894.

Smith, T. W., Aberger, E. W., Follick, M. J., & Ahern, D. K. (1986), Cognitive distortion and psychological distress in chronic low back pain. *J. Consult. & Clin. Psychol.*, 54:573–575.

Smith, W. L., & Duerksen, D. L. (1980), Personality and the relief of chronic pain: Predicting surgical outcome. In: *Pain: Meaning and Management*, eds. W. L. Smith, H. Merskey & S.C. Gross, Jamaica, New York: Spectrum, pp. 119–126.

Snyder, D. K., & Power, D. G. (1981), Empirical descriptors of unelevated MMPI profiles among chronic pain patients: A typological approach. *J. Clin. Psychol.*, 37:602–607.

Sovak, M., Kunzel, M., Sternbach, R. A., & Dalessio, D. J. (1981), Mechanism of the biofeedback therapy of migraine: Volitional manipulation of the psychophysiological background. *Headache*, 21:89–92.

Spergel, P., Ehrlich, G. E., & Glass, D. (1978), The rheumatoid arthritic personality: A psychodiagnostic myth. *Psychosom.*, 19:79–86.

Spielberger, C. D., Gorsuch, R. L., Lushene, R., Vagg, P. R., & Jacobs, G. A. (1983), *Manual for the State-Trait Anxiety Inventory.* Palo Alto, CA: Consulting Psychologists Press.

Sternbach, R. A. (1974), *Pain Patients: Traits and Treatment.* New York: Academic Press.

———(1976), Psychological factors in pain. In: *Advances in Pain Research and Therapy* Vol. 1, eds. J. J. Bonica & D. G. Albe-Fessard. New York: Raven Press, pp. 293–299.

———(1977), Psychological aspects of chronic pain. *Clin. Orthopaed. & Rel. Res.*, 129:150–155.

———(1982), The psychologist's role in the diagnosis and treatment of pain patients. In: *Psychological Approaches to the Management of Pain*, eds. J. Barber & C. Adrian. New York: Brunner/Mazel, pp. 3–20.

———Dalessio, D. J., Kunzel, M., & Bowman, G. E. (1980), MMPI patterns in common headache disorders. *Headache*, 20:311–315.

———Wolf, S. R., Murphy, R. W., & Akeson, W. H. (1973), Traits of pain patients: The low-back "loser." *Psychosom.* 14:226–229.

Strassberg, D. S., Reimherr, F., Ward, M., Russell, S., & Cole, A. (1981), The MMPI and chronic pain. *J. Consult. & Clin. Psychol.*, 49:220–226.

Swanson, D. W., Swenson, W. M., Maruta, T., & McPhee, M. C. (1976), Program for managing chronic pain. I. Program description and characteristics of patients. *Mayo Clinic Proc.*, 51:401–408.

Swenson, W. M., Pearson, J. S., & Osborne, D. (1973), *An MMPI Source Book.* Minneapolis: University of Minnesota Press.

Trief, P. M., & Yuan, H. A. (1983), The use of the MMPI in a chronic back pain rehabilitation program. *J. Clin. Psychol.*, 39:46–53.

Turner, J. A., Herron, L., & Weiner, P. (1986), Utility of the MMPI pain assessment index in predicting outcome after lumbar surgery. *J. Clin. Psychol.*, 42:764–769.

———McCreary, C. (1978), Short forms of the MMPI with back pain patients. *J. Consult. & Clin. Psychol.*, 46:354–355.

———Romano, J. M. (1984), Self-report screening measures for depression in chronic pain patients. *J. Clin. Psychol.*, 40:909–913.

Waring, E. M., Weisz, G. M., & Bailey, S. I. (1976), Predictive factors in the treatment of low back pain by surgical intervention. In: *Advances in Pain Research and Therapy*, Vol. 1, eds. J. J. Bonica & D. Albe-Fessard. New York: Raven Press, pp. 939–942.

Watson, D. (1982), Neurotic tendencies among chronic pain patients: An MMPI item analysis. *Pain*, 14:365–385.

Webb, J. T. (1970), The relation of MMPI two-point codes to age, sex, and educational level in a representative nationwide sample of psychiatric outpatients. Paper presented at the meeting of the Southeastern Psychological Association, Louisville, KY, April.

Werder, D. S., Sargent, J. D., & Coyne, L. (1981), MMPI profiles of headache patients using self regulation to control headache activity. Paper presented at the meeting of the American Association of Biofeedback Clinicians, Kansas City, KS, October.

Wiener, D. (1952), Personality characteristics of selected disability groups. *Gen. Psychol. Monogr.*, 45:175–255.

Wiggins, J. S. (1973), *Personality and Prediction: Principles of Personality Assessment.* Reading, MA: Addison-Wesley.

Wilfling, F. J., Klonoff, H., & Kokan, P. (1973), Psychological, demographic, and orthopaedic factors associated with prediction of outcome of spinal fusion. *Clin. Orthopaed. & Rel. Res.*, 90:153–160.

Wiltse, L. L., & Rocchio, P. D. (1975), Preoperative psychological tests as predictors of success of chemonucleolysis in the treatment of the low-back syndrome. *J. Bone & J. Surg.*, 57A:478–483.

Zaretsky, H. H., Lee, M. H., & Rubin, M. (1976), Psychological factors and clinical observations in acupuncture analgesia and pain abatement. *J. Psychol.*, 93:113–120.

8

Diagnostic Considerations in Management of Patients with Cancer Pain

STEVEN F. BRENA, M.D. AND
STEVEN SANDERS, PH.D.

INTRODUCTION

Estimates of the prevalence of pain associated with malignancy range from 60 to 82 percent (Foley, 1979; Bonica, 1982). During 1981 and 1982, a survey of 120 patients referred to the University of California, Los Angeles (UCLA) Cancer Pain Clinic indicated that pain secondary to tumor invasion occurred in 61.7 percent of patients. Bone metastasis was the most common (18.3%), followed by neural invasion (15.8%) and visceral invasion (10%) (Cohen, Breckner, and Reeding, 1982). Almost one-third of the patients in the UCLA survey had pain secondary to oncological therapy for cancer control and not due to tumor invasion. Under this category, 16.6 percent of patients had postsurgical pain, 5.8 percent due to postherpetic neuralgia, 5 percent due to chemotherapy, and 4.2 percent due to radiation injury. Despite the prevalence of pain in cancer patients, little attention has been given to structured pain control programs for cancer patients. With the exception of a

259

few highly sophisticated cancer pain control centers, the over-whelming majority of cancer patients are still treated within an acute medical model, mostly with random prescriptions of various drugs, many of them habit-forming, leading to physical dependence and tolerance. Even less attention is paid to the possibility of rehabilitation for nonterminal cancer patients, despite the fact that research data have indicated that over 40 percent of patients with cancer in all sites do have physical and psychological impairments which can be corrected through rehabilitation medicine (Lehman, DeLisa, Warner, 1978). To design a quality pain management program for cancer patients, knowledge of the physical and psychological factors contribut-ing to the pain problem is necessary. This chapter provides a brief overview of the physical and psychological factors com-monly associated with pain in adult cancer patients, and current management strategies for health care support of these pa-tients within the framework of structured, long-range treat-ment programs.

COMMON PHYSICAL FACTORS IN CANCER PAIN

Tissue Invasion from a Malignant Pathological Process

A malignant growth involving any tissue of the body is likely to cause pain whenever it involves nerve structures, peripheral vessels, or bones. Quite often the invasion involves all of these structures. By far the most common cause of cancer pain is destruction of bone with neurological complications from metastatic diffusion.

Painful Syndromes Caused by Medical Interventions

Almost paradoxically, medical and surgical interventions for cancer disease may cause as much pain and suffering as the disease itself. A common denominator for pain following cancer therapy is nerve damage and circulatory disturbances from damage to peripheral vessels.

Pain from Irradiation and Chemotherapy. Irradiation therapy often results in extensive fibrosis of the connective tissue, with secondary damage to peripheral nerve structures, and sometimes to the central nervous system (CNS) itself. Postchemotherapy pain is caused by several lesions, which include peripheral neuropathy, bone necrosis, and herpetic infection. Mostly in elderly people the herpetic infection may result in postherpetic neuralgia.

Pain Caused by Surgical Procedures. Several painful syndromes have been described following the surgical removal of a tumor (Foley, 1979). Surgical amputation of a limb may result in pain in a stump or in phantom limb pain. Various neuralgias may develop following a surgical procedure which has caused peripheral nerve damage, mostly when a thoracotomy has been performed. Finally, extensive destructive surgery, such as radical neck dissection, may lead to severe pain both from direct nerve and vascular damage and from nerve and vascular compressions from the extensive scar tissue.

COMMON PSYCHOLOGICAL FACTORS IN CANCER PAIN

Behavioral and Interpersonal Deterioration

In addition to the physical contributors in cancer pain, general reduction in activity level, loss of ability to engage in activities of daily living, and reduction in interpersonal contact and social stimulation can significantly exacerbate the patient's level of pain and distress. This is particularly true during the latter stages of the disease process (Black, 1979; Bond, 1979). Patients experience a gradual deterioration in ability to engage in normal activity, as well as deterioration in social contacts and recreational activities. The end result is less emotional and physical resistance to the stresses of cancer and its treatment, as well as more time and opportunity to focus on the pain experience. Both such consequences within and outside the cancer pain arena have been shown to exacerbate the overall pain experience (Turk and Rennert, 1983; Mount, 1984; Brena and Chapman, 1985). These factors play an important part in the patient's initial reaction to and subsequent coping with the prospect of cancer and the pain thereof.

Stress

The exacerbatory effects of stress on clinical pain have long been appreciated and empirically demonstrated (Sanders, 1985). There are a host of potential stressors for the cancer patient that can significantly contribute to the pain experience. These include disruption in daily routine, deteriorating interpersonal interactions, family discord, work demands and modifications, economic hardships, physical and emotional demands of the disease process itself and related pain, and the demands and side effects from physical evaluation and treatment (e.g., bone marrow aspirations, radiation therapy, and chemotherapy, etc.). Such multifocal stress can be a major determinant regarding the quantity and quality of pain experienced with cancer, with a tendency to escalate in magnitude as the disease progresses. Even with remission, there can be an ongoing residual level of stress associated with the fear of disease return and possible permanent loss of significant function in the various areas.

Mood Disturbances

As with stress, the presence of significant levels of anxiety, anger, or depression all have demonstrable exacerbatory effects on clinical pain (Sanders, 1985). These mood disturbances are quite common with cancer patients (Lewis, Gottesman, and Gutstine, 1979; Gottesman and Lewis, 1982; Ahles, Blanchard, and Ruckdeschel, 1983) and further add to the pain experience. In the early stages of the disease process, anxiety and anger appear to dominate mood disturbances, with depression more predominant as the disease process develops. Commonly, specific mood disturbances are embedded in a more general grief reaction (Kübler-Ross, 1969; Averill and Wisocki, 1983) experienced in one form or another by the cancer patient. Regardless of the context, such mood dysfunction adds to the pain experience and may become a significant problem in itself (e.g., major depression or generalized anxiety disorder).

MANAGEMENT STRATEGIES FOR PAIN CONTROL IN CANCER PATIENTS

Over the last decade, a large body of clinical knowledge has accumulated documenting the effectiveness of interdisciplinary, goal-oriented treatment programs for chronic pain patients in structured medical facilities, known around the world as "pain clinics" and "pain centers" (Chapman, Brena, and Bradford, 1981; Aronoff, Evans, and Enders, 1983; Brena, 1985b). Because the experience of pain is a multidimensional physiological and psychosocial phenomenon, the basic philosophy of pain control programs is that proper management of pain, mostly in its chronic form, should identify, address, and possibly correct all physical, behavioral, and psychosocial malfunctions associated with each person in pain. Specifically, for the cancer patient, this multidimensional strategy should be diversified in three stages of intervention.

Stage 1

During the earlier stages of malignancy, along with the oncological treatment of the malignancy itself, attempts should be made to minimize the responses of patients to early painful perceptions and to avoid the formation of multiple vicious cycles of pain and suffering. These goals can be accomplished through information and communication as well as the use of psychological–behavioral treatment.

Information and Communication. A major factor in minimizing the amount of pain and discomfort experienced by cancer pain patients in stage 1 is the ongoing delivery of important information regarding the disease process and its treatment, as well as continual communication with the patient regarding con-

cerns, needs, and expectations. Unfortunately, providing information and establishing good communication can be
overlooked in the zeal to establish a differential diagnosis and
implement oncological treatment for the malignancy. The
patient and family need to have verbal and written (if possible)
information regarding the type of cancer, treatment options,
probable treatment side effects and complications, expected
course of the disease and treatment if known, and realistic
information regarding prognosis as it becomes available (Turk
and Rennert, 1983; Mount, 1984). While there may be some
reluctance to share this information with patients and family
for fear of producing more problems, it is typically the case that
not sharing information produces many more difficulties and
problems than being open and honest with the patient and
family. Initial information should be followed with updates on
a regular basis by the physician and other health care professionals. Likewise, regular contact with the patient by the
physician to discuss concerns and issues and to answer questions is vital for minimizing the degree of pain and distress.
Without such ongoing communication and interaction the
patient and family are left to their own imagination and fears
regarding their future. More often than not, this results in
marked exacerbation and general fear, anxiety, and a sense of
loss of control. All of these reactions can significantly exacerbate the level of pain and distress.

Psychological–Behavioral Treatment. For maximum benefit and
ongoing usage, it is crucial that psychological–behavioral treatment be implemented during stage 1 of the disease process.
Too often, these "nonmedical" techniques which can be very
helpful in overall management are not considered or withheld
until the end of stage 2 and into stage 3 of a disease process. If
one waits to implement psychological–behavioral treatment
until these more advanced stages, the patient and family are
many times so consumed with the disease process and its
treatment, that they cannot take full advantage of these very
useful techniques. As with many medical interventions, the
general rule of thumb is the sooner psychological–behavioral
treatment can begin the more benefit can be derived from such

intervention (Sobel, 1981a). In general, the interventions are focused on minimizing and/or eliminating those psychological factors delineated earlier in the chapter (i.e., loss of activity and social stimulation, increase in stress, and mood disturbances) that can significantly exacerbate pain. The ultimate goal is to significantly improve the patient's ability to effectively cope with the pain and distress associated with the disease itself, as well as those oncological treatment interventions employed.

Relaxation Therapy, Biofeedback and Hypnosis. The utility of relaxation therapy, biofeedback, and hypnosis in cancer pain management is increasingly being recognized and empirically supported in the literature (Sobel, 1981b; Mount, 1984; Jay, Elliott, and Varni, 1986). All three techniques have been successfully utilized to enhance ability to reduce the subjective pain experienced from the cancer, as well as from those medical diagnostic and therapeutic methods (e.g., bone marrow aspirations, radiation therapy, and chemotherapy) utilized in management (Burish, Carey, Krozely, and Greco, 1987; Jay et al., 1986). While research to date does not offer adequate guidelines as to which patients may respond to which of the three procedures, data clearly indicate that their usage can be quite helpful for patients in reducing the pain and distress associated with cancer. As a clinical note, it is recommended that whenever possible emphasis be placed on those techniques that can be self-applied by the patient after initial intervention. Thus, relaxation training may prove to be superior over the course of treatment for many patients. (This needs additional empirical scrutiny before definitive conclusions can be drawn.)

Cognitive and Behavioral Activity Management. It is also quite important to address the patient's and family's cognitive (thinking and self-statements) and overt behavioral patterns in reducing the level of pain and distress. In concert with information sharing and communication described earlier, identification and rehearsal of adaptive self-statements that can be utilized by the patient and family can be quite helpful (Ellis, 1981; Turk and Rennert, 1983). For example, a simple exercise of having patients and family read adaptive self-statements such as "I am not helpless and can help manage my problem through my own actions"; or "In spite of the pain, I still can function and find pleasure each day" can have significant effects. Through self-directed rehearsal of appropriate and stress-reducing self-statements the patient and family can reduce pain and distress. These self-statements should be applied frequently (as often as every hour) and be rehearsed and reinforced by health care professionals involved in the patient care.

The establishment of a therapeutic behavioral routine is also vital for pain and distress management. This is particularly true given evidence demonstrating that overt pain behavior is clearly a part of the cancer pain experience (Ahles et al., 1983; Ahles, Cohen, Little, Balducci, Dubbert, and Keane, 1984) and may tend to increase over the course of the disease process and treatment intervention (Keefe, Brantley, Manuel, and Crisson, 1985). Specific attention should be given to maximizing and stabilizing the patient's activity level, trying to establish a predictable and set daily routine, and maximizing pleasurable activities on a regular basis. In other words, patients should stay as active as possible, establish a preset and planned routine that is predictable, and engage in both solitary and social activities that historically are, or have been, pleasurable. The same advice should also be given and supported with regard to the patient's family. It is crucial that the patient be actively involved with the decision-making process regarding the quantity and quality of those activities just outlined. However, even if there is resistance and a tendency for the patient to retreat and significantly reduce behavioral activity, after allowing a short period of time to overcome the initial shock and distress associated with the discovery of the cancer, the patient should be strongly encouraged to engage in the preceding overt behavioral regimen. If compliance with this recommendation becomes problematic, family members should be enlisted to enhance carrying out such a program during the initial stages. For ultimate success, however, the patient should eventually commit to this activity schedule.

Group Therapy. In keeping with the overall approach of reducing stress—distress in both the patient and family, participation in an ongoing support group should also be considered. While specific empirial demonstration of the efficacy for such intervention has yet to be established, at the clinical level it appears therapeutic. Such group involvement can effectively address stress issues within and outside the family, offer suggestions regarding more effective coping at work and with financial issues, and provide effective modeling of adaptive thinking and behavior for patients and family regarding treatment methods and changes in the course of the disease. Obviously, these stressful issues should be addressed on an individual basis as well; however, group participation can facilitate this process. Likewise, group therapy can facilitate the more generalized anticipatory grief reaction exhibited by patients and family alike. It is typically wise to make patient and family groups as homogeneous as possible regarding the level of the disease process. The segregation of stage 1, 2, and 3 patients and family members into separate groups, respectively, is typically advantageous and enhances therapeutic value. (It should be noted that recommendations regarding group segregation of patients and families by stage is based purely on clinical observation and has not undergone empirical scrutiny.)

Stage 2

Tumor-directed therapy may result in pain reduction by reducing the size of the tumor. However, during the more advanced stages of the disease, further diminution of the tumor is no longer feasible by tumor-directed therapy. At this stage, pain becomes a disease entity in itself and further modalities must be aimed at managing pain as a disease.

Analgesic Drug Management. Proper analgesic drug therapy should be carefully tailored to each individual, with careful consideration of the nociceptive mechanisms, levels of physical and psychosocial functioning, and the pharmacodynamic of the prescribed drug (Brena, 1984). Because every patient with terminal illness has easy access to well-meaning physicians ready to prescribe medication, the responsibility of analgesic drug intake should ultimately be the patient's. Consequently, he needs access to information about the effects, adverse reactions, and correct use of drugs for pain. A large number of drugs with different pharmacodynamic actions are presently available.

Peripheral Analgesics. Drugs in this group include acetaminophen, aspirin, and the nonsteroidal anti-inflammatory drugs (NSAIDs). Aspirin remains probably one of the best and most economical of these drugs. Both aspirin and acetaminophen are equally effective at 650 mg dosage; both have a ceiling effect of 600 to 900 mg. Above this dosage peak effectiveness increases slightly, but side effects and toxic reactions become likely. The average duration of effect of both drugs is around three to six hours. Equipotent doses of NSAIDs have a greater peak effect and longer duration than aspirin. All peripheral analgesics, with different degrees, demonstrate similar side effects on various bodily systems. The use of aspirin in patients receiving other NSAIDs should be avoided since aspirin lowers the concentration of the NSAIDs by displacing them from plasma proteins. Peripheral analgesics are probably the drugs of first choice in stage 2 cancer patients with recurrently acute episodes of pain.

Central Analgesics (Opiates and Opioids). Drugs in this group produce analgesia by binding to opiate receptors in the CNS. Onset, peak, and duration of analgesic effects vary with each drug and its route of administration. For instance, both for morphine and hydromorphone (Dilaudid) an analgesic effect can be demonstrated within fifteen minutes of parenteral administration and within thirty minutes following oral administration. However, hydromorphone is six times more potent than morphine but has the same duration of action, averaging four to five hours. Regularly scheduled drug administration on a time contingency is better than PRN administration, allowing for variations in potency, efficacy, and duration of actions of the central analgesic drugs. A regular dosage schedule minimizes peaks and valleys in pain intensity. However, when methadone is used, a fixed schedule should be carefully titrated with continuous monitoring of the patient's vital signs, since the plasma half-life of methadone is seventeen to twenty-four hours, thus leading to accumulation of blood levels and overdosage. The oral route of opiates has a lower onset of action than the intramuscular (IM) and intravenous (IV) routes, but a longer duration of analgesic affect. Tolerance develops in all patients who take central analgesics habitually, the earliest sign being decreased duration of analgesic effects. Tolerance develops at different speeds according to the route of administration; the IV route produces tolerance more quickly than the IM and oral routes, respectively. Since cross-tolerance among opiates is not complete, analgesic protection may be achieved by switching a patient from a large dose of one opiate to a smaller dosage of another. In cases of terminal cancer disease, tolerance can be overcome by increasing the frequency of the administration and the amount of each dose. All central analgesics produce adverse effects, such as constipation, sedation, nausea, and vomiting. Management of these side effects includes proper bowel regimen, dosage adjustments to minimize sedation while preserving analgesia, and wise use of antiemetics. Tolerance and physical dependence can be minimized and corrected through skillful drug management, education and open communication with patients.

Tricyclic Antidepressants. Recent evidence indicates that these drugs may actually have a specific effect on certain serotonergic pain pathways within the CNS. Presumptive evidence also indicates that the tricyclic antidepressants may interreact with opiate receptors directly to produce analgesia and indirectly to increase morphine analgesia (Malseed and Goldsdein, 1979; Biegon and Samwel, 1980). Actually an analgesic effect with the tricyclic drugs is usually achieved long before the dosage reaches antidepressant levels. Among the many tricyclic antidepressant drugs, when an analgesic effect is the primary pharmacological target, preference should be given to those drugs such as doxepin and amitriptyline, with higher affinities for serotonin receptors. Unfortunately, doxepin also demonstrates the highest affinity for histamine receptors, leading to clinical drowsiness. On the other side amitriptyline has less histamine affinity; for these reasons, amitriptyline is probably the tricyclic antidepressant of choice whenever such medication is prescribed primarily for analgesia. Common side effects with tricyclic compounds include blurred vision, constipation, urinary retention, and dryness of the mouth. Tricyclic drugs are particularly useful in stage 2 management, since they may provide adequate analgesic protection, with far less risk of developing physical dependence and tolerance.

Nonchemical Supportive Therapy for Pain: Sensory Stimulation

Sensory stimulation of peripheral nerves has been demonstrated repeatedly to provide mild to moderate pain reduction (Melzack, 1985). Although peripheral stimulation can be achieved through thermal and mechanical devices, the most commonly used technique for sensory stimulation is the transcutaneous electrical nerve stimulation (TENS), which involves application of both high- and low-intensity electrical current to selected bodily areas. Although TENS is a noninvasive, nonchemical analgesic method with minimal risks; the pain reduction is transient, and tolerance to its effect is known to develop. In cancer patients few attempts have been made to provide neural stimulation through electrical devices implanted in certain selected areas of the CNS and operated by an external transmitter. Release of endogenous opiates by stimulation of the periventricular gray (PVG) has been effective in cancer-related pain (Meyerson Boethius, and Carlsson, 1978). More recent studies, however, have questioned the opioid mechanism of PVG stimulation since no difference was found between sham and actual stimulation in patients with chronic pain (Wolskie, Gacely, and Greenberg, 1982). Moreover, deeper brain stimulation is often associated with increased hormone serum release, such as growth hormone and prolactin. These hormonal changes may have an effect on the growth of tumors sensitive to the released hormones, such as the prolactin-sensitive mammary tumor (Breckner, Motyka & Sherman, 1983).

Neural Blockade

Blockade of nociceptive pathways is probably the most popular form of treatment in cancer patients. The use of nerve blocks for pain control dates back to the early years of the twentieth century (Bonica, 1953; Brena, 1985). When a local anesthetic agent is used, the pain reduction may be expected to last between eight and twelve hours. In cancer patients, attempts have been made to prolong the duration of nerve blocks by injecting a neurolytic agent, such as alcohol or phenol, which causes the potential destruction of nerve structures. Early literature on pain is rich in descriptive reports extolling the great usefulness of nerve blocks in controlling all pain syndromes, including cancer pain (Bonica, 1959). However, the majority of these optimistic reports have not been able to withstand the test of controlled research, and the use of nerve blocks has somewhat fallen out of use. More so, the use of many neurolytic nerve blocks has been discontinued, as the painful consequences of nerve damage and subsequent deafferentiation syndromes have been recognized. At present, a few selective nerve blocks have passed the test of time and accountability.

Sympathetic Nerve Blocks. Blocks of the sympathetic system may be useful to increase bloodflow in cases where impaired circulation has been documented. Repeated sympathetic nerve blocks may result in prolonged pain reduction lasting much longer than the chemical duration of the anesthetic agent; the causes of this paradoxical clinical analgesia are not clear. Blockade of the celiac plexus is particularly useful for temporary control of the pain associated with malignancy in upper abdominal organs, since most of the nociceptive stimulation from this viscera cross the celiac plexus. The neurolytic block of the celiac plexus may provide up to six months of significant pain reduction; this neurolytic block has passed successfully the scrutiny of time and criticism, with no apparent risk of serious complications. Such blocks should be attempted and eventually repeated as needed in most patients with terminal disease of the upper abdominal organs (Thompson, Moore, and Bridenbaugh, 1977).

Epidural Blocks. Most of the analgesic effects of an epidural block are similar to those obtained through sympathetic nerve block, mainly blocking the preganglionic sympathetic fibers as they leave the spinal cord and cross the epidural space. The main advantage of an epidural block over a sympathetic nerve block is that a catheter can be placed in the epidural space safely, affording continuing pain control by periodic injection of an anesthetic agent through the catheter. Epidural blocks are highly invasive and their use should be restricted to selected cases of extremely painful metastatic syndromes, involving the lumbosacral plexuses (Cousins and Bridenbaugh, 1980).

Psychological–Behavioral Treatment

Upon entering stage 2 of the disease process, the potential utility of psychological—behavioral treatment to reduce the pain and distress experience becomes even more significant. It is hoped that during stage 1 of the disease, the patient and family were sufficiently provided with those basic psychological and behavioral techniques necessary to effectively utilize during stage 2. If not, all those methods described in the preceding section should be implemented as quickly as possible during stage 2. In general, psychological–behavioral treatment during stage 2 involves continuation of those techniques employed during stage 1 in concert with increase in more aggressive pharmacological pain control at the systemic and regional levels. Particular emphasis should be given to titration of patients' behavioral activity schedules in keeping with the need to maximize activity level, and the reality that movement to stage 2 inevitably results in some reduction in activity and loss of function. Likewise, a marked focus on increasing pleasurable activities on a daily basis and emphasizing daily accomplishments is quite important to offset the escalation in mood disturbance typically observed during this stage. Revisions in adaptive self-statements and cognitive activity should be done and include incorporating the idea that moving closer to a terminal state does not mean a subsequent loss of control and ability to manage pain and distress effectively. Finally, with the passage to stage 2, attention should be more directly given to death and dying issues inherent in such progression. This can be addressed at the individual and group level, with both typically necessary (Sobel, 1981a).

Stage 3

The terminal phase of cancer disease is reached when a patient's life expectancy is no greater than a few months. At this stage usually the oncological treatment is discontinued, while all the supportive and analgesic treatment modalities already in use during stage 2 must be reassessed and readjusted.

Adjusted Analgesic Drug Therapy

Routes and choices for drug therapy must be adapted to the needs of stage 3 terminal patients. For patients plagued with nausea and vomiting, certain opiates, such as Numorphan and morphine are available for rectal use and may be useful in patients with gastrointestinal obstructions, limited venous access, and reduced muscular mass. Routes and modes of administration for central analgesic drugs are not limited to intermittent oral, rectal, or IM and IV routes. Intragastric administration through an existing nasogastric tube, continuous subcutaneous infusion, epidural and intrathecal routes are alternates that have been used. A few studies have compared the difference in plasma levels according to the route of administration; one of these studies has compared the difference in plasma levels between deltoid and gluteal intramuscular injections and has indicated peak levels 2.5 times higher with deltoid injections (Grabinski, Kaiko, and Rogers, 1983). Further studies need to be made comparing effective plasma levels between various routes of opiate administration.

Besides adjustment of routes of administration, changes in drug regimens may also be considered. Aspirin and hydroxyzine HC1 have additive analgesic affects on central analgesics drugs, while the additive analgesic properties of chlorpromazine HC1 and other phenothiazines are questionable (Halpern and Bonica, 1979). In a double-blind crossover study,

Breckner and Gantz (1984) have demonstrated that the combination of ibuprofen with methadone 2.5 and 5 mg significantly increased the analgesic potency of the same dose of methadone, mostly in patients with bone metastasis. Other drugs suggested for control of bone pain, include L-dopa steroids (Minton, 1974), mitramycin (Davies, Trask, and Souhami, 1979), and fluoride (Scott, 1968). Heroin does not offer an advantage over morphine in terms of analgesic and mood effects (Kaiko, Wallenstein, and Rogers, 1981). Brompton mixtures (alcohol, cocaine, phenothiazine, chloroform, water, and morphine or heroin) are popular for pain control in terminal cancer patients. However, a double-blind comparison of morphine in solution versus morphine in the Brompton mixture has shown no difference in analgesic potency and side effect (Melzack et al., 1979).

Continuous epidural infusions of an anesthetic agent may be useful in patients with severe metastatic pain in the lower spine and limbs, as already mentioned. The main advantage is that the resultant analgesia is not cross-tolerant with opiate analgesic, thus allowing some reduction in dosages of central analgesics.

Ablative Neurosurgical Procedures

In the unfortunate case where a patient's life expectancy has outlasted conservative drug therapy and block therapy, physical tolerance to opiates cannot be overcome, and the painful experience is out of proportion to a patient's capability of managing himself, several neuroablative surgical procedures are now available. All of them result in destruction of nerve fibers and structures, and have clinical indication only in patients with short life expectancy, before painful complications from iatrogenic nerve damage can develop. Cordotomy remains the most useful and well-documented approach. New surgical techniques include radiofrequency lesions in the dorsal horn of the spinal cord and hypophysectomy. Radiofrequency lesions are supposed to destroy those central neurons which are involved in the transmission of nociceptive stimulation (Sweet, Polletti, and Challis, 1984). Removal of the hypophysis was introduced as part of the therapy for treating carcinomas of the breast and of the prostate (Moricca, 1974). Remission of symptoms and dramatic decrease in pain intensity has been documented in about 40 percent of patients. The mechanism by which analgesia is produced in these cases is not clear.

Psychological–Behavioral Treatment

During the end stage of cancer, all of the psychological–behavioral strategies and ongoing information and communication should be continued, with the following modifications and focus. Relaxation techniques, biofeedback, and hypnosis can be maintained and utilized as part of the overall pain management regime, with specific focus on more imaginal techniques. Cognitive activity management should be focused on helping the patient and family utilize self-statements to intellectually reconcile the inevitability of death and the quality of living at that point (Ellis, 1981). Behavioral activity management should center around stabilization of routine and assisting the patient in taking care of those activities in preparation for death (e.g., preparing a will, communicating with loved ones and saying good-bye, obtaining and sustaining spiritual support). Such activity can significantly reduce stress and mood disturbance which exacerbate the general pain and distress levels. Finally, increased attention to the grief process of family members through individual and group intervention may be necessary and useful to offset distress and mood disturbance in patients (who are quite often very concerned and distressed about grief in the family).

Thus, psychological–behavioral treatment can significantly enhance overall pain and distress management in stage 3 of the disease process, as well as the earlier stages of cancer. In concert with oncological, pharmacological, and on occasion, surgical, pain management methods, psychological–behavioral treatment and enhanced information and communication with patients and family can significantly improve the quality of existence.

CONCLUSION

Clinical research data clearly indicate that in complex cases of prolonged illness, disease-oriented medical intervention must be supplemented by psychological–behavioral supportive techniques to provide patients with skills to cope with the chronic illness process and the related changes in life-style, family relationship, work functioning, and so on. At present, the management of cancer patients is heavily tilted toward oncological intervention to control tumor growth. In the process, the concept of comprehensive, total patient management is often overlooked. As a consequence, patients often experience emotional and social "death" long before the biological end occurs. Control of neoplastic growths should be matched by the equally crucial control of pain, with both integrated so that the patient's overall state of mental and social functioning is protected as much as possible. Every effort should be made to maintain the patient's capability to endure and cope. These goals can best be accomplished through interdisciplinary and goal-oriented health care, such as that offered in accredited, quality pain control facilities.

REFERENCES

Ahles, T.A., Blanchard, E.B., & Ruckdeschel, J.C. (1983), The multi-dimensional nature of cancer-related pain. *Pain*, 17:277–288.
———Cohen, R.E., Little, D., Balducci, L., Dubbert, P.M., & Keane, T.M. (1984), Toward a behavioral assessment of anticipatory symptoms associated with cancer chemotherapy. *J. Behav. Ther. & Experiment. Psychiat.*, 15:141–145.
Aronoff, G.M., Evans, W.O., & Enders, P.L. (1983), A review of follow-up studies of multidisciplinary pain units. *Pain*, 16:1–11.
Averill, J.R., & Wisocki, P.A., (1983), Some observations on behavioral approaches to the treatment of grief among the elderly. In: *Behavior Therapy in Terminal Care: The Humanistic Approach*, ed. H.J. Sobel. Cambridge, MA: Ballinger.
Biegon, A., & Samwel, D. (1980), Interaction of tricyclic antidepressants with opiate reception. *Biochem. Pharmacol.*, 29:460–465.
Black, P. (1979), Management of cancer pain: An overview. *Neurosurgery*, 5:507–518.
Bond, M. (1979), Psychological and emotional aspects of cancer pain. In: *Advances in Pain Research and Therapy*, Vol. 2, eds. J. Bonica & V. Ventafridda. New York: Raven Press.
Bonica, J.J. (1953), *The Management of Pain*. Philadelphia: Lea & Febiger.

————(1959), *Clinical Applications of Diagnostic and Therapeutic Nerve Blocks.* Springfield, IL: Charles C. Thomas.

————(1982), The management of cancer pain. *Acta Anesthesiol. Scand. (Suppl.),* 74:75–82.

Breckner, F.T., & Gantz, P. (1984), Combination therapy with ibuprofen and methadone for chronic cancer pain. *Amer. J. Med.,* 77:78–83.

————Motyka, D., & Sherman, J. (1983), Growth enhancement of prolactin-sensitive mammary tumor by periacquiductal grey stimulation. *Life Sci.,* 32:525–530.

Brena, S.F. (1984), Chronic pain: A structured approach to drug therapy. *Mod. Med.,* 12:124–144.

————1985a. Nerve blocks and chronic pain states: An update. *Post Grad. Med.,* 78 4:64–85.

————1985b. Pain control facilities: Patterns of operation and problems of organization. In: *Clinics in Anaesthesiology. Chronic Pain: Management Principles,* eds. S.F. Brena & S.L. Chapman. London: W.B. Saunders.

————Chapman, S.L. (1985), Acute versus chronic pain states: "The learned pain syndrome." In: *Clinics in Anaesthesiology. Chronic Pain: Management Principles,* eds. S.F. Brena & S.L. Chapman. London: W.B. Saunders.

Burish, T.G., Carey, M.P., Krozely, M.G., & Greco, F.A., (1987), Conditioned side effects induced by cancer chemotherapy: Prevention through behavioral treatment. *J. Consult. & Clin. Psychol.,* 55:42–48.

Chapman, S.L., Brena, S.F., & Bradford, L.A. (1981), Treatment outcome in a chronic pain rehabilitation program. *Pain.* 11:255–268.

Cohen, R.S., Breckner, T.F., & Reeding, A.E. (1982), A survey of the subjective parameters of pain in cancer patients. *Amer. Pain Soc. Abstr.* 18:187–93.

Cousins, M.G., & Bridenbaugh, P.L. (1980), *Neural Blockade Clinical Anesthesia and Management of Pain.* Philadelphia: J.B. Lippincott.

Davies, J., Trask, C., & Souhami, R.L. (1979), Effect of mitramycin on widespread painful bone metastasis in cancer of the breast. *Cancer Treat. Rep.,* 63:1835–1838.

Ellis, A. (1981), Behavioral approaches to chronic pain. In: *Behavior Therapy in Terminal Care: The Humanistic Approach,* ed. H.J. Sobel. Cambridge, MA: Ballinger.

Foley, K.M. (1979), Pain syndromes in patients with cancer. In: *Advances in Pain Research and Therapy,* Vol. 2, eds. J.J Bonica & V. Ventafridda. New York: Raven Press.

Gottesman, D., & Lewis, M.S. (1982), Differences in crisis reactions among cancer and surgery patients. *J. Consult. & Clin. Psychol.,* 50:381–388.

Grabinski, P.Y., Kaiko, R.F., & Rogers, A.G., (1983), Plasma levels in analgesia following deltoid and gluteal injections of methadone and morphine. *J. Clin. Pharmacol.,* 23:48–55.

Halpern, L.M., & Bonica, J.J. (1979), Analgesics. In: *Drugs of Choice,* ed. P.V. Modell. St. Louis: C. V. Mosby.

Jay, S.M., Elliott, C., & Varni, J.W. (1986), Acute and chronic pain in adults and children with cancer. *J. Consult. & Clin. Psychol.,* 54:601–607.

Kaiko, R.F., Wallenstein, S.L., & Rogers, A.G., (1981), Analgesic and mood effects of heroin and morphine in cancer patients with postoperative pain. *New Eng. J. Med.,* 304:1501–1505.

Keefe, F.J., Brantley, A., Manuel, G., & Crisson, J.E. (1985), Behavioral assessment of head and neck cancer pain. *Pain,* 23:327–336.

Kübler-Ross, E. (1969), *On Death and Dying.* New York: Macmillan.

Lehman, J.F., DeLisa, G.A., & Warren, C.G., (1978), Cancer rehabilitation: Assessment of need, development and evaluation of a model care. *Arch. Phys. Med. & Rehab.*, 59:410–419.

Lewis, M., Gottesman, D., & Gutstine, S. (1979), The course and duration of crisis. *J. Consult. & Clin. Psychol.*, 47:128–134.

Malseed, R.T., & Goldsdein, F.G. (1979), Announcement of morphine analgesia by tricyclic antidepressant. *Neuropharmacol.*, 18:827–830.

Melzack, R. (1985), Hyperstimulation analgesia. In: *Clinics in Anaesthesiology. Chronic Pain: Management Principles*, eds. S.F. Brena & S.L. Chapman. London: W.B. Saunders.

Melzack, R.L. (1979), The Brompton mixture versus morphine solution given orally: Effects of pain. *Can. Med. Assn., J.*, 120:435–445.

Meyerson, B.A., Boethius, J. & Carlsson, A.M. (1978), Periventricular central grey stimulation from cancer pain. *Appl. Neurophysiol.*, 41:57–65.

Minton, J.P. (1974), The response of breast cancer to L-Dopa. *Cancer*, 33:358–363.

Moricca, G. (1974), Chemical hypophysectomy for cancer pain. In: *Advances in Neurology*, Vol. 4, ed. J.J. Bonica. New York: Raven Press.

Mount, B.W. (1984), Psychological and social aspects of cancer pain. In: *Textbook of Pain*, eds. P.D. Wall, & R. Melzack. New York: Churchill Livingston.

Sanders, S.H. (1985), The role of learning in chronic pain states. In: *Clinics in Anaesthesiology: Chronic Pain: Management Principles*, eds. S.F. Brena & S.L. Chapman. London: W.B. Saunders.

Scott, W.P. (1968), Fluoride therapy for pain in malignant bone disease. *Radiol.*, 90:588–590.

Sobel, H.J. (1981a), Toward a behavioral thanatology in clinical care. In: *Behavior Therapy in Terminal Care: A Humanistic Approach*, ed. H.J. Sobel. Cambridge, MA: Ballinger.

———ed. (1981b), *Behavior Therapy in Terminal Care: A Humanistic Approach*. Cambridge, MA: Ballinger.

Sweet, W.H., Polletti, E.C., & Challis, C.E. (1984), Operations in the brain stem and spinal canal, with an appendix on open cordotomy. In: *Textbook of Pain*, eds. P.D. Wall & R. Melzack. London: Churchill-Livingston.

Thompson, G.E., Moore, D.C., & Bridenbaugh, L.D. (1977), Abdominal pain and alcohol celiac plexus nerve blocks. *Anesthes. & Analges.*, 56:1–5.

Turk, D.C., & Rennert, K. (1983), Pain and the terminally ill cancer patient: A cognitive-social learning perspective. In: *Behavior Therapy in Terminal Care: A Humanistic Approach*, ed. H.J. Sobel. Cambridge, MA: Ballinger.

Wolskie, P.G., Gacely, R.H., & Greenberg, R.P. (1982), Comparison of effects of morphine and deep brain stimulation in chronic pain. *Amer. Pain Soc., Abstr.* 36:45–49.

9

Diagnostic Issues and Personality Variables in Coping with Treatment For Life-Threatening Illness

MARK B. WEISBERG, PH. D. AND STEWART PAGE, PH. D.

INTRODUCTION

Why do some patients get well and others die when the prognosis is the same for both? Is there a scientific basis for the will to live? One finds the above questions on the back cover of the book *Getting Well Again* by Simonton, Mathews-Simonton, and Creighton (1981). In the book, Simonton et al. describe a

The present chapter is based in part on a doctoral dissertation conducted by the first author in the Department of Psychology, University of Windsor, in 1984, and also in part upon a journal article (Weisberg and Page, 1988). We would like to thank the *Journal of Social and Clinical Psychology*, James Maddux, Associate Editor, and the Guilford Press, New York City, for kindly granting permission to include portions of this paper in the present chapter, and for other assistance to us.

We would like also to acknowledge the assistance of Drs. Kevin Moreland, Catherine Green, William Balance, Robert Fehr, and Sidney Baskin, M. D., in various phases of this research, as well as the Kidney Unit Staff of Mt. Carmel Mercy Hospital, Detroit, Michigan.

Complete descriptions of all measurement instruments used in the present research are available upon request or may be found in Weisberg (1984). Also, several analyses concerning choice of the various dialysis submodalities (i.e., home hemodialysis, home intermittent peritoneal dialysis (IPD), home continuous ambulatory peritoneal dialysis CAPD, hospital hemodialysis, and hospital IPD), not fully reported herein, are also available upon request.

recent research program, focusing on cancer patients, in which
the personality and general character of the supposedly cancer-
prone person is identified and described. The Simonton et al.
program is indeed an outgrowth of "wholistic" medicine; that is,
the belief that the mind influences bodily processes, for better
or worse. This occurs not only in terms of differential susceptibility to certain disorders, but also in terms of variations in
recuperative or self-restorative powers in individuals, once a
disease process has taken effect. The Simonton program, as
described in *Getting Well Again*, has indeed provided evidence
that treatment regimens based on enhancing the beneficial
effects of positive expectations, relaxation, exercise, pain management, and so on, appear likely to increase cancer patient
survival rates considerably, in comparison to the national norm.

The common thread running through the Simonton et al.
program has its academic roots primarily in attribution theory
(Strickland and Janoff-Bulman, 1981), learned helplessness
theory (Seligman, 1975), and in Rotter's (1954) theory of
learning and reinforcement. Even before Seligman's influential
research on the learned helplessness concept became prominent, the American physiologist Curt Richter (1957) had made
a number of dramatic observations about animal behavior
which were harmonious with Seligman's later work. As described in Rosenhan and Seligman (1984), Richter observed
that a state of apparent "hopelessness" could be created in
laboratory animals and that such a state generally led to an
animal's demise. Richter studied the behavior of rats placed in
a tank of water, over which strong jets of water shot downward,
preventing the struggling animal from floating. If Richter
placed a wild rat directly into the tank, it would typically
struggle against the water jet for sixty to eighty hours, before
finally expiring. If, however, Richter first restrained such an
animal in his hand until it stopped struggling, and then placed
it in the tank, it would typically struggle to survive only for a
three-to five-minute period. If Richter held the rat in his hand
before immersion, but then released it briefly to show it there
was "hope," it would typically struggle, upon immersion, for
sixty to eighty hours. Richter also had found that some wild
rats, when held captive in his hand for a short time, would die

there, without release and without participating in any experimental task whatsoever.

Julian Rotter (1954) was indeed one of the first to describe, in terms of formal psychological theory, the process by which individuals develop generalized expectancies concerning the extent to which they can exert control over their own life events. Those with "internal" locus of control, for example, were described by Rotter as feeling essentially in command of their lives, and as believing in their own ability to exert some effect or control upon life events. The individual with "external" locus of control, by contrast, is described by Rotter as feeling no such sense of control, or feeling he has the ability to influence life events; for example, believing that life was in effect a gamble to which one must defer, and over which one has little or no control. The common theme again is that while some patients feel negative and pessimistic, and remain passive recipients of medical treatment, there are others, by contrast, who possess a strong sense of alliance with a treatment program. These individuals thus actively participate in—indeed often enhance and modify—a treatment regimen. It is this sense of active personal participation in one's treatment, its presence in some and its relative absence in other patients, which appears critical in maximizing the patient's progress in recovery and resistance to the disease process.

A second general perspective on the importance of psychological or personality factors in response to the stress of disease may also be drawn from the relevant literature on the self-fulfilling prophecy (Rosenthal and Jacobson, 1968; Rosenthal, 1969; Rosenthal and Rubin, 1978) and the related phenomenon of medical placebo effects (Shapiro, 1960, 1964). Shapiro (1960), for example, in his detailed review of the placebo effect, indicates that, until relatively late in the nineteenth century, most if not all medical treatment exerted its beneficial effects largely through operation of the placebo effect. That is, treatments capitalized on the self-fulfilling effects of the patient's own optimism, faith in the medical profession, and belief that medical intervention would be helpful. Usually, the medical procedures available did indeed precipitate recovery. In most such cases, where improvement seems attributable to genuine placebo effects, the patient is able, once again, to participate as a catalyst in his or her recovery. Although we must not accept anecdotal evidence alone as definitive, there in fact exists a large collection of descriptions and first-hand observations of how patient optimism and expectations for improvement may work to bring about actual improvement. We cite here a brief example from the writings of Allport (1964), concerning a hospitalized (male) patient suffering from an apparently terminal illness, whose diagnosis was unfortunately unknown to the physicians involved. As Allport's report is described in Rosenthal and Jacobson (1968):

> The attending physicians told him quite frankly that he could not expect to be cured since the diagnosis was unknown. The only hope they offered him was a distinguished diagnostician had been called in and was soon to give his expert opinion. The specialist arrived but needed only a little time to reach his conclusion. To the physicians in attendance and almost out of the patient's earshot he pronounced: "moribundus". After some years, our patient, who did not die, called on the specialist to report on his good health and to thank the physician for saving his life. The ex-patient explained how the medical staff had told him that he could be cured only if the disease could be diagnosed. Therefore, he explained, he knew that he would recover as soon as he heard the consultant's diagnosis of "moribundus" [pp. 14–15].

Allport's anecodote is instructive, since once again we see strong evidence of patient participation as a positive force toward recovery. Although the expert "diagnosis" of moribundus was in fact a statement about the patient's apparent incurability, it served to mobilize hope, even enthusiasm, for recovery, in a patient who sincerely interpreted its content in a positive fashion.

A third perspective on personality-related factors in adjustment, as background for the research to be described below, concerns the rapidly escalating popular and academic literature on stress, its origins, effects, and alleviation. This literature of course owes much of its impact to the original theory and research of Selye (1956) and to that of Friedman and Rosenman (1974). The latter writers, in their book *Type A Behavior and Your Heart*, first described the "Type A" personality, its apparent vulnerability to stress, and indeed its increased likelihood of precipitating ulcers, hypertension, psychosomatic problems, as well as cardiovascular disease. Since the appearance of Friedman and Rosenman's influential research, the Type A person has become the object of considerable attention from both clinicians and academicians. The Type A syndrome of impatience, anxiety, overemphasis on job advancement, and so on, now is commonly described in abnormal psychology texts (e.g., excellent descriptions appear in Rosenhan and Seligman [1984]; Sue, Sue, and Sue [1986]) and in numerous other texts dealing with the issues of anxiety, neurosis, adjustment to life's hassles (Lazarus, 1984), and so on. In this latter area, we might also include recent studies on biofeedback (Kobler, 1978), on the effects of life events (Holmes and Rahe, 1967; Gibbs, 1981; Johnston, 1986), on the issue of whether perhaps men (or women) are generally more vulnerable to Type A stresses (Greenglass, 1982; Basow, 1986), and on predicting individual differences in amount and type of response to stress (Sue and Zane, 1981). An even more recent development, here with particular reference to Alzheimer's disease, is the current attempt to develop assessment instruments with which to measure personality-related factors affecting the quality of care provided by relatives, friends, and dependents of Alzheimer's patients and of the elderly infirm patient generally (Kosberg and Cairl, 1986; Zarit, Todd, and Zarit, 1986).

While the above perspectives each merit much additional research, again their common theme is relatively clear. The majority of studies show that patients who "participate" in treatment seem to do better, live longer, and generally respond more adequately to bodily stress. The present research, which concerned personality factors in adjustment to dialysis treatment for end-stage renal disease (ESRD), further explored this theme. Our approach and philosophy in this research, however, was to consider that while ESRD was itself an obvious stressor in terms of its immediate medical ramifications and effects, the necessary treatment for ESRD, that is, dialysis, itself constituted a major additional stress with which ESRD patients must cope. Phrased in its most general form, our overall goal in the study was therefore to examine personality-related factors in dialysis patients, of whom some preferred to receive the treatment in a hospital setting in which they were required to accommodate themselves to hospital rules and procedures, and of whom some preferred to dialyze in their own homes, in which case they were able to maintain virtually complete control over the necessary medical procedures.

PERSONALITY AND DIALYSIS: THE PRESENT STUDY

As emphasized in the recent review by Binik (1983), ESRD has been long neglected by researchers concerned with psychological factors in illness.

As described by several writers (Evans, Garrison, and Manninen, 1982; Weisberg, 1984) such disease is, however, a major health problem. According to Cummings (1970), more than 50,000 persons die annually from kidney disease in the United States alone. While dialysis, the removal of toxins and excess fluid from the system, is the most common treatment method for ESRD, its effectiveness remains limited by the fact that development of its technical aspects has grown faster than has understanding of its psychological aspects and ramifications (Simmons, 1977). Kidney disease seriously disrupts the lives of patients and their families, socially, sexually, and financially, hence the need for investigation of psychological factors which might enhance (or impede) adjustment to a dialysis regime. End-stage renal disease patients undergoing dialysis treatment encounter several broad areas of stress (Mock, 1976; Kaplan De-Nour, 1981). These include physiological fluctuation, deterioration, and discomfort, as well as strict dietary restrictions. With a life-threatening chronic illness, patients must also confront such issues as their mortality, fear of death, and, in fact, fear of life (Beard and Sampson, 1981; Devins, 1981). The presence of serious emotional and psychological turmoil in ESRD patients has thus precipitated development of the field of psychonephrology, the study of psychological factors in dialysis and transplantation (Drees and Gallagher, 1981).

HEMODIALYSIS AND PERITONEAL DIALYSIS

In hemodialysis, the most frequent form of dialysis, blood is passed through a cleansing system to remove toxins and excess fluid. The blood is filtered through semipermeable membranes in the dialyzing machine, thus removing water, salt, and waste products. Access to the circulatory system is usually through an arteriovenous fistula. The procedure must be used an average of two or three days weekly. This may be done, however, either in the patient's home or in a hospital setting. In the former type, the patient works with spouse or partner in using, monitoring, and operating the equipment correctly, preceded by a necessary training program. In the latter type, the patient receives the treatment passively, with hospital staff monitoring details of machine maintenance and operation, as well as monitoring of blood pressure, fluid, and chemical levels. Both home and hospital hemodialysis patients must also learn the necessary medical and dietary restrictions.

An alternative treatment is peritoneal dialysis, in which no blood is removed from the body. Tubing is inserted just inside the peritoneum (the sac surrounding the abdomen), and dialysate fluid introduced through the tubing into the peritoneum, causing dialysis of water and waste material to occur through the peritoneal sac. Fluid and waste are later drained through the same tubing. There are two commonly used forms of peritoneal dialysis. Intermittent peritoneal dialysis (IPD) can be performed either in the patient's home or in the hospital. If performed at home, both patient and partner require special training in proper use of IPD equipment. Another option for home peritoneal patients is continuous ambulatory peritoneal dialysis (CAPD), which functions similarly to IPD but on a continuous (24-hour) basis. In this procedure, the patient is essentially free to continue normal activities while dialyzing continuously by means of a portable dialysate container. Although there are disadvantages to CAPD treatment, there are fewer nutritional and dietary restrictions than with other procedures. Both hemodialysis and peritoneal dialysis appear equally effective physiologically; detailed descriptions of these procedures are found in sources such as Friedman (1978) and Weisberg (1984).

Thus, more important than the distinction between the various treatment procedures, for present purposes, was the issue of whether the treatment is experienced in one's home or in a hospital. The choice of whether to dialyze in the hospital or at home has physiological, psychological, and economic ramifications, both for ESRD patients and medical ESRD staff. At present, however, little is known as to personality factors enhancing or inhibiting success with these different modalities. Also, little is known as to the effects of personality and personal coping styles of ESRD patients on the efficacy of dialysis treatment. End-stage renal disease staff frequently see patients with equivalent degrees of organ pathology and physiological deterioration who nevertheless show considerable variability in their response to ESRD treatment. Greater understanding of such processes would thus be valuable to such staff. Personality differences between those adjusting better to hospital, versus those adjusting better to home dialysis, have been claimed (Friedman, 1978; Lowry and Atcherson, 1980) but very few studies have been able to gather empirical data on this issue directly from ESRD patients. The present study therefore studied the relationship to dialysis adjustment of the personality styles and psychogenic attitudes (patient perceptions of current stresses) of ESRD patients undergoing home as opposed to hospital dialysis treatment.

THE MILLON BEHAVIORAL HEALTH INVENTORY

To date, studies of personality factors with renal patients have utilized instruments such as the MMPI (Ziarnik, Freeman, Sherrard, and Calsyn, 1977), Sentence Completion Test (Kaplan De-Nour, 1981), or Rorschach (Rabinowitz and Van Der Spuy, 1978). Such tests were developed for use mainly with psychiatric populations. Problems thus exist regarding appropriateness of test content, norms, and interpretation of results. The Millon Behavioral Health Inventory (MBHI) (Millon, Green, and Meagher, 1979), developed with nonpsychiatric medical populations, was therefore used in the present study.

The MBHI is a 150-item true–false psychodiagnostic inventory, which possesses superior psychometric properties in terms of reliability, validity, and yield of clinically useful information (Millon et al., 1979; Schmidt, 1981). The MBHI assesses: (1) *Patient Personality or Coping Styles*. Eight dimensions of personality style are measured (Millon et al., 1979). These are: patient introversion–extroversion, inhibition, cooperation, sociability, confidence, forcefulness, respect, and sensitivity; (2) *Psychogenic Attitudes*. These refer to the patient's current perceptions of present and future stressors, and are labeled by Millon et al. as: chronic tension, recent stress, premorbid pessimism, future despair, social alienation, and somatic anxiety; and (3) a two-dimension *Prognostic Index*. These dimensions, life-threat reactivity and emotional vulnerability, assess likelihood of dysfunctional reaction to stress or illness, and likelihood of developing dysfunctional emotional reactions, such as depression or apathy, in response to major medical treatment. Thus, the coping style scales measure general characteristics or traits reflecting personal functioning before as well as subsequent to treatment. The psychogenic attitude and prognostic index scales serve as "state" measures of current responses to stress and of emotional well-being which are largely coincident with onset of dialysis treatment. An outline of the MBHI scales appears in Table 9.1.

TABLE 9.1

DESCRIPTIONS OF HIGH SCORERS ON CLINICAL SCALES OF THE MILLON
BEHAVIORAL HEALTH INVENTORY[1]

Scale	Description
Personality Style (Coping Style)	
Introversive Personality	Keeps to self, quiet, unemotional, not easily excited, rarely gets socially involved, lacks energy, vague about symptoms

Inhibited Personality	Shy, avoids close relationships, fears rejection, distrustful, easily hurt, socially ill at ease
Cooperative Personality	Soft hearted, submissive with others, lacks initiative, is dependent, nonassertive
Sociable Personality	Charming, histrionic, capricious in affect, talkative, attention seeking, unreliable
Confident Personality	Self-centered, narcissistic, is exploitive, takes others for granted, egocentric
Forceful Personality	Domineering, abrasive, blunt, aggressive, impatient, easily angered, intimidating
Respectful Personality	Serious minded, rule conscious, emotions constrained, avoids the unpredictable, socially conforming
Sensitive Personality	Unpredictable, moody, negativistic, guilt ridden, anticipates disappointment, displeased with self and others

Psychogenic Attitude

Chronic Tension	Under self-imposed pressure, has difficulty relaxing
Recent Stress	Life routine has been unset by unanticipated tensions and problems
Premorbid Pessimism	Is disposed to interpret life as a series of misfortunes
Future Despair	Displays a bleak outlook, anticipates the future as distressing or potentially threatening
Social Alienation	Feels isolated, perceives minimal family and social support
Somatic Anxiety	Is hypochondriacally concerned with bodily functions, fears pain and illness

Prognostic Index

Life-Threat Reactivity	Is empirically similar to patients with chronic or progressive life-threatening illnesses, such as renal failure, who display a more troubled course than is typical of patients with chronic illness
Emotional Vulnerability	Is empirically similar to patients with chronic or progressive life-threatening illnesses, such as renal failure, who exhibit severe depression, disorientation, or psychotic episodes as a result of treatment

[1]Higher scores indicate greater prominence of the trait.

No previous study has assessed ESRD patients, using the MBHI. The present study thus investigated its validity and clinical usefulness by examining patient responses on its coping style scales and also on the scales measuring current adjustment and satisfaction with dialysis treatment; that is, the psychogenic attitude and prognostic index scales. Further, these relationships were examined in relation to patient choice of home versus hospital dialysis.

METHOD

Subjects

Forty-two patients of the Kidney Unit at Mt. Carmel Mercy Hospital, Detroit, participated as subjects, as did thirty-seven partners. Subjects were selected randomly from lists of patients dialyzing at home or in the hospital. Most of the common renal diagnoses were equally represented, both in patients dialyzing in hospital and in the group choosing home dialysis. Such diagnoses included glomerulonephritis, pyelonephritis, hypertensive renal failure, polycystic renal failure, and nephrosclerosis. Mean age for the total sample was 48.42 years for patients and 42.18 years for partners. Twenty-nine patients were female, thirteen were male. Mean length of time on dialysis at the time of the study was 18.21 months. Most patients earned $10,000 or less annually, and had at least a high school education, but 80 percent were unemployed at the time of the study. Also, 65 percent of the patients' partners were unemployed. Forty-three percent of the partners were spouses, with the remainder being a son, daughter, sibling, parent, or friend.

Chi-square tests indicated no significant differences between the home and hospital patients in income, marital status, number of available support persons, or employment status. The home group contained six males and sixteen females; the hospital group contained seven males and thirteen females. A t-test indicated that the hospital group was significantly older (M = 55.75 yrs.) than the home group (M = 41.77 yrs.), $t (40)$ = 3.74 p <0.006. All analyses of variance, reported in the

"*Results*" section below, were therefore also performed with patient age as a covariate. In all cases, the obtained p levels for these analyses remained as reported below. Both groups had been determined by unit medical staff to be comparable in overall medical status; that is, apart from ESRD symptoms. Three patients were diabetic in each group. It should be noted also that the use of home versus hospital dialysis was a result primarily of the patient's own decision, and not of medical or other factors. It was the policy of the Mt. Carmel Kidney unit staff to present new ESRD patients with complete verbal and written descriptions of both home and hospital dialysis procedures, including advantages and disadvantages of each, from which patients freely chose their preferred modality. The present home and hospital groups were thus constituted in this fashion. A t-test indicated no significant difference between the groups in number of months on dialysis at the time of the present study.

Procedure

Eligible patients were contacted initially by letter, and then by telephone. All completed a form acknowledging free and informed consent for participation. MBHI (coping style, psychogenic attitude, and prognostic index scales) plus patient and partner rating scales were completed, by appointment, at the Kidney Unit, Mt. Carmel Mercy Hospital, Detroit, under the supervision of the first author. Certain demographic and medical information was also obtained from patient charts.

Additionally, both patients and their partners in the present study completed a series of five-point Likert rating scales, referred to hereafter as patient (and partner) rating scales. These scales gathered educational and demographic information as well as additional information on general emotional factors and current adjustment to dialysis. The patient rating scales assessed degree of: patient comfort with partner's involvement in treatment; patient desire for control over the disease; feeling less like a man or woman; satisfaction with dialysis modality chosen; being influenced by others in choice of modality; conceiving of one's self as "sick"; closeness to partner since onset of treatment; sexual satisfaction since onset of treatment; change in sexual satisfaction from before treatment; estimated degree of responsibility for treatment requirements as compared to partner; and perceived increase or decrease in family closeness since onset of dialysis. Partner rating scales required the partner (usually a spouse) to respond to each issue as above, but to do so from his or her perception of the patient, for example, "How much does your partner think of himself/herself as a sick patient?"

Results

Results were examined specifically in terms of relationships between (1) treatment modality and MBHI psychogenic attitude/prognostic index scales; (2) treatment modality and MBHI coping style scales; (3) MBHI psychogenic attitude /prognostic index and patient/partner scales; and (4) MBHI coping style scales and the patient/partner rating scales. Lastly, some additional comparisons concerning involving demographic variables are reported.

Treatment Modality and MBHI Psychogenic/Prognostic
Index Scales

Home and hospital patients were compared on the MBHI psychogenic attitude and prognostic index scales. As described, these scales assessed patient perceptions of current and future stressors, perceptions along a general hopelessness–helplessness dimension, and included the two-scale prognostic index.

Mean scores for hospital patients, on all eight of the above scales, were consistently higher than those for home dialysis patients, as shown in Table 9.2. This pattern indicated greater psychological maladjustment, more intensely perceived current stressors, and poorer prognosis for adjustment to treatment and rehabilitation.

TABLE 9.2

MEAN MBHI PSYCHOGENIC ATTITUDE AND PROGNOSTIC INDEX SCORES
FOR HOME (N = 22) AND HOSPITAL PATIENTS (N = 20)[1]

Psychogenic Attitude Scales	Hospital Mean	SD	Home Mean	SD
Chronic Tension	64.75	21.42	42.05	22.63
Recent Stress	68.05	20.42	34.64	23.98
Premorbid Pessimism	69.75	21.53	44.55	23.61
Future Despair	67.15	21.42	45.59	21.48
Social Alienation	51.35	19.23	38.41	20.76
Somatic Anxiety	79.90	18.86	50.27	19.74
Prognostic Index Scales				
Life Threat Reactivity	77.00	11.45	55.45	19.59
Emotional Vulnerability	45.95	24.74	26.14	23.60

[1]Means refer to MBHI T-scores.

Using the SAS (1982) General Linear Models (GLM) procedure, a multivariate analysis of variance (MANOVA) was performed, with choice of home versus hospital dialysis as the nominal variable and the psychogenic attitude and prognostic index scales as continuous variables. MANOVA is a statistical procedure in which the relationship between one or more nominal variables and two or more continuous variables may be assessed. In effect, MANOVA groups the continuous variables (Millon scales in the present research) together and then analyzes the degree of relationship between this composite measure and the nominal variable. A common practice, if the MANOVA results are significant, is to follow up with individual analyses of variance on each of the dependent variables (i.e., scales). A further option is to conduct a discriminant function analysis (see below) in which the goal is generally to ascertain which dependent measures appear most strongly related to the nominal variable. Using the Hotelling-Lawley Trace criterion, the MANOVA was significant, $F(8,33) = 4.28$, $p < 0.001$. Subsequent univariate analyses of variance of each scale, by dialysis modality, were all significant; that is, for Chronic Tension, $F(1,41) = 11.10$, $p < 0.01$, Recent Stress, $F(1,41) = 23.40$, $p < 0.001$, Premorbid Pessissism, $F(1,41) = 12.98$, $p < 0.01$, Future Despair, $F(1,41) = 10.58$, $p < 0.01$, Social Alienation, $F(1,41) = 4.37$, $p < 0.05$, Somatic Anxiety, $F(1,41) = 27.08$, $p < 0.001$, Life Threat Reactivity, $F(1,41) = 18.44$, $p < 0.001$, and Emotional Vulnerability, $F(1,41)) = 7.05$, $p < 0.05$. Using the SAS (1982) STEPDISC procedure, the MBHI scales were also entered into a stepwise discriminant analysis, with modality of dialysis as the classification variable. One variable only, somatic anxiety, was selected by the stepwise procedure, producing an R^2 of 0.40 with an F, for all scales considered together, of 27.08, $p < 0.0001$; no other scales improved this model. Higher levels of somatic and hypochondriacal concerns thus were particularly associated with greater likelihood of hospital rather than home dialysis.

Treatment Modality and MBHI Coping Style Scales

As described before, the eight MBHI Coping Style scales measure relatively stable, health-related personality dispositions. The mean scale scores of hospitalized patients were again higher than those of home patients on all scales, except for Introversion and Sociability, as shown in Table 9.3. Such a pattern indicated that the hospital patients generally showed less constructive, more deferential, and more compliant, personality patterns.

Using the SAS (1982) GLM procedure, a multivariate analysis of variance (MANOVA) was performed, with MBHI coping style scales as continuous variables and choice of home versus hospital dialysis as the nominal variable. Using the Hotelling-Lawley trace criterion, the MANOVA was significant, $F(8.33) = 3.80$, $p < 0.002$. Subsequent univariate analyses of variance indicated that the MBHI respectful scale, a measure of conformist, submissive tendencies, significantly discriminated between modalities, $F(1.40) = 10.85$, $p < 0.002$, with hospital patients scoring higher. Using the SAS (1982) STEPDISC procedure, significant discrimination between modalities (Wilks' Lambda $= 0.55$, $p < 0.0004$) was achieved, with the respectful, sensitive, cooperative, confident, and sociable scales selected as predictors (listed in order of selection).

TABLE 9.3
MEAN MBHI COPING STYLE SCALE SCORES FOR HOME (N = 22)
AND HOSPITAL PATIENTS (N = 20)[1]

Coping Style Scale	Hospital		Home	
	Mean	SD	Mean	SD
Introversive	47.20	15.65	54.77	24.63
Inhibited	54.25	23.76	45.64	29.04
Cooperative	35.00	17.48	31.82	23.55
Sociable	27.25	18.93	39.41	26.19
Confident	60.30	19.16	54.73	22.24
Forceful	58.90	17.64	54.82	19.55
Respectful	81.10	19.40	62.77	16.65
Sensitive	55.75	24.25	43.50	29.45

[1]Means refer to MBHI
T-scores.

MBHI Psychogenic Attitude/Prognostic Index and Patient/Partner Scales

Intercorrelations were computed between MBHI psychogenic attitude/prognostic index scales, as measures of adaptation to current life stressors, and the patient/partner scales, as measures of current adaptation to ongoing dialysis treatment as seen by both patient and partner.

Seven of the scales involving patient evaluations of current treatment procedures showed significant correlations (at p <0.05; N = 42) with various MBHI psychogenic attitude/prognostic index scales. Patients less able to accept help from partners, for example, showed elevations on scales measuring chronic tension ($r = -0.39$), recent stress ($r = -0.37$), and premorbid pessimism ($r = -0.33$). Patients viewing themselves as less masculine or less feminine as a result of ESRD scored more highly on the emotional vulnerability scale ($r = -0.33$). Patients less satisfied with their chosen dialysis modality were elevated on recent stress ($r = -0.37$), premorbid pessimism ($r = -0.44$), Future Despair ($r = -0.46$), Somatic Anxiety ($r = -0.42$), Life Threat Reactivity ($r = -0.36$), and emotional vulnerability ($r = -0.33$). Subjects likelier to view themselves as "sick patients" scored more highly on premorbid pessimism ($r = -0.33$), future despair ($r = -0.35$), social alienation ($r = -0.36$), life threat reactivity ($r = -0.36$), and emotional vulnerability ($r = -0.43$). Patients reporting greater loss of sexual functioning were elevated on both the chronic tension ($r = -0.36$ and life threat reactivity ($r = -0.35$) scales. Patients reporting feeling more in charge of daily treatment responsibilities than their partners scored at lower levels on chronic tension ($r = -0.35$), recent stress ($r = -0.36$), and future despair ($r = -0.35$).

Patients showing greater satisfaction with the type of dialysis modality chosen, that is, as perceived by partners, scored lower on the social alienation ($r = -0.36$) and life threat reactivity ($r = -0.34$) scales. Patients whose choice of treatment modality was influenced more highly by partners, as judged by partners, scored more highly on scales measuring recent stress ($r = -0.36$), premorbid pessimism ($r = -0.42$), and life threat reactivity ($r = -0.38$). Patients viewing themselves as "sick," as perceived by partners, scored higher on emotional vulnerability ($r = -0.39$). Patients with diminished sexual satisfaction since dialysis, as perceived by partners, showed higher scores on emotional vulnerability ($r = 0.44$). Also, partners themselves reporting diminished sexual satisfaction since the patient's dialysis, tended to be spouses of patients scoring higher on social alienation ($r = 0.38$), life threat reactivity ($r = 0.41$), and emotional vulnerability ($r = 0.44$).

MBHI Coping Style and Patient/Partner Scales

Correlations were computed between the MBHI coping style scales, as measures of stable personality dispositions, and patient/partner scales, as measures of adjustment to ongoing dialysis treatment.

Results ($p \geqslant 0.05$) for patient scales showed that patients feeling less masculine or feminine since dialysis scored higher on the inhibited scale ($r = -0.35$) as did patients tending to view themselves as "sick" ($r = -0.40$). Those who experienced difficulty accepting partner help tended to be lower on the cooperative scale ($r = 0.35$), as did those feeling less close to their partners since onset of ESRD ($r = 0.27$). Patients scoring higher on the sociable scale were less likely to feel less masculine or feminine since dialysis ($r = 0.28$), tended to be more satisfied with treatment ($r = 0.29$), tended less to see themselves as sick ($r = 0.40$), reported somewhat less satisfactory sexual adjustment ($r = 0.30$), and tended to feel more in charge of their own treatment than their partner ($r = 0.28$). Those scoring higher on the confident scale tended less to view themselves as sick ($r = 0.37$). Those scoring higher on the forceful scale tended to experience more difficulty accepting partner help ($r = - 0.29$). Those scoring higher on the respectful scale tended to be less satisfied with treatment modality chosen ($r = -0.30$), less satisfied with sexual adjustment ($r = 0.28$), to report lower sexual satisfaction before dialysis ($r = -0.32$), and to feel less in control of treatment procedures than partner ($r = -0.37$). Patients scoring higher on the sensitive scale tended not to feel less masculine or feminine ($r = 0.32$), but tended to view themselves as sick ($r = -0.49$).

The results for partner scales showed that higher patient scores on the introversive scale were associated with less partner influence upon choice of modality, as perceived by partners ($r = 0.43$). Patients scoring higher on the inhibited scale tended to show greater partner influence as to modality, as seen by partners ($r = -0.33$), and to be perceived by partners as showing lower satisfaction with chosen modality ($r = -0.33$). Patients higher on the cooperative scale tended to be seen by partners as having less need to exert control over their disease and treatment ($r = 0.37$). Those scoring higher on the sensitive scale were seen by partners as more dissatisfied with treatment ($r = -0.28$), as accepting of more partner influence as to chosen modality ($r = -0.43$), and as more likely to view themselves as sick patients ($r = -0.31$).

MBHI Psychogenic Attitude/Prognostic Index and Demographic Variables

Finally, correlations were computed between the MBHI psychogenic attitude/prognostic index scales and the demographic variables of marital status, income, education, and employment status. Patient income correlated negatively with somatic anxiety ($r = -0.32$). Patient marital status (using point biserial correlation) correlated significantly at $p \geqslant 0.05$ with all but one scale; that is, chronic tension ($r = 0.59$), recent stress ($r = 0.59$), premorbid pessimism ($r = 0.51$), future despair ($r = 0.42$), social alienation ($r = 0.30$), somatic anxiety ($r = 0.48$), and life threat reactivity ($r = 0.32$). Thus, married patients consistently scored less pathologically on these scales than did single patients. Patients having fewer or no children tended to score lower on the chronic tension scale ($r = 0.37$). Patients with more years of formal education scored consistently lower, less pathologically, on all scales. These correlations were: chronic tension ($r = -0.44$); recent stress ($r = -0.41$); premorbid pessimism ($r = -0.37$); future despair ($r = -0.44$); social alienation ($r = -0.38$); somatic anxiety ($r = -0.45$); life threat reactivity ($r = -0.46$); and emotional vulnerability ($r = -0.40$). (Five of these scales, chronic tension, recent stress, future despair, social alienation, and life threat reactivity, also correlated significantly, in the same direction, with partner's years of formal education). Patients unemployed during dialysis procedures scored higher on five scales, that is, future despair ($r = 0.33$), social alienation ($r = 0.30$), somatic anxiety ($r = 0.31$), life threat reactivity ($r = 0.51$), and emotional vulnerability ($r = 0.51$), as compared to employed patients. Lastly, it appeared that experience with the dialysis procedure itself may exert some salutory effect in terms of the patient's sense of current well-being and adjustment. Patients who had been on dialysis for longer periods as of the time of study, showed lower scores on four scales, that is, recent stress ($r = -0.40$), premorbid pessimism ($r = -0.39$), social alienation ($r = -0.36$), and life threat reactivity ($r = -0.36$).

Discussion

Overall, in our opinion, the results indicated substantial predictive and construct validity for the MBHI, and gave evidence also that the instrument has potential use in medical settings as a measure and predictor of adjustment to treatment for life-threatening sickness. More specifically, in the present study, the choice of receiving treatment at home or in hospital was significantly related to patient scores on all psychogenic attitude scales and to the two-scale prognostic index. These differences consistently favored those using home dialysis, in that these patients exhibited less tension, more constructive coping with stress, less anxiety about bodily symptoms, and more optimistic patterns of attitudes, as compared to those dialyzing in the hospital. Those with fewer hypochondriacal concerns were more likely to have chosen home dialysis. The pattern of mean scores on the MBHI coping style scales also generally favored the home dialyzing group, in that patients dialyzing in the hospital were found to have less constructive, more conformist, and more submissive characteristics in terms of overall personality functioning.

The patient/partner scale data also showed that scores on the psychogenic attitude/prognostic index scales were predictive, in many instances, of patient self-reports about ongoing treatment progress as well as of partner evaluations of patient progress. With few exceptions, these relationships were consistent with the theoretical or conceptual meaning of the MBHI scales involved. Patients less satisfied with their chosen modality, for example, were higher on several scales, as were those tending to view themselves as sick patients, having diminished sexual satisfaction, tending to see themselves as less masculine or feminine, tending to see themselves as not "in charge" of their lives, or who gave considerable responsibility to partners for choice of dialysis modality and for day-to-day help with treatment procedures. As described above, many of the patient/partner scales also correlated significantly with one or more of the MBHI coping style scales.

In general, the MBHI appeared to be of considerable

usefulness regarding the major treatment choice of home versus hospital dialysis. Mean T-scores on all but two scales were higher, indicating greater psychological disturbance, for those dialyzing in hospital. Most of the scale means for these patients, unlike those for home patients, also approached or surpassed Millon's T-score criterion of 70; that is, an approximate point beyond which the measured characteristic may become clinically problematic (Millon et al., 1979). Clearly, patients choosing hospital dialysis perceived greater stress in their current situation and showed a less hopeful outlook for the future, both according to their own self-reports and to the MBHI Prognostic Index scales. It should be noted that analyses of variance of the patient rating scales, by modality, confirmed that home patients were significantly more satisfied with their chosen treatment modality than were hospital patients, felt significantly closer to their partners, and also experienced (as did their partners) more satisfactory sexual adjustment as compared to hospital patients. Further, the most salient coping style scale for the present patient sample was the MBHI respectful scale (Table 9.1). Millon et al. (1979) describe high scorers on this scale as markedly serious minded, rule conscious, unexpressive, socially conforming, disliking of unpredictability, and emotionally constrained. Such a pattern seems to typify many chronically ill patients in general, as well as, in the present study, patients dialyzing in the hospital. In knowingly choosing hospital dialysis, such patients must adhere to hospital routines and rules, and must generally behave in a deferential fashion. They seem in fact more hesitant to entrust their own care to either self or spouse, in comparison to those dialyzing at home. This general pattern also included the somatic anxiety scale, on which patients dialyzing in hospital were elevated. In our opinion, the data indicate that choice and level of functioning on a particular dialysis modality is related to both ongoing and reactive, as well as to more stable, personality dimensions. Indices of adjustment to treatment and of patient satisfaction with dialysis also seem related both to modality choice and to many MBHI subscales. As such, psychologists employed in medical settings should be able to utilize MBHI information both as a predictor of treatment success and as a source of practical information as to the nature and efficacy of different modalities. Although the choice of dialysis modality also depends somewhat on personal, family, and economic factors (Perras and Zappacosta, 1980; Weisberg, 1984), psychometric information based on personality and coping style factors should be uniquely useful to ESRD staff, particularly since advising new ESRD patients on treatment options, and so on is a practical task for which many such staff report being in need of data-based assistance. Knowledge of patient characteristics likely to facilitate or impede various aspects of treatment thus should enable more informed and efficacious treatment strategies. The present results also supported Kaplan De-Nour's (1981) position that adjustment to ESRD and to dialysis treatment is related to clinically important personality and coping style characteristics in patients, especially those involving hypochondriacal or somatic concerns.

Implications for Psychological Intervention Within Dialysis Settings

The results of the present study indicated that hospitalized patients were generally at somewhat greater risk psychologically. They were more likely than patients at home to experience high levels of chronic stress, depression, hopelessness, and sex role adjustment to treatment. They were more likely to identify themselves as "sick patients" and more likely to be hypochondriacally concerned, with resulting adverse effects both physically and psychologically. We found that families of these patients tended to lack flexibility and expressiveness, and this appeared to interfere with their ability to make the difficult adjustment to a treatment regimen. In the present study, high levels of family rigidity and control were also correlated with high levels of self-imposed pressure and chronic tension in the patient.

The status of the marital or other primary relationship, between patient and significant other, appeared to be of some importance in the present study. For all participants, the patient's level of satisfaction with the marriage (or other significant-other relationship) correlated significantly with overall treatment satisfaction.

Certain demographic factors seem to place some patients at greater risk for maladjustment. In the present study, patients who were older, single or divorced, unemployed, or who had received less education, generally experienced a more difficult adjustment to the dialysis regimen and appeared worse in regard to long-term prognosis, both physically and emotionally.

Given the styles of personality functioning and types of symptomatology found in patients like those in the present study, the need for various types of psychological intervention becomes more apparent. Psychological assessment (intellectual, personality, vocational, and neuropsychological) is needed: (1) to identify which patients may be at risk emotionally; (2) to evaluate individuals as to emotional preparedness for transplant in live related donor situations; (3) to provide relevant data in helping patients cope with treatment in the inpatient and home settings; and (4) assess loss of cognitive function due to uremia or other causes.

Implications for the Psychologist in Settings Treating
Chronic Illness and Pain

The health care psychologist must be not only competent in psychological methods, but also must be sensitive to a larger domain in which physical, social, and psychological factors interface and can only be understood in relationship to one another.

Degood (1983) addresses these issues in connection with the functions of a psychologist in a medical setting. The contemporary medical psychologist is likely to be faced with requests to identify, and modify, cognitive, physiological, and social behaviors that have become part of an illness pattern.

According to Degood, a psychologist working in such medical settings is well advised to be cognizant of certain strategies. First, the psychologist should disavow the "organic versus functional" myth held by the patient and health care team, emphasizing that psychological issues are also consequences of physical symptoms. Most complaints indeed involve a combination of physiological and psychological factors. The psychologist should indeed avoid premature efforts to "psychologize" the patient's symptoms, since it is often easier to establish rapport with a patient if one initially goes along with their symptom-focused presentation. Degood stresses that the patient should be required to make an active decision to participate in a treatment program. Psychologists in medical settings are usually part of a multidisciplinary team, and need to be supportive and express the importance of various dietary, exercise, and medication strategies in the overall care of the patient. Such cooperation also "prevents the patient from playing one profession against another, a game in which psychologists all too often become spirited participants" (1983, p. 576).

Assessment instruments used in nonpsychiatric medical settings must be sensitive to issues such as the ones outlined above; that is, if the psychologist is to make an informed contribution. The construction of instruments such as the MBHI acknowledges the intricate interplay of physiological, emotional, and cognitive factors which affect the chronically ill patient. More attention needs to be directed toward the use and further development of appropriate assessment tools in medical settings. Straightfaced adherence to traditional personality assessment instruments in evaluating the complex problems of the chronically ill medical patient "contradicts every major principle of sound test use" (Millon et al., 1979, pp. 530–531). Most importantly, such adherence prevents the health care psychologist from making the contribution of which he or she is capable, in terms of expediting the rehabilitation of chronically ill patients.

Lastly, economic factors are relevant, in that, for example, home dialysis is being increasingly advocated as a preferred treatment modality in order to reduce government costs for maintenance of hospitalized patients (Inglehart, 1982). In the United States, Medicare payments for dialysis have been recently reduced. Further investigation of home versus hospital modalities, and, conceivably, of strategies aimed at expediting home dialysis with patients for whom hospital care might normally be chosen, is therefore vital. The MBHI thus appears to have potential as a useful instrument for the medical psychologist, that is, as one who is likely to be faced with requests to identify and deal with cognitive, psychophysiological, and social dysfunction in the chronically ill patient.

CONCLUSION

Although our immediate research concerns were those specifically involving personality characteristics of ESRD patients and choice of dialysis modality, we generally interpret our overall results within the framework of health-related personality research described at the outset. That is, our results with the MBHI appeared, in our view, generally consistent with the emerging pattern of two basic patient responses to illness—one being constructive, of internal locus of control, even optimistic, the other being relatively less constructive, of external locus of control, and more pessimistic in general prognostic outlook. We look forward therefore to future research in which this general view may be further evaluated and tested.

We conclude with a brief comment on a recent and provocative statement by Angell (1985). In Angell's view, the evidence that personality factors or mental status can affect the onset, treatment, or cure, of disease is subjective and without scientific foundation. Angell thus claims that such evidence is mostly anecdotal, and portrays it as "largely folklore" (1985, p. 1572). She claims further that an emphasis on personality factors in disease is a form of victim-blaming, in that patients, already ill with serious disease, should not be held accountable or given personal responsibility for the outcome. Angell thus cites the example of artificial heart recipient William Schroeder, who was criticized, even by physicians, for showing withdrawn, timid behavior following a stroke, therein implying that Schroeder's personal characteristics were impeding or preventing more satisfactory medical progress.

We do not feel, however, that the moral concept of blame is an accurate description for patients whose personality characteristics, objectively measured and factually described, may be dysfunctional in terms of coping with disease, no more than we could wish to "blame" individuals of short stature for not being basketball stars. We would also point out that there does in fact exist a considerable body of evidence that a patient's belief in his or her ability to influence the disease process often itself serves to precipitate improvement or recovery, as in the case of Allport's dramatic example, which we described earlier in the context of medical self-fulfilling prophecies. We do agree somewhat with Angell, in the sense that perhaps the psychological or personality perspective on disease has indeed been overemphasized. Perhaps we are thus witnessing a "bandwagon effect," as hastened by the much publicized comments of individuals such as Norman Cousins or by the attention given to the Simonton et al. (1981) cancer treatment program described earlier. We offer one further point, however. In her article, Angell (1985) does recognize that people do retain some "responsibility" for their health (p. 1572). She recognizes therefore that certainly such behaviors as smoking, drinking alcohol, eating foods rich in cholesterol or saturated fats, have great impact on one's health. We would note here that Angell restricts her interpretation of this impact, since she limits her view to the biochemical or physiological effects upon the body of these agents, and does not consider the quickly accumulating evidence that engaging in such health-enhancing practices is itself related to measureable personality dispositions. Many relevant studies, for example, are summarized in Ryckman (1985), in connection with Rotter's locus of control formulation, as described earlier (Strickland, 1979). Together, these studies generally indicate that individuals with internal locus of control, and associated personal characteristics, show heightened concern for, and more frequently engage in, a variety of behaviors leading to better health. They also show more effective preventive health care, as well as more effective efforts to cope with sickness if and when it does occur. The most tragic, most extreme, and most dramatic examples of these phenomena are summarized in Seligman's (1975) description of hopelessness-induced death, both in animals and human beings. Among other goals, a worthwhile objective for future research, with dialysis specifically, would be to assess the possibility that different personality dispositions may be related to differences in ESRD mortality rates.

REFERENCES

Allport, G. (1964), Mental health: A generic attitude. *J. Religion & Health*, 4:7–21.

Angell, M. (1985), Disease as a reflection of the psyche. *New Eng. J. Med.*, 312: 1570–1573.

Basow, S., (1986), *Gender Stereotypes*. Monterey, CA: Brooks Cole.

Beard, B., & Sampson, T. (1981), Denial and objectivity in hemodialysis patients: Adjustments by opposite mechanisms. In: *Psychonephrology: Psychological Factors in Hemodialysis and Transplantation*, ed. N. Levy. New York: Plenum Press, pp. 300–330.

Binik, Y. (1983), Coping with chronic life threatening illness: Psychosocial perspectives on end stage renal disease. *Can. J. Behav. Sci.*, 15:373–391.

Cummings, J. (1970), Hemodialysis: Facts, feelings, and fantasies. *Amer. J. Nurs.*, 1: 70–75.

Degood, D. (1983), Reducing patient reluctance to participate in therapy. *Profess. Psychol.*, 14: 570.

Devins, G. (1981), Helplessness and depression in end stage renal disease. *J. Abnorm. Psychol.*, 90:531–537.

Drees, A., & Gallagher, E. (1981), Hemodialysis, rehabilitation, and psychological report. In: *Psychonephrology: Psychological Factors in Hemodialysis and Transplantation*, ed. N. Levy. New York: Plenum Press, pp. 210–220.

Evans, R., Garrison, L., & Manninen, D. (1982), The national kidney dialysis and transplantation study II: Study description, statement of objectives and project significance. *Contemp. Dial.*, 9:38–51.

Friedman, E. (1978), *Strategy in Renal Failure*. New York; John Wiley.

——— Rosenman, R.H. (1974), *Type A Behavior and Your Heart*. New York: Alfred A. Knopf.

Gibbs, M. (1981), Social class, mental disorder, and implications for community psychology. In: *Community Psychology*, eds. M. Gibbs, J. Lachenmeyer, & J. Sigal. New York: Gardner Press.

Greenglass, E. (1982), *A World of Difference*. New York: Wiley Press.

Guest, C. (1986), *Investigation of Caregiver Burden in Family Members of Alzheimer's Patients*. Unpublished master's dissertation, University of Windsor, Windsor, Ontario.

Holmes, T., & Rahe, R. (1967), The social readjustment rating scale. *J. Psychosoma. Rese.*, 11:213–218.

Inglehart, S. (1982), Health policy report: funding the end-stage renal disease program. *New Eng. J. Med.*, 306:406–410.

Johnston, M. (1986), *Life Stress Theory and Role Stereotypes As Predictors of Psychological Adjustment*. Unpublished doctoral dissertation. University of Windsor, Windsor, Ontario.

Kaplan De-Nour, A. (1981), Prediction of adjustment to chronic hemodialysis. In: *Psychonephrology: Psychological Factors in Hemodialysis and Transplantation*, ed. N. Levy. New York: Plenum Press, pp. 35–51.

Kobler, J. (1978), Can blood pressure be self-controlled? *Esquire*, July 18:91–94.

Kosberg, J., & Cairl, R. (1986), The cost of care index: A case management tool for screening informal care providers. *Gerontologist*, 26:273–278.

Lazarus, R. S. (1984), Puzzles in the study of daily hassles. *J. Behav. Med.*, 7:375–379.

Lowry, M., & Atcherson, E. (1980), A short-term follow-up of patients with depressive disorder on entry into home dialysis. *J. Affect. Disord.*, 3:341–345.

Millon, T., Green, C., & Meagher, R. (1979), The MBHI: A new inventory for the psychodiagnostician in medical settings. *Profess. Psychol.*, 10:529–540.

Mock, L. (1976), Psychosocial aspects of home and in-center dialysis. *Diss. Abstr. Internat.*, 36:5810.

Perras, S., & Zappacosta, A. (1980), Identifying candidates for continuous ambulatory peritoneal dialysis. *Dial. & Transplant.*, 12:108–109.

Rabinowitz, S., & Van Der Spuy, H. (1978), Selection criteria for dialysis and renal transplant. *Amer. J. Psychiat.*, 135:861–870.

Richter, C. (1957), On the phenomenon of sudden death in animals and men. *Psychosom. Med.*, 19:191–198.

Rosenhan, D., & Seligman, M. (1984). *Abnormal Psychology*. New York: W. W. Norton.

Rosenthal, R. (1969), Unintended effects of the clinician in clinical interaction: A taxonomy and review of clinician expectancy effects. *Austral. J. Psychol.*, 21:1–20.

———Jacobson, L. (1968), *Pygmalion in The Classroom*. New York: Holt, Rinehart, & Winston.

———Rubin, D. (1978), Interpersonal expectancy effects: The first 345 studies. *Behav. & Brain Sci.*, 3:377–387.

Rotter, J. (1954), *Social Learning and Clinical Psychology*. Englewood Cliffs, NJ: Prentice-Hall

Ryckman, R. (1985), *Theories of Personality*. Monterey, CA: Brooks Cole.

Schmidt, A. (1981), *Application of the Social Ecological Approach to Compliance with Hemodialysis Treatment*. Unpublished doctoral dissertation, University of Windsor, Windsor, Ontario.

Seligman, M. (1975), *Helplessness: On Depression, Development, and Death*. San Francisco: W. H. Freeman.

Selye, H. (1956), *The Stress of Life*. New York:McGraw-Hill.

Shapiro, A. (1960), A contribution to the history of the placebo effect. *Behav. Sci.*, 5: 109–135.

———(1964), Factors contributing to the placebo effect. *Amer. J. Psychother.*, 18:73–88.

Simmons, R. (1977), *The Gift of Life: The Social and Psychological Impact of Organ Transplantation*. New York: John Wiley.

Simonton, C., Mathews-Simonton, S., & Creighton, J. (1981), *Getting Well Again*. New York: Bantam Books.

Strickland, B. (1979), Internal external expectancies and health-related behaviors. *J. Consult. & Clin. Psychol.*, 46:1192–1211.

———Janoff-Bulman, R. (1981), Expectancies and attributions: implications for community mental health. In: *Community Psychology*, eds. M. Gibbs, J. Lachenmeyer, & J. Sigal. New York: Gardner Press.

Sue, S., & Zane, N. (1981), Learned helplessness theory and community psychology. In: *Community Psychology*, eds. M. Gibbs, J. Lachenmeyer, & J. Sigal. New York: Gardner Press.

———Sue, D., & Sue, S. (1986), *Understanding Abnormal Behavior*. Boston: Houghton Mifflin.

Weisberg, M. (1984), *Personality, Marital, and Family Characteristics of Patients Receiving Dialysis In-Center or at Home*. Unpublished doctoral dissertation, University of Windsor, Windsor, Ontario.

———Page, S. (1988), The Millon Behavioral Health Inventory and perceived efficacy of home and hospital dialysis. *J. Soc. Clin. Psychol.*, 6:408–422.

Zarit, S., Todd, P., & Zarit, J. (1986), Subjective burden of husbands and wives as caregivers: a longitudinal study. *Gerontol.*, 26:260–266.

Ziarnik, J., Freeman, C., Sherrard, D., & Calsyn, D. (1977), Psychological correlates of survival on renal dialysis. *J. Nerv. & Ment. Dis.*, 164:210–220.

10

Chronic Pain: A Multiaxial Approach to Psychosocial Assessment and Intervention

DAN BLAZER, M.D.

With the advent of new and improved psychiatric treatment of chronic pain, and new treatment facilities, such as pain clinics and pain rehabilitation wards, increased interest has been directed toward those psychosocial factors that contribute to chronic pain. Although acute symptomatic pain is important as a warning of disease or injury and for guiding the physician to the underlying illness, chronic pain has no biologic value. (Bonica, 1977). Yet chronic pain is one of the most difficult problems for the modern physician. This report presents a conceptual framework for the psychosocial assessment and treatment of chronic pain.

Management of chronic pain has been an enigma for many years because of the multiple factors contributing to the presentation of the pain. Chronic pain has, on different occasions, been linked to personality problems (Engel, 1959), "pay offs" in the home and job situation (Sternbach, 1968), communication problems (Sternbach, 1968), abuse of medication or other forms of treatment such as surgery, and underlying neurotic conflict. A number of authors have therefore suggested a

Reprinted by permission of the author, and the publisher of the *Southern Medical Journal*, 1981, 74(2):203–207, 214.

multidimensional approach to the assessment of chronic pain
(Melzack, 1973; Chapman 1977). The literature contains reports of successful treatment by nerve blocks, transcutaneous
stimulation, analgesics, psychoactive drugs, behavior modification, biofeedback, and psychotherapy (Engel, 1959; Bonica,
1977; Orne 1977).

Considerable attention has been directed toward operational assessment of chronic pain, which is an attempt to
reliably describe aspects of the pain. Although its etiology is
frequently unknown, the nomenclature of chronic pain (*psychogenic pain, supratentorial pain,* etc.) suggests a knowledge of
cause. Yet these terms are not used uniformly. Pain therapy and
research can be assisted by a consistent, reliable nomenclature
that describes the pain accurately without implying an etiology.
This approach to diagnosis has been manifested in the new
psychiatric nomenclature, DSM-III (1980). Melzack (1975) has
developed an excellent descriptive questionnaire for the assessment of acute or chronic pain, paralleling developments in the
assessment of depression (Zung, 1965), anxiety (Zung, 1971),
self-care capacity (Duke University Center for the Study of
Aging, 1978), and personality (Cattell, Eber, Tatzsuokas, 1970).
The purpose of this report is to present a conceptual framework for assessing chronic pain which incorporates the principles of operational assessment into a comprehensive assessment
procedure, and to present techniques of psychosocial management of chronic pain. The conceptual framework can be used
to select and evaluate the various forms of treatment. This
approach has been used in the Pain Clinic of Duke University
Medical Center.

ETIOLOGY AND DEVELOPMENT OF CHRONIC PAIN

In contrast to acute pain, such as pain secondary to a
myocardial infarction, rupture of an intervertebral disc, or
trauma, chronic pain can rarely be described in neurophysiologic terms alone. Even if the pain follows the expected
dermatome map or a recognizable pattern of visceral pain,
other factors have become important (Table 10.1). Individual

factors include the pain syndrome proper, physical disability, and psychologic dysfunction associated with the pain syndrome, defined as that constellation of symptoms that describe the intensity, quality, duration, and location of the pain. Rather than visualize a series of unique chronic pain syndromes along a single axis, such as causalgia, atypical facial pain, or low back pain, the clinician should conceptualize every presentation of chronic pain along three dimensions simultaneously, each being orthogonal or perpendicular to one another. Therefore the "diagnosis" for a given individual's chronic pain falls somewhere within this three-dimensional space. The common fallacy of excluding one factor if another is present is avoided; for example, "psychogenic" pain has no physical component. Rarely are one or two of these factors in chronic pain seen without all three being present simultaneously.

TABLE 10.1

PSYCHOSOCIAL ASSESSMENT OF CHRONIC PAIN SYNDROMES

I. Prepain Factors
   A. History of previous painful or serious illness
   B. Experience with significant others who have had a serious or painful illness
   C. Psychiatric history
   D. Childhood illness behavior
   E. Childhood emotional trauma
II. Pain Syndrome
   A. History of present pain
      1. Duration
      2. Suggested cause
      3. Interval between cause and onset
   B. Description of present pain
      1. Location
      2. Verbal description
      3. Change with time and situation
      4. Severity
      5. Pain tolerance
III. Physical Disability
   A. Work history
      1. Employment before onset of pain
      2. Change, if any, since onset of pain
   B. Activities of daily living
      1. Use of leisure time before and after onset of the pain syndrome
      2. Instrumental self-care capacity
      3. Physical self-care capacity
IV. Psychologic Dysfunction
   A. Affect

       1. Anger
       2. Depression
       3. Anxiety
       4. Suicidal ideation
    B. Personality factors
       1. Dependent—self-sufficient
       2. Trusting—suspicious
       3. Assertive—accommodating
       4. Intelligent and insightful—less intelligent, concrete in thinking
       5. Spontaneous—controlled
       6. Emotionally labile—emotionally stable
       7. Forthright—shrewd, manipulative
    C. Perception of the meaning of the pain
V. Person-Environment Interaction
    A. Social environment
       1. Social and economic resources
          a. Social interactions
          b. Income
          c. Presence or absence of continuing support in the social environment
       2. Social interaction
          a. Reaction and attitude of others to the pain syndrome
          b. Reaction of health care personnel to requests for pain alleviation
    B. Personal reaction to the social environment
       1. Reaction to stimuli and feedback from the social environment
       2. Pain behavior
       3. Expression and direction of anger
VI. Development
    A. Evaluation of the change in II–V from onset of pain to first evaluation session
    B. Evaluation of the change in II–V from the onset of therapy to predetermined
       point of follow-up, e.g., e months or 6 months

Other factors are involved in the pain syndrome as well. These include factors that existed before the onset of the pain, such as previous health, affect, and person–environment interactions. For example, childhood trauma or abuse may contribute significantly to the development and progression of chronic pain later in life. Interactional factors include those transactions by the person with the social environment at the onset of the chronic pain syndrome. This transaction involves the behavior of the individual toward the environment plus the stimuli and feedback received from the environment.

Initial interactional factors are most important in assessment. Frequently the first interaction between the patient with chronic pain and his physician and the perceived concern by the physician for the patient determines, to a great extent, future patient–physician interactions. The key to the understanding of chronic pain, however, is development. Chronic pain is a dynamic phenomenon, and change in any factor must be accommodated by change in other factors. For example, increased intensity of low back pain may lead to decreased activity, increased withdrawal, and subsequent depressive symptoms.

During the first appointment with the patient, the treatment team must evaluate individual and interactional factors occurring at the time of evaluation as well as the developmental history of these factors. Important elements to be included in the psychosocial assessment of chronic pain are also listed in Table 10.1. Many of these elements are included in already existing questionnaires. For example, the pain syndrome can be assessed by the Melzack Pain Questionnaire (Melzack, 1975). Activities of daily living, especially instrumental and physical self-care capacity can be assessed with the OARS Multidimensional Functional Assessment Questionnaire (Duke University Center for the Study of Aging and Human Development, 1978). Affect can be assessed by using scales already available, such as the Zung Self-Rating Depression and Anxiety scales (SDS) (Zung, 1965; 1971). Given the nature of chronic pain, the activity and affect scales may be of more value (because of their linear construction) than the usual diagnostic procedures. Change in affect can be monitored by repeated use of such instruments. Personality factors can be measured by a number of scales, including the Minnesota Multiphasic Personality Inventory and the Cattell 16-PF (Cattell et al., 1970). We have found the Cattell 16-PF to contain a series of seven scales (Table 10.1, under IV.B) that appear to be particularly helpful in assessing patients with chronic pain. Social and economic resources can be measured by the Social Resources section of the OARS Multidimensional Functional Assessment Questionnaire (1978).

The assessment of chronic pain is a long, involved task. The procedure can be made easier for the patient by using a variety of techniques and extending the evaluation over one or two days, either on an outpatient or inpatient basis. Much of the information can be obtained by having the patients fill out self-rating questionnaires in the waiting room. Questionnaires can also be sent to the patient before the first evaluation, filled out at leisure, and returned by mail or at the first visit. Information obtained by these questionnaires can then be placed in an information retrieval system, such as a computer data bank, and profiles of patients can be generated for the clinician. This follows the development of information systems in assessing other chronic illnesses, such as cardiovascular disease (Rosati, McNeer, and Starmer, 1975) and the chronic illnesses of later life (Blazer, 1979).

TREATMENT OF CHRONIC PAIN SYNDROMES

If the assessment of chronic pain is to be of value, it must facilitate the selection of proper therapy and its evaluation. As shown in Table 10.2, treatment of chronic pain can be directed toward a variety of factors (e.g., the pain syndrome proper may be alleviated through a nerve block, physical disability can be improved through physical therapy, or psychologic dysfunction may be alleviated by psychotherapy). The respective goals of these therapeutic methods are pain alleviation, physical rehabilitation, and psychologic adaptation, following the multiaxial approach. Social stimuli may be changed through methods such as family therapy, and behavior therapy leads to modification in behavior. Just as time is a significant factor in the development of chronic pain, its treatment also evolves over time. The experience of many clinicians suggests that treatment and rehabilitation must take place over a number of months or even years. Therapy may be instituted at different points during the progress of treatment, and a logical approach to the timing of treatment as well as the treatment per se should follow from the assessment data and a knowledge of the nature of the treatment. For example, psychotherapy may be an important therapeutic adjunct but would not be appropriate until the patient–physician relationship has been firmly established and more conventional physical therapies have been instituted.

TABLE 10.2
PSYCHOPHARMACOLOGIC TREATMENT OF CHRONIC PAIN SYNDROME

Drug Class	Axis of Intervention	Comments
1. Analgesics:		
a. Narcotic analgesics. Examples: morphine, meperidine (Demerol), oxycodone (Percodan), codeine, pentazocine (Talwin)	Pain alleviation	Chronic use indicated only secondary to cancer (Holden, 1976) Frequently prescribed in inadequate dosage for acute pain Side effects include hallucinations (Blazer and Haller, 1975) Must assess the "cost-benefit" of withdrawal Withdraw in the hospital with the patient's compliance (Fordyce, 1976) Avoid PRN doses in chronic pain patients (Fordyce, 1976)
b Nonnarcotic analgesics. Examples: aspirin, acetaminophen	Pain alleviation	Usually of little or no benefit in moderate to severe chronic pain syndromes. Side effects can be dangerous if used chronically (e.g., gastric bleeding) Aspirin remains the most effective
c. Endogenous opioid compounds. Example:B-endorphin	Pain alleviation? Psychologic adaptation?	Experimental use only at present (Snyder, 1975)
2. Tricyclic Antidepressants: Examples: amitriptyline (Elavil, Endep), doxepin (Sinequan, Adapin), nortriptyline (Aventyl, Pamelor)	Psychologic adaptation Pain alleviation?	Indicated for depressive symptoms accompanying chronic pain syndromes (Wilson et al., 1976) Increases monoaminergically mediated pain-inhibiting structures in the CNS (Sternbach et al., 1976) Significant side effects and withdrawal effects
3. Antipsychotic Agents: Examples: fluphenazine (Prolixin), perphenazine (Trilafon), chlorpromazine (Thorazine), chlorprothixene (Taractan), thioridazine (Mellaril), haloperidol (Haldol)	Psychologic adaptation Pain alleviation?	May block arousal of the RAS (Adler, 1978) May potentiate narcotic analgesia in cancer pain (Adler, 1978) Alleviates somatic delusions of pain Haloperidol particularly indicated in cancer pain

4. Combinations of Antipsychotic Agents and Tricyclic Antidepressants	Pain alleviation?	Effective specifically in treatment of postherpetic neuralgia (Taub and College, 1974) May aid the withdrawal of narcotic analgesics Neurophysiologic mechanisms unknown
5. Antianxiety Agents: Examples: diazepam (Valium), lorazepam (Ativan), chlordiazepoxide (Librium)	Psychologic adaptation	Effective in relieving anxiety associated with pain syndromes Potentially addicting
6. Sedative-Hypnotic Agents	Psychologic adaptation?	There are no specific indicators for these agents in the management of chronic pain Frequent side effects Potentially addicting

The psychopharmacologic treatment of chronic pain syndromes is outlined in Table 10.2 (Taub and College 1974; Blazer and Haller, 1975; Snyder, 1975; Fordyce, 1976; Wilson, Blazer, and Nashold, 1976; Sternbach, Janowski, and Huey, 1976; Long, 1976; Holden, 1976; Adler, 1978). Notice that the axis of intervention remains unclear for a number of these agents, though their role in pain therapy is well established. Future psychopharmacologic studies will eliminate many of the question marks and enable clinicians to better determine which psychopharmacologic agents are of value. Nevertheless, the present-day physician should carefully identify the target symptoms for a given agent. If a means for objectively assessing the benefit of the medication is available (e.g., the use of the Zung SDS for assessing depressive symptoms), such techniques should be instituted. The clinician must remember, however, that the peripheral assessment of the sensation of pain in a depressed patient is not a valid means of evaluating the effectiveness of medication. Specifically, pain thresholds may be increased in depressed patients while the subjective experience of suffering is also increased (Davis, Buschbaum, and Bunney, 1979).

Different types of behavior and milieu therapy are outlined in Table 10.3 (Rolpe, 1969; Budzynski, Stoyva, & Adler, 1978; Newman, Painter, and Seres, 1978). The most important advances in the psychosocial management of chronic pain during the past fifteen years have been in the development of effective behavioral and milieu therapeutic techniques. These are directed toward pain alleviation less often than the psychopharmacologic agents, but are successful because of the breadth of the axis of intervention. They are useful adjuncts to more specific methods for pain relief, such as nerve blocks, and therefore must be coordinated with these specific techniques and with each other.

TABLE 10.3

BEHAVIOR AND MILIEU THERAPY

Therapy	Axis of Intervention	Comments
1. Biofeedback	Pain alleviation Psychologic adaptation	Most effective in pain syndromes secondary to muscle tension Especially effective with headache (Budzynski et al., 1978). Useful adjunct to other therapeutic modalities
2. Pain Rehabilitation Ward (milieu therapy)	Physical rehabilitation Stimulus modification Behavior modification	Behavioral techniques coupled with a realistic approach to the pain syndrome (Newman et al., 1978) Must include work with the family to insure lasting results Withdrawal from narcotic analgesics best accomplished in this treatment setting
3. Assertiveness Training	Psychologic adaptation Behavior modification	An important adjunct to other therapeutic modalities Diffuses "stored-up" hostility (Rolpe, 1969)
4. Family Therapy	Stimulus modification Behavior modification Psychologic adaptation	Establishes patient–family interactions that reward "healthy" rather than "pain" behavior

Psychotherapy has been prescribed for many years for the treatment of chronic pain. Psychiatrists who have treated chronic pain can attest to the benefit of psychotherapy in given

TABLE 10.4

PSYCHOTHERAPY FOR CHRONIC PAIN SYNDROMES

Medication

Pain associated with obvious intrapersonal conflict and/or psychosocial stress

Axis of Intervention

Psychosocial adaptation, pain alleviation (?), behavior modification

Factors Suggesting a Positive Response to Psychotherapy

Pain-free intervals

Significant affective component to the pain syndrome

Maintenance of usual activities of daily living

Intelligence and insight

Motivation

Guidelines

Supportive and empathic with few attempts at interpretation initially

Limited to once a week or less but continued over a number of months

Attention paid to issues other than description of pain

TABLE 10.5

OTHER TREATMENT METHODS

Therapy	Axis of Intervention	Comments
1. Self-hypnosis and Relaxation Techniques	Pain alleviation Psychologic adaptation	Select suitable patients with "hypnotic talent" Teach muscle relaxation techniques Hypnotic suggestion of progressively increased pain-free intervals Move to self-hypnosis techniques after adequate training (Orne, 1977; Spiegel, 1979)
2. Physical Therapy	Physical rehabilitation Psychologic adaptation Pain alleviation?	Include ROM exercises, gait training, etc. A useful adjunct to other therapies
3. Recreational Therapy	Physical rehabilitation Psychologic adaptation	A useful adjunct to other therapies Insures patient that the treatment team is "person" oriented rather than "pain" oriented

situations. Yet the nonpsychiatric physician frequently has difficulty in determining under what circumstances psychotherapy is valuable. Table 10.4 presents the indications for psychotherapy in chronic pain and factors that might predict a positive response. Other treatment modalities for chronic pain are listed in Table 10.5 (Orne, 1977; Newman et al., 1978; Spiegel, 1979). Although these lists do not exhaust the possibilities, they show the variety of approaches available to the clinician. The selection of a "treatment package" is the most important task in prescribing psychosocial therapy for chronic pain. If treatment is logically coupled with assessment, the selection of this treatment package will not be a haphazard endeavor.

REFERENCES

Adler, R.H. (1978), Psychotropic agents in the management of chronic pain. *J. Hum. Stress*, 4:13–17.

American Psychiatric Association, (1980), *The Diagnostic and Statistical Manual of Mental Disorders*, 3rd ed. Washington, DC: American Psychiatric Press.

Blazer, D. (1979), The living textbook of geriatric care: An overview. Paper presented at the 34th Annual Scientific Meeting of the Gerontological Society, Washington, DC, November 27.

———Haller, L. (1975), Pentazocine psychosis: A case of persistent delusions. *Dis. Nerv. Syst.*, 36:404–405.

Bonica, J.J. (1977a), Introduction to symposium on pain. *Arch. Surg.*, 112:749–754.

———(1977b), Symposium on pain: Part I. *Arch. Surg.*, 112:749–787.

Budzynski, T.H., Stoyva, J.M., & Adler, C.S., (1978), EMG, biofeedback and tension headache: A controlled outcome study. *Psychosomat. Med.*, 36:484–496.

Cattell, R.B., Eber, H.J., & Tatzsuokas, M. (1970), *The Sixteen Personality Factor Questionnaire*, 3rd ed. Champaign, IL, Institute for Personality and Ability Testing.

Chapman, C.R. (1977), The psychological aspects of pain patient treatment. *Arch. Surg.*, 112:767–772.

Davis, G.C., Buschbaum, M.S., & Bunney, W.E. (1979), Analgesia to painful stimuli in affective illness. *Amer. J. Psychiat.*, 136:1148–1151.

Duke University Center for the Study of Aging and Human Development (1978), *Multidimensional Functional Assessment: The OARS Methodology*. Durham, NC: Duke University Center for the Study of Aging and Human Development.

Engel, G.L. (1959), "Psychogenic" pain and the pain prone patient. *Amer. J. Med.*, 26:899–918.

Fordyce, W.E. (1976), *Behavioral Medicine for Chronic Pain and Illness*. St. Louis: C.V. Mosby.

Holden, C. (1976), Hospices: For the dying, relief from pain and fear. *Sci.* 193:389–391.

Long, D.M. (1976), Use and misuse of drug therapy in chronic pain. In: *Proceedings of the First World Congress on Pain*, eds.J.J. Bonica & D. Albe-Fessard. New York: Raven Press, pp. 226–227.

Melzack, R. (1973), *The Puzzle of Pain*. New York: Basic Books.

——(1975), The McGill Pain Questionnaire: Major properties and scoring methods. *Pain*, 1:277–299.

Newman, R.I., Painter, J.R., & Seres, J.L. (1978), A therapeutic milieu for chronic pain patients. *J. Hum. Stress*, 4:8–12.

Orne, M.T. (1977), New studies challenge old concepts of hypnosis and relief of pain. *Front. Psychiat.* 7:5–7.

Rolpe, J. (1969) *The Practice of Behavior Therapy*. New York: Pergamon Press, pp. 61–68.

Rosati, R.A., McNeer, J.F., & Starmer, F. (1975), A new information system for medical practice. *Arch. Intern. Med.*, 135:1017–1024.

Snyder, S.H. (1975), Opiate receptor in normal and drug altered brain function. *Nature*, 257:185–189.

Spiegel, D. (1979), Hypnosis. In: *Psychiatry for the Primary Care Physician*. eds. A.M. Freeman, R.L. Sack, & T.A. Berger. Baltimore, Williams & Wilkins.

Sternbach, R.A. (1968), *Pain: A Psychophysiological Analysis*. New York: Academic Press.

——Janowski, D.S., & Huey, L.Y. (1976), Effects of altering brain serotonin activity on human chronic pain. In: *Proceedings of the First World Congress on Pain*. eds. J.J. Bonica, & D. Albe-Fessard. New York: Raven Press, p. 249.

Taub, A., & College, W.F. (1974), Observation on the treatment of denervation, dysesthesia with tri-psychotropic drugs: post-herpetic neuralgia, anesthesia, dolorosa, peripheral neuropathy. In: *Advances in Neurology*, Vol. 4, ed. J.J. Bonica. New York: Raven Press, pp. 309–315.

Wilson, W.P., Blazer, D.G., & Nashold, B.S. (1976), Observation on pain and suffering. *Psychosomat.*, 17:73–76.

Zung, W.W.K. (1965), A self-rating depression scale. *Arch. Gen. Psychiat.*, 12:63–70.

——(1971), A rating instrument for anxiety disorders. *Psychosomatics*, 12:371–379.

11

Behavioral Assessment and Treatment of Recurrent Headache

CRAIG D. WAGGONER, PH.D. AND
FRANK ANDRASIK, PH.D.

Headaches are among the most commonly presented symptoms in outpatient medical clinics (Delozier and Gagnon, 1975; Leviton, 1978). Although they are not life-threatening disorders, their prevalence, along with the assumption that certain types have strong psychological factors influencing them, have resulted in much attention from behavioral scientists. Approximately 42 million of the U.S. population suffer from headaches, almost 12 million of which are considered some form of migraine (Adams, Feuerstein, and Fowler, 1980). European surveys have provided estimates that 14 percent to 70 percent of individuals in their samples suffered from some form of headache (Waters and O'Connor, 1975; Leviton, 1978; Ziegler, 1978). These large-scale surveys indicate that muscle-contraction, migraine, and combined headaches are the most common types and, according to the Ad Hoc Committee on Classification of Headache (1962), are not the result of permanent structural abnormalities.

The most common type of headache is the muscle-contraction or "tension" headache, thought to account for approximately 80 percent of all headaches (Ostfeld, 1962;

Waters and O'Connor, 1971). The Ad Hoc Committee (1962) defined this type of headache as:

> Ache or sensations of tightness, pressure, or constriction, widely varied in frequency, intensity, and duration, sometimes long-lasting, and commonly suboccipital. It is associated with sustained contraction of skeletal muscles in the absence of permanent structural change, usually as part of the individual's reaction during life stress [p. 717].

These headaches are usually bilateral (but can be unilateral), with the pain generally located in the occipital regions but also radiating to the frontal, parietal, and temporal regions (Friedman, 1979; Diamond and Dalessio, 1986).

> The Ad Hoc Committee defines migraine headaches as: Recurrent attacks of headache, widely varied in frequency, intensity, and duration. The attacks are commonly unilateral in onset; are usually associated with anorexia and, sometimes, with nausea and vomiting; in some, are preceded by, or associated with, conspicuous sensory, motor, and mood disturbances; and are often familial [p. 718].

A migraine attack is usually characterized by a pulsating pain that has a sudden unilateral onset (but may also be bilateral), is often accompanied by increased sensitivity to light, sound, and some odors, and sometimes accompanied by diarrhea or constipation (Diamond and Dalessio, 1986). The head pain, which is usually located in the temporal, orbital, supraorbital, or occipital regions, typically lasts from six to eight hours but can last up to several days (Adams, Feuerstein, and Fowler, 1980; Diamond and Dalessio, 1986). The Ad Hoc Committee (1962) also made a distinction between "classic" and "common" migraine, the former being preceded by a prodromal phase, ten to thirty minutes prior to the onset of head pain, during which visual disturbances, auditory disturbances, and paresthesias are reported. Common migraine headaches are less often unilateral than classic migraine headaches, and comprise approximately 85 percent to 90 percent of all migraine cases (Friedman, 1978; Kudrow, 1978).

The descriptions of tension and migraine headaches, presented above, represent the typical clinical pictures. In reality, there is considerable overlap of symptoms between them (Appenzeller, Feldman, and Friedman, 1979; Ziegler, 1979). Acknowledging the fact that many individuals experience headaches presenting with both muscle-contraction and migraine symptoms, the Ad Hoc Committee (1962) established the category of "combined headache" (also called "mixed") defined as: "Combinations of vascular headache of the migraine type and muscle-contraction headache prominently coexisting in an attack" (p. 718).

The considerable overlap of symptoms among headache types has led some to view headache disorders as lying on the same etiological continuum with purely muscle-contraction and purely migraine symptoms positioned at opposite ends (Philips, 1978; Bakal and Kaganov, 1979; Drummond and Lance, 1984). Taking this continuum view one step further, Bakal (1982) has proposed that there is only one disorder of "chronic headache" rather than distinct categories. While the continuum hypothesis has received support, the major purpose of delineating subgroups of headache sufferers, as for any physical disorder, is to develop treatments that may be more effective for one type of disorder than another. The available literature addressing the psychological or "nonpharmacological" treatment of headache disorders indicates that several approaches work equally well with tension, migraine, and mixed headache disorders, but some approaches are differentially effective. Thus, there is clinical utility in differentiating among headache types to guide treatment (Blanchard and Andrasik, 1982). Before turning to the psychological assessment and treatment of headache disorders, a brief review of the biological and psychological accounts of headache will be helpful. The clinician must be familiar with these factors in order to accurately assess the causes of a particular patient's headaches and to design an effective treatment approach.

BIOLOGICAL ACCOUNTS OF MIGRAINE AND TENSION HEADACHES

Migraine Headaches

Biological investigations of migraine headaches have explored vasomotor functioning, biochemical factors, hormonal factors, electroencephalographic (EEG) abnormalities, and genetic contributions.

Vasomotor Functioning. Alterations in cerebral blood flow have been well documented during migraine attacks (Tunis and Wolff, 1952; Skinhoj, 1973; Sakai and Meyer, 1978). Research reported by Wolff (1963) and later, Dalessio (1987), delineated a distinct progression of vasomotor changes just before, during, and following a migraine headache. Their research showed that just prior to the painful attack there is vasoconstriction of the cranial arterial beds, followed by vasodilation and the subjective experience of pain during the attack, and the eventual return to normal vasomotor tone of the cranial vasculature as the headache subsides. Such observations have led to the postulation of the presence of an overreactive vasoconstrictor mechanism (Appenzeller, 1969) or a more general problem with autonomic stability (Tunis and Wolff, 1953) that could produce the abnormal vasomotor activity.

Biochemical Factors. Various vasoactive humoral agents have been implicated in the pathogenesis of migraines based on observed excesses or deficiencies of them during and following attacks. Histamine (Horton, 1956), acetylcholine (Kunkle, 1959), and serotonin (Sicuteri, 1959; Anthony, Hinterberger, and Lance, 1967) have received the most attention in studies. For example, Anthony and associates (1967) estimated that serotonin levels fall to 60 percent of preheadache levels during the attack itself. In addition, they found injections of serotonin improved headaches (Sacks [1970], Appenzeller, [1976]; and Botney [1981], for extensive reviews). Adenosine triphosphate (Burnstock, 1981), substance P (Moskowitz, Reinhard, Romero, Melamed, and Pettibone, 1979), one of the most powerful vasodilating substances known, and the plasma kinins (Dalessio, 1978) have more recently been implicated in migraines.

Appenzeller (1969) has suggested that excessive amounts of certain humoral vasoconstrictors produce the initial excessive cranial vasoconstriction and subsequent prodromata as a result of ischemia. When the concentration of these humoral agents changes again, the vasoconstriction gives way to vasodilation of the cranial arteries. According to this theory, the rapid change in the diameter of the cranial vessels causes the pain associated with migraine headaches (Appenzeller, 1969). An alternate theory has been proposed by Diamond and Dalessio (1986): Their "Unified Theory of Migraine" holds that various stimuli and environmental stressors produce the initial constriction of the extracranial blood vessels. These vessels are innervated by adrenergic fibers that are respondent to catecholamines. This vasoconstriction is thought to produce the prodromata in classic migraines as a result of anoxia and acidosis and, through hemodynamic effects, to lead to vasodilation of the intracranial blood vessels. If the intracranial vessels react to the metabolic needs of the brain and constrict, a rebound dilation of the extracranial vasculature ensues, causing the release of vasoactive substances, which, in turn, produces a sterile inflammation, edema, and the throbbing pain characteristic of migraine headache.

Botney (1981) hypothesizes that cerebral hypoxia and ischemia result in an inhibition of serotonin synthesis that leads to an increased perception of pain. The theories described above differ mainly in the ordering of the events that are postulated to occur. Whether vasoactive substances produce the initial vasoconstriction, are released subsequent to vasodilation, or are inhibited by vasomotor changes remains a focus of study (Williamson, 1981).

Dietary Factors. The ingestion of alcohol, foods containing tyramine (e.g., some cheeses and chicken livers), sodium nitrite (found in cured meats), monosodium glutamate, and carbohydrates have been found to be associated with the occurrence of migraine headaches (Johnson, 1978; Diamond and Dalessio, 1986). Selby and Lance (1960) estimated that the ingestion of certain foods such as chocolates, fats, oranges, and those fried in oil, elicited headache attacks in 25 percent of 339 migraine sufferers. Controlled research on dietary factors is scant and conclusions stem mostly from clinical observations.

Hormonal Factors. Changes in the patterns of migraine attacks have been observed as a result of pregnancy, menstruation, and the use of oral contraceptives (Waters and O'Connor, 1971; Somerville, 1972; Kudrow, 1978). Reports have indicated that many women who suffer from migraines cease to have them while pregnant, with increased levels of estrogen during the menstrual cycle, and by the use of oral contraceptives containing estrogen (Lance and Anthony, 1966; Blau, 1971; Carroll, 1971; Kudrow, 1975; Saper, 1978). Menstrual migraines occur most commonly during the premenstrual period, when estrogen levels have reached their peak and are rapidly declining (Somerville, 1972).

EEG Abnormalities. Early studies reported that many migraine sufferers' EEGs demonstrated excessive fast-wave activity, excessive slow-wave activity, or asymmetrical slow-wave activity (Strauss and Selinsky, 1941; Engel, Ferris, and Romano, 1945; Selby and Lance, 1960). Excessive positive spikes, resembling epileptiform patterns have also been found in the EEGs of migraine headache sufferers (Whitehouse, Pappas, Escala, and Livingston, 1967). As others have pointed out, however, there is not much evidence to suggest that a specific relationship exists between vascular headaches and EEG abnormalities because such abnormalities have been found to exist equally often in tension headache sufferers (in at least one study) and they occur in several other behavioral disorders as well (Masland, 1978; Adams et al., 1980; Diamond and Dalessio, 1986).

Genetic Contributions. Some studies have found as many as 50 to 60 percent of migraine headache sufferers to have a family history for vascular headaches (Selby and Lance, 1960; Lance and Anthony, 1966; Drummond, 1983). Further, one study found that migraine onset was earlier if there was a "strong" family history for migraines and that a maternal history appeared to be more important than a paternal history (Steiner, Guha, Capildeo, and Rose, 1980). More systematic investigations, however, have found lower overall incidence rates. Lucas (1977) studied 1800 pairs of twins from the London Register and found 26 percent and 13 percent concordance rates for monozygotic and dizygotic twins, respectively. Waters (1971) directly interviewed relatives of migraineurs, rather than relying upon the recall of headache patients, in his investigation of migraine heritability. When he did this he found a prevalence rate of only 10 percent in the families of migraine patients. The strength of any genetic influence, thus, is still in question (Adams et al., 1980).

Tension Headaches

Research investigating the biological etiology of tension headaches is much less specific and less molecular than the research on migraine headaches. This research has advanced relatively little since the pioneering work of Wolff and his associates, which implicated sustained (voluntary or involuntary) muscle contractions of the scalp and neck musculature and, possibly, a vascular component, in the etiology of this type of head pain (Tunis and Wolff, 1954; Wolff, 1963). Unlike migraine headaches, dietary and genetic influences are not commonly believed to be as important in the development of tension headaches (Drummond, 1983; Diamond and Dalessio, 1986).

Sustained Muscle Contractions. The early conclusions drawn by Wolff (Tunis and Wolf, 1954; Wolff, 1963) were based on the observations that increases and decreases in pain were related to increases and decreases, respectively, in electromyographic (EMG) activity in reactions to various chemical and physical agents. Some studies, investigating the relationship between reports of head pain and head and neck EMG activity, have found higher EMG levels during headache states (Friedman, 1963; van Boxtel and van der Ven, 1978), while others have not found such a relationship (Pozniak-Patewicz, 1976; Philips, 1977; Martin and Mathews, 1978) nor significant correlations between pain reports and EMG activity (Bakal and Kaganov, 1977; Holroyd, Andrasik, and Westbrook, 1977; Hart and Chichanski, 1981). The results of these studies lead to the conclusion that muscle-contraction, alone, cannot account for this type of head pain (Andrasik, Blanchard, Arena, Saunders, and Barron [1982] for a more detailed review). The recent findings of Haber, Kuczmierczyk, and Adams (1985) suggest that some of the contradictory results of these studies may be due to researchers failing to distinguish between tension headache sufferers and psychogenic pain patients. Their findings suggest that the EMG activity of psychogenic pain patients does not correlate with pain, while that of tension headache sufferers does. Dalessio (1978) has offered that a local pathologic process could initiate the cephalic muscle spasm causing continuous stimulation of the gamma efferent neurons. According to Dalessio, the stimulation of these neurons causes the affected muscles to remain contracted and enhances muscle contractions by way of the spinal ventral horn. This theory, while plausible, is in need of supporting data.

Vasomotor Changes. Wolff's (1963) original conceptualization of the etiology of tension headaches also included observations that these headache sufferers displayed higher pulse-wave amplitudes during headache-free states (relative to nonheadache controls) and that vasoconstriction of various nutrient arteries occurred with increases in EMG activity (Tunis and Wolf, 1954). Others, however, have observed vasodilations of additional, unrelated, arteries during headache attacks, thus raising problems for Wolff's original theory (Williamson, 1981).

Biochemical Factors. A survey of the literature of the etiology of tension headaches reveals only sparse attention to biochemical factors. The early work of Ostfeld and associates (Ostfeld et al., 1957; Ostfeld, 1962) led them to postulate a role for norepinephrine. They suggested that local and circulating norepinephrine increases with feelings of tension and leads to vasoconstriction of the nutrient arteries of relevant head and neck muscles. Pain is increased as a result of ischemia when sustained muscle contraction occurs. Twenty years later,

Mathew, Weinman, and Largen (1982) also postulated that epinephrine is released in response to acute stress and that norepinephrine is released in response to sustained emotional tension as mechanisms of migraine headache. Interestingly, their suggestion pertained to the role of these neurotransmitters for the production of migraines. Should additional data arise supporting the role of these humoral agents in tension headaches, the hypothesis that these headaches lie on a "continuum" would also receive further support.

Mixed Migraine and Muscle-Contraction Headache

Perusal of the literature quickly reveals an absence of data on the etiology of mixed headaches. The only conclusions that can be drawn to date suggest that headaches with mixed symptoms are the result of a combination of factors believed to be involved in both migraine and tension headaches. As mentioned earlier, some authors have suggested that headache symptoms fall on a continuum, and that as initial tension headaches become more severe and long-standing, they take on an increasing number of vascular components (Bakal, 1975; Philips, 1978; Martin, 1983).

PSYCHOLOGICAL CONCEPTUALIZATIONS OF HEADACHES

Personality Traits as Causes of Headaches

Various psychological accounts of migraine and tension headaches have been offered. The oldest, based on psychodynamic theory postulates that individuals with certain personality traits and unconscious conflicts will, especially at times of inordinate stress, develop specific physical disorders (Alexander, 1950; Dunbar, 1954). For migraine sufferers, the unconscious conflicts have been hypothesized to be related to hostility, guilt, dependency needs, problematic identifications, and psychosexual adjustment difficulties (Fromm-Reichman, 1937; Friedman, Von Storch, and Merritt, 1954). Similarly, the unconscious conflicts leading to tension headaches have been hypothesized to be related to dependency needs, sexuality, and anger control (Friedman et al., 1954; Martin, 1966). The specific personality traits are thought to cause weakness in specific biological systems and result in the specific physical disorder. These conceptualizations give psychological factors a causal role in the production of headaches.

One cannot help but notice the striking similarity in the personality descriptions of migraine and tension headache sufferers. Philips (1976) has noted, "although two distinct types of common headache are recognized—migraine and tension—they are not predicted to differ in personality characteristics" (p. 535). In the search for specific personality traits causing different types of headaches, researchers have turned to objective personality measures and have compared headache groups to nonheadache populations and to each other.

In most instances, headache sufferers have been found to have mild elevations on the "neurotic" scales of objective personality tests such as the MMPI, Eysenck Personality Inventory, and Maudsley Personality Inventory (Howarth, 1965; Henryk-Gutt & Rees, 1973; Harrison, 1975; Kudrow and Sutkus, 1979; Andrasik, Blanchard, Arena, Teders, Teevan, and Rodichok, 1982). In addition, Anderson and Fanks (1981) found both migraine and tension headache sufferers to exceed normals in anxiety and sympathy seeking. They also provided evidence to support the notion that migraine sufferers were overly competitive and perfectionistic and that tension headache sufferers were excessively anxious and insecure. When compared to nonheadache control groups, most studies report that at least one headache group has scored significantly different (Kudrow and Sutkus, 1979; Anderson and Fanks, 1981; Andrasik, Blanchard, Arena, Teders, and Rodichok, 1982). Although headache groups typically score higher than normals on personality measures, these elevations rarely reach clinical significance (Sternbach, Dalessio, Kunzel, and Bowman, 1980; Andrasik, Blanchard, Arena, Teders, and Rodichok, 1982; Blanchard and Andrasik, 1982). In addition, the personality scores of headache sufferers have not been found to be significantly different from other medical populations (e.g.,

Blanchard and Andrasik, 1982; Watson, 1982). Further, the scores of migraine sufferers have been found to be essentially normal in some studies (Kudrow and Sutkus, 1979; Sternbach et al., 1980; Weeks, Baskin, Rapoport, Sheftell, and Arrowsmith, 1983). Similarly, Henryk-Gutt and Rees (1973) and Philips (1976) did not find the personality scores of their tension headache sufferers to differ from normals.

In general, the available evidence provided by researchers using objective personality measures agrees with the conclusions of Harrison (1975) that, more often than not, headache sufferers as a group evidence more psychopathology than normal samples, particularly on scales 1, 2, and 3 of the MMPI. They probably do not, however, significantly differ from other medical populations.

There is some evidence that migraine and tension headache sufferers present themselves differently on psychological measures. Different headache types have been found to score differently on scales 1, 2, 3, and 7 of the MMPI (Kudrow and Sutkus, 1979; Sternbach et al., 1980; Andrasik, Blanchard, Arena, Teders, and Rodichok, 1982; Weeks et al., 1983). In these studies, the mixed and tension headache groups tended to exhibit more psychopathology than the migraine groups. In contrast, however, at least two studies have found migraine groups to score significantly higher than tension headache groups on scales measuring anxiety, somatization, and neuroticism (Maxwell, 1966; Henryk-Gutt and Rees, 1973). Further, other studies have not found differences in scores between headache groups (Philips, 1976; Andrasik, Blanchard, Arena, Teders, and Rodichok, 1982). Blanchard and Andrasik (1982) have noted that statistical analyses may not reveal differences between headache groups due to great within-group variability and considerable overlap in the groups' distributions of scores. Heightened variability in the personality scores of headache groups has been reported by others (Bakal, 1975).

More recent studies, employing multivariate statistical procedures, have attempted to discriminate between headache groups on the basis of patterns of scores on various subscales of the MMPI and other measures (Multiple Affect Adjective Checklist, Beck Depression Inventory). The results of three such attempts generally concur that headache groups can be placed on a continuum according to the degree of psychopathology they evidenced. Migraine groups tend to be at the "normal" end, followed by the mixed groups and, at the most psychologically distressed end, the tension headache groups (Kudrow and Sutkus, 1979; Andrasik, Blanchard, Arena, Teders, and Rodichok, 1982; Pratt, Williamson, Cohen, Granberry, and Jarrel, 1982). In further support of a continuum of psychopathology, Drummond (1983) observed 600 cases of headaches of varying types and found that as headaches became more frequent, the number of social problems and amount of reported depression also increased. He noted that symptoms of muscular contraction were reported more often by the subjects with more frequently occurring headaches.

In summary, the results of studies comparing headache groups on psychological characteristics remain unclear. On the one hand, the majority of studies have found statistically significant differences between the scores on psychological measures produced by different headache groups—with the balanced tipped toward the tension headache sufferers—as evidencing the greatest psychological disturbance. On the other hand, the differences, when found, are probably not of clinical significance and may be mostly due to the frequency of headache symptoms rather than constitutional personality differences. Longitudinal studies tracing headache parameters and psychological disturbance could shed some light on the cause–effect issue. Sovak, Kunzel, Sternbach, and Dalessio (1981) addressed this issue with an innovative approach. These researchers gave MMPIs to two groups of migraineurs both before and after receiving either a standard drug regimen (propanalol and analgesics) or thermal biofeedback. Although individuals improved from each treatment, only the group receiving biofeedback showed significant improvement on their MMPI scores. Based on these findings, the authors suggested that the psychoneurotic characteristics of migraineurs may be etiological factors and not just a product of head pain. These results are certainly compelling but we cannot rule out the possibility that the psychological disturbance observed in these headache groups initially resulted from living with headaches. Biofeedback may simply be a more effective treatment for anxiety and depression than are propranolol and analgesics.

The Psychobiological Formulation of Headaches

In recent years, behavioral scientists have developed "working models" to aid the understanding of how psychological factors may be involved in headache disorders. In general, psychobiological theorists believe that constitutional physiological differences exist, which are activated when the individual is exposed to stress, to produce different headache syndromes (Bakal, 1975; Cinciripini, Williamson, and Epstein, 1980; Bakal, Demjen, and Kaganov, 1981; Epstein and Cinciripini, 1981; Blanchard and Andrasik, 1987). The likelihood of an individual experiencing a headache is dependent upon the specific pathophysiological mechanisms that are "triggered" by the interplay of an individual's physiological status (e.g., level of autonomic arousal), environmental factors (e.g., toxins, some foods, alcohol, light, odors, stressful circumstances, hormonal fluctuations, etc.), the individual's ability to cope with these factors, both cognitively and behaviorally, and consequential factors that may serve to reinforce, and thus increase, an individual's likelihood of reporting head pain. The main determinant for the type of headache experienced is the pathophysiological response system that is activated. Psychological factors do not play a causal role in the production of headaches. Rather, psychological factors are involved in three primary ways: (1) as triggering factors, many of which are considered to be under the direct control of the patient (i.e., the interpretation of, and reaction to, stress); (2) as maintaining factors, many of which are also considered to be under the direct control of the patient (i.e., stress-coping abilities and reinforcement for reports of headache symptoms); and (3) as symptoms as a result of continued head pain and subsequent life disruption (e.g., of depression). The psychodynamic and the psychobiological formulations of headaches, although at odds, do agree on two basic points, however: (1) that stressful situations are important precipitating factors in headaches, and (2) that stress can produce aberrant psychological and physiological reactions in headache sufferers.

The Role of Stress in Headache Disorders. Stress is frequently reported to be a major contributing factor in both tension (Friedman et al., 1954; Ad Hoc Committee, 1962; Friedman, 1979; Drummond, 1983) and migraine headaches (Friedman et al., 1954; Selby and Lance, 1960; Dalsgaard-Nielsen, 1965; Henryk-Gutt and Rees, 1973; Parnell and Cooperstock, 1979; Drummond, 1983). One early survey concluded that emotional factors were contributory in all of the 2,000 cases of chronic tension and migraine headaches studied (Friedman et al., 1954). Henryk-Gutt and Rees (1973) found that one-half of their migraine headache sufferers reported the initial onset of their headache problem to coincide with a period of emotional stress. Further, Feuerstein, Bush, and Corbisiero (1982) found that approximately 64 percent, 87 percent, and 100 percent of their migraine, tension, and mixed headache subjects, respectively, reported stress as a precipitating factor of headaches.

All of the above studies obtained their results from retrospective, nonstandardized and, often, unstructured interviews and none of them reported information on the amount of stress present in a comparison population. As a result, we cannot determine whether headache sufferers experienced greater amounts of stress than other groups. In addition, these studies did not attempt to determine the strength or nature of the relationship between stress and various headache disorders. More current methods in use for measuring the stress–headache relationship concern assessment of physiological and subjective reactions to stressors presented in the laboratory and quantification of the amount/number of stressful life events to which headache sufferers have been exposed.

There is no question that stressful stimuli, presented in controlled laboratory settings, produce changes in physiological responses indicative of autonomic arousal in both headache and nonheadache control populations (Pozniak-Patewicz, 1976; Bakal and Kaganov, 1977; Vaughn, Pall, and Haynes, 1977; Cohen, Rickles, and McArthur, 1978; Anderson and Franks, 1981; Andrasik, Blanchard, Arena, Teders, Teevan, and Rodichok, 1982; Feuerstein, Bush, and Corbisiero, 1982; Passchier, van der Helm-Hylkema, and Orlebeke, 1984; Haber et al., 1985). Most often, however, no differences are observed between headache and control groups in the magnitude of physiological reactivity to laboratory stressors. When differences are observed, they reflect different *patterns* of physiological responding, providing evidence for response stereotypy, the notion that physiological responses will be the greatest in those systems believed to be related to the patient's somatic complaints (Malmo and Shagass, 1949; Lacey and Lacey, 1958), rather than differences in the *reactivity* of responses (Bakal and Kaganov, 1977; Gannon, Haynes, Safranek, and Hamilton, 1981; Cohen, Williamson, Monguillot, Hutchinson, Gottlieb, and Waters, 1983). However, differences in patterns of physiological responses have not always been found (Brantley, 1980; Anderson and Fanks, 1981; Andrasik and Blanchard, 1987). In conclusion, laboratory studies fail to unequivocally support the notion that headache sufferers physiologically overreact to stressors presented in the laboratory as compared to controls.

Of three studies that have examined subject ratings of subjectively experienced stress in response to laboratory stressors, none found the ratings of subjective stress for headache subjects to exceed that reported by control subjects (Brantley, 1980; Feuerstein et al., 1982; Passchier et al., 1984). Passchier and associates (1984) did find, however, that both migraine and tension headache subjects reported more subjective tension than headache-free controls during relaxing imagery and recovery-from-stress periods. Headache subjects have also been found to request the premature termination of a physical stressor, the inflation of an occlusion cuff, more often than controls, suggesting that they may have experienced the same physical stressor more intensely (Gannon et al., 1981). Further, migraine subjects have been found to prefer situations and activities with less intense levels of stimulation than those preferred by a comparison group (Klein, 1983). Based on these findings, Klein (1983) concluded that migraine sufferers are stimulus intensity "augmenters" and may be hypersensitive to environmental stress. On the other hand, Martin and Mathews

(1978) found a slightly higher pain threshold for their headache subjects when compared to controls. Taken together, these studies suggest that various headache and control groups may experience stressful events differently; however, no consistent trend in the direction of this difference has emerged.

Another approach to studying the stress–headache relationship has been through the objective and standardized assessment of the "real" life stress or major life events experienced by headache sufferers (via instruments such as the Social Readjustment Rating Scale [SRRS] [Holmes and Rahe, 1967] and the Life Experiences Survey [LES] [Sarason, Johnson, and Seigel, 1978]). The hypotheses of researchers using these scales is that headache sufferers will report experiencing more stress than the normal population. Studies comparing scores on these measures for headache and control groups have not found headache subjects to report increased exposure to stress (Andrasik and Holroyd, 1980a; Brantley, 1980; Andrasik, Blanchard, Arena, Teders, Teevan, and Rodichok, 1982; Waggoner, 1986). An additional issue addressed by researchers has been whether or not the severity of a headache problem is related to being exposed to life stress outside of the laboratory. Blanchard, Andrasik, Arena, Neff, Jurish, Teders, Saunders, Pallmeyer, Dudek, and Rodichok (1984) performed separate stepwise multiple regression equations with scores from psychological, biological, and sociodemographic measures, both separately and combined, to predict the headache activity of migraine, mixed, and tension headache groups. They found when all measures were included in the equations, the scores from the SRRS did not account for a significant amount of variance in headache activity for any group. When only the psychological scores were entered into the equations, however, life events scores accounted for more of the variance in the headache activity of the migraine group (16%) than any other score that entered the equation, including scores from scales 6 and 7 of the MMPI and trait anxiety. The stress score did not significantly predict the headache activity of the mixed and tension headache groups however. It is tempting to speculate that because headache subjects experience similar exposure to stressful events, that the reaction of headache patients to a particular stressful event may be of greater magnitude than the reaction of a nonheadache individual. This conclusion must await more data because the use of life-event scales, such as the SRRS, for measuring stress has been debated (Rabkin and Streuning, 1976; Cleary, 1980; Miller, 1988).

To account for the minimal findings to date, some researchers have suggested that measures such as the SRRS and LES measure "major" life events and may not adequately assess the possible universe of stressful events (Kanner, Coyne, Schaefer, and Lazarus, 1981; DeLongis, Coyne, Folkman, and Lazarus, 1982; Lake, Yeglic, and Saper, 1986; Levor, Cohen, Naliboff, McArthur, and Heuser, 1986; Brantley, Waggoner, Jones, and Rappaport, 1987). These researchers suggest that consideration of relatively minor, day-to-day "hassles," such as arguments, social pressures, and job strains, may lead to more illuminating relationships. The occurrence of such minor events have been shown to correlate significantly with negative affective states and to account for a significant portion of the variance in the presentation of psychological and physical symptoms over and above the variance accounted for by major life events in other areas of research. One recent study, which compared the predictive ability of scores from a major life-events scale and a standardized measure of daily stress, found that daily stress scores predicted headache activity significantly and accounted for significantly more variance than scores from the major life-events scale (Waggoner, 1986).

The role of stress in the stress–headache relationship remains an enigma. Although evidence is accumulating to suggest that stress plays a role, it is probably only a modest one when compared to the role of biological factors (Blanchard, Andrasik, Arena, Neff, Saunders, Jurish, Teders, and Rodichok, 1983). The fact that nonpharmacological treatments, directed at reducing the effects of stress, are effective for reducing headache symptoms, however, is the impetus for continued research in this area.

BEHAVIORAL ASSESSMENT OF HEADACHES

The preceding review indicates that chronic headaches are a ubiquitous disorder with numerous possible factors contributing to their etiology and perpetuation. There are three major goals when evaluating a patient's headache problem. The first is to confirm or establish a diagnosis. Although most patients have had thorough medical evaluations and have received diagnoses for their headaches in the past, the reliability of independent diagnoses is less than perfect (refer to Andrasik and Baskin [1987], for a recent review of this research). In addition, many patients have never been evaluated by a psychologist, who may be in a better position to examine symptoms of stress and the relationship between stress and the onset of headache difficulties. The literature on the psychological treatment of headaches, reviewed in a later section, suggests that different types of headaches respond differentially to treatments, and a number of variables have been suggested to predict success or failure in response to particular treatments. The second major goal of assessment is to determine if and how psychological factors contribute to a patient's headaches. The task here is to discover whether psychological factors serve to trigger or maintain the headaches, or are a symptom of something else; for example, depression. This is probably the most important goal of assessment because once achieved, the clinician should be able to make treatment recommendations, the third and final goal of assessment. Although predetermined and uniform treatment programs are the rule for research purposes, not every patient will receive or need the same treatment components in the clinical setting. In order to achieve these goals, the assessment process should include: (1) a detailed headache history; (2) self-monitoring data; (3) psychological testing data; (4) psychophysiological data; and (5) a clinical interview. The utility of these strategies in assessment is presented below.

The Headache History

The headache history is an essential first step in the evaluation process. Questions pertaining to the circumstances of the initial onset, patterning, and recent changes in symptoms or pattern are sought, in addition to questions designed to facilitate diagnosis. Because, as nonmedical professionals, psychologists are not equipped to diagnose and treat headaches due to organic causes, patients need to be evaluated by a physician experienced with the diagnosis and treatment of headaches, prior to being evaluated by a psychologist. While taking the headache history, particular attention must be given to symptoms which do not fit the "typical" symptom presentation of migraine, tension, and mixed headaches and which may, instead, be indicative of an organic process. Various types of head pain are associated with metabolic disease (e.g., hypothyroidism), hypertension, ocular disease, cerebral vascular disease, anueurysm, and tumor (Diamond and Dalessio, 1986). Immediate referral to a physician is made when atypical symptoms are found. Most patients will have had multiple medical examinations, which typically include a skull X-ray, CT scan, and an EEG, prior to being referred to a nonmedical practitioner. Organic pathology, when present, is considered a contraindication for biofeedback (Diamond and Montrose, 1984).

A behavioral analysis of antecedents of headaches will aid in identifying variables which patients may have associated with their onset, such as situational stress, maladaptive thoughts, weather, weekends, menses, changes in activity levels or moods, and the ingestion of certain foods. If the patient habitually uses medications to cope with the headache, the possibility exists that the effects of analgesic withdrawal or ergotamine "rebound" headaches are perpetuating the problem (Saper, 1987). The discontinuation of analgesics, alone, may improve headache symptoms (Andrasik and Baskin, 1987). A poor prognosis for improvement in headache symptoms, from behavioral treatment, is expected when a patient is overutilizing medications. In such circumstances the physician should consider discontinuing medications prior to, or during, the early stages of behavioral treatment (Diamond, Diamond-Falk, and DeVeno, 1978; Diamond and Montrose, 1984). For these reasons, a close collaborative relationship should be maintained with the patient's physician. In addition to asking questions pertaining to current headache symptoms and medication usage, it is also useful to inquire about past exacerbations and remissions of headaches and factors related to these fluctuations in symptoms. Particular attention is given to incidents of head trauma, major life changes (e.g., change in job, moving, divorce), and changes in marital relations, social relations, and recreational pursuits that are associated with changes in symptoms. A careful analysis of how past problematic events were handled by the patient may provide insight to important maintaining factors for headaches.

In clinical practice, it is common for patients to have difficulty answering many of the questions asked during the headache history because they "have never noticed" whether or not particular symptoms or events have preceded or followed their headaches, or the pattern, if any, of when their headaches occur. This type of information is usually obtained through the examination of self-monitoring data.

The Role of Self-Monitoring in Assessment

Self-monitoring data serve several functions, depending on what symptoms, behaviors, thoughts, and events are chosen for the patient to monitor. Self-monitoring data can be used to assist with diagnosing headaches if the headache symptoms themselves (e.g., throbbing pain, photophobia, tightness, aching) and their pattern of occurrence are recorded. If the patient has difficulty relating headaches to potential triggering factors or noticing the consequences of headaches, these can be monitored as well. Factors which have been found to precipitate migraine headaches, and can be included on this monitoring form, are exposure to bright light, glare, loud noise, odors, noxious chemicals (e.g., ozone, alcohol), consumption of vasoactive substances, such as tyramine, sodium nitrite, and monosodium glutamate, found in some foods (Diamond and Dalessio, 1986), menses (Somerville, 1972), sleep patterns (Moss, Lombardo, Villarosa, Cooley, and Gramling, 1987), and the ingestion of alcohol. As previously discussed, exposure to stressful life events is often considered to be a precipitant of both migraine and tension headaches (Henryk-Gutt and Rees,

1973; Feuerstein et al., 1982; Drummond, 1983) and the relationship of such events to the occurrence of headaches, and how the patient copes with them, are important to monitor.

The most common use of self-monitoring data in assessment is for determining the baseline severity of the headache problem. Research has shown that the self-report of headache parameters (frequency, intensity, and duration), as obtained in the headache history, does not highly correlate with self-monitoring data (Andrasik and Holroyd, 1980b; Cahn and Cram, 1980). The typical procedure requires the patient to rate the intensity of headaches on a Likert-type scale, along with medication consumption (Budzynski, Stoyva, and Adler, 1970; Haynes, Griffin, Mooney, and Parise, 1975; Blanchard and Andrasik, 1985). Others have also required patients to monitor the degree of disability or impairment due to the headaches (Sargent, Walters, and Greene, 1973; Kewman and Roberts, 1980). Headache activity self-monitoring is initiated during the assessment phase and continues through treatment and serves as the yardstick for monitoring the success of treatment. Blanchard and Andrasik (1985), suggest using a zero (no headache) to five (extremely intense headache) scale of headache intensity requiring patients to rate their headaches four times a day to yield three scores: (1) a headache index score; (2) the number of headache-free days; and (3) a peak headache rating. They suggest that the headache index score is the most sensitive to treatment effects because it incorporates the frequency, intensity, and duration parameters of a patient's headaches.

The Role of Psychological Tests in Assessment

Most of the research examining psychological functioning of headache patients has been concerned with finding basic personality differences that would distinguish between diagnostic groups. Of more importance to clinicians, however, is the use of psychological tests to: (1) screen for psychological problems needing more immediate attention, (e.g., depression, symptoms of psychosis); (2) assist with the development of an overall formulation of the way in which psychological factors are involved in an individual's headaches; and (3) assist with the selection of the treatment strategy most likely to result in the improvement in headache symptoms (i.e., prediction of outcome).

Psychological tests are used to supplement, and not replace, the clinical interview when screening for major psychopathology. Certain patterns of scores on psychological tests, for example the MMPI, are expected for someone who presents with headaches. The clinical elevation of scores on the "neurotic triad" (scales 1, 2, and 3) of the MMPI would be expected (Kudrow and Sutkus, 1979; Andrasik, Blanchard, Arena, Teders, Teevan, and Rodichok, 1982), whereas the elevation of other scales would not be expected. Other tests often included in the assessment of psychological factors contributing to a headache problem measure depression (e.g., Beck Depression Inventory), anxiety (e.g., State-Trait Anxiety Inventory), problems with asserting oneself (e.g., Rathus Assertiveness Scale), life stress (e.g., SRRS), and the tendency toward experiencing a variety of psychosomatic symptoms (e.g., Psychosomatic Symptom Checklist). Clinically significant scores on these tests suggest a relationship exists but provide little information of the exact nature of this relationship for the particular headache problem under study. Scores suggesting that a significant problem in one of these areas exists warrants further investigation through the clinical interview.

The role of psychological measures in the prediction of treatment outcome has begun to receive some attention in the more recent literature. Results of studies using the MMPI suggest that scales L, F, K, 2, 3, 4, 7, 8, and 9 have some power for predicting outcome from relaxation and biofeedback (Werder, Sargent, and Coyne, 1981; Blanchard, Andrasik, Neff, Arena, Ahles, Jurish, Pallmeyer, Saunders, Teders, Barron, and Rodichok, 1982; Blanchard, Andrasik, Arena, Neff, Saunders, Jurish, Teders, and Rodichok, 1983). Blanchard et al. (1983) provide tables for using scores from various tests, in equations derived through canonical analyses, to predict the likelihood of success with biofeedback and relaxation. The test scores included in each equation are different for migraine, tension, and mixed headache sufferers. In general, these studies suggest that patients reporting more distress or psychological symptoms do not do as well with relaxation or biofeedback when compared to patients with less psychological distress. Patients evidencing serious depression do poorly with biofeedback (Billings, Thomas, Rapp, Reyes, and Leith, 1984; Diamond and Montrose, 1984). One study, however, found that a higher depression score on the MMPI (scale 2) was associated with a better outcome for vascular patients who received biofeedback (Blanchard, Andrasik, Arena, Neff, Jurish, Teders, Barron, and Rodichok, 1983). Taken together, the results of these studies emphasize the need for a thorough clinical interview to assist in treatment planning. Individuals reporting a higher level of psychological distress may well benefit from an initial course of treatment focusing on precipitating factors, or for depression, prior to initiating relaxation or biofeedback to decrease autonomic activity.

The Role of Psychophysiological Measurements in Assessment

Like the researchers investigating psychological factors in headaches, psychophysiological investigators had hopes of delineating clear differences in autonomic responses as a function of headache diagnosis. Unfortunately, as previously discussed, these differences have not yet emerged. Assessing autonomic functioning, however, has been used in two primary ways in assessment: (1) to examine if a patient exhibits excessive activity/reactivity in a particular response system; and (2) to predict patients' responses to treatment. For both purposes, the patient is situated in a sound and light attenuated room while measures of autonomic activity (e.g., EMG, heart rate, skin resistance, and skin temperature), are measured during resting states and during and following the presentation of various stimuli (e.g., mental arithmetic, loud noise, stressful mental imagery).

Although headache sufferers, as a group, have not been found to differ in autonomic reactivity to stress, there is an appeal for assessing the individual case because much variability in these measurements occur within diagnostic groups. The practice of assessing a patient's autonomic responses to stress-full stimuli is called "Stress Profiling" and has been suggested as a needed prerequisite for selecting a response and site for biofeedback training (Philips, 1977; Belar, 1979). There is little published data to support this practice at present, however. An interesting approach has recently been taken by Ahles, King, and Martin (1984). They evaluated frontal and trapezius EMG responses of a tension headache patient while the patient was ambulating on a treadmill and subsequently taught him to decrease these EMG levels during this activity to decrease his headache symptoms. The present authors have found similar procedures useful (i.e., providing a tension headache patient with trapezius EMG biofeedback while she ambulated through-out the hospital-based pain program; providing patients with feedback in the office while simulating working conditions and subsequently practicing biofeedback in vivo at work).

The second way psychophysiological assessments have been used is in the prediction of treatment outcome. Although the data are meager, several studies suggest that higher resting EMG levels are associated with poorer outcomes for tension headache sufferers receiving EMG biofeedback (Epstein and Able, 1977; Bruhn, Olesen, and Melgaard, 1979) and relaxation training (Blanchard, Andrasik, Arena, Neff, Jurish, Ted-ers, Barron, and Rodichok, 1983). Blanchard, Andrasik, and associates (1983) have published the results of multivariate analyses of the autonomic responses of ninety-three chronic headache sufferers for predicting their response to relaxation training and biofeedback treatment. They found they could correctly classify an average of 80 percent of their subjects as improved or unimproved, based on these equations. Their classification scheme awaits cross-validation, however. In con-clusion, the data available suggest that the psychophysiological assessment of headache patients has practical value both for targeting autonomic responses for biofeedback treatment and for selecting patients likely to receive benefits from relaxation and biofeedback treatment.

The Role of the Clinical Interview in Assessment

The functions of a good clinical interview cannot be duplicated by any number of tests or measurements. Its most obvious functions are to screen for major psychological problems and to follow up on problem areas identified through the results of testing. At a very rudimentary level, just by knowing that a patient is young, female, and not married has been suggested to indicate that she is likely to improve with biofeedback or relaxation training (Diamond, Diamond-Falk, and DeVeno, 1978; Blanchard et al., 1982; Diamond and Montrose, 1984). Of more importance, however, is its use for assisting the clinician in determining the cause–effect relationship between psychological problems and headaches and, thus, arriving at a formulation of a patient's headache problem. For example, knowing that a patient has "always been a depressed person," long before a problem with headaches surfaced, might suggest that headaches are a symptom of depression. Depression might be the better target of treatment in this case rather than the headaches. A headache problem that fluctuates over time with the amount of marital discord present may suggest that the patient is really dissatisfied with the relationship and is considering dissolving the marriage, and headaches are one way to temporarily fend off the spouse. This observation may instead be one instance of a more general problem of poor stress-coping skills or poor problem-resolution skills. Other observations of past stressful circumstances, other than marital problems, or of a relationship between stress and the exacerbation of headache symptoms would reinforce the second hypothesis. Answers to additional questions regarding the style with which problems are solved (e.g., passive avoidance and withdrawal, punitive and aggressive) and how these problem-solving strategies may be serving to prolong autonomic arousal and eventually lead to a headache, would also be desirable. Marital therapy might be more beneficial in the former instance while stress-coping skills (including relaxation or biofeedback) or problem-solving skills training would be indicated in the latter instance (Holroyd and Andrasik, 1982).

Another line of inquiry that assists in formulating the

causes and, therefore, the treatment of a particular headache problem, is concerned with the hypothesis that illness behavior may play a role in the development and maintenance of chronic headache in the same manner as those observed in chronic pain patients (Demjen and Bakal, 1981; Philips and Hunter, 1981). These researchers suggest that an inordinate amount of pain behavior (e.g., resting, avoiding activity, taking time away from work, verbally complaining of pain, rubbing/holding head, taking pills), may be presented in the absence of physiological indications of headaches, such as muscle tension and vascular changes and, consequently, may be a better target of treatment than relaxation or biofeedback. Questionnaires have been developed to assess the amount of illness behavior displayed by a patient in general (e.g., Illness Behavior Questionnaire, Illness Behavior Inventory, UAB Pain Behavior Scale) and with headache populations specifically (Philips and Hunter, 1981). However, determining if and how pain behaviors are maintaining complaints of chronic pain are left to interview data. A careful behavioral analysis of operant conditioning factors, that is, factors which may increase illness behavior and/or decrease "well" behaviors, is used to gather this information. Fordyce (1976) presents a detailed format for questions to ask patients (and family members) presenting with chronic pain which are also appropriate to ask when interviewing chronic headache patients. In general, if a significantly greater amount of reinforcement is available for a patient's headaches than are reasons to eliminate–reduce them, little benefit is expected from providing the patient with relaxation treatment. This set of circumstances will usually be observed as a "motivation problem" (assuming the case formulation does not indicate that depression is causing headaches). In this case, altering the consequences of a patient's headaches (e.g., the spouse's reinforcing reactions to the patient's complaints of headaches), may be the target of choice for treatment.

In conclusion, the interview plays the most important role in the assessment process. If used properly, it allows the clinician to connect all of the other parts of the assessment process together—headache history, self-monitoring data, psychological testing data, and psychophysiological testing data—

to determine if predisposing, precipitating, maintaining, or consequential factors (any or all) are involved in a particular patient's headache problem. This overall formulation can then be used to select the most efficient and potentially beneficial treatment program.

BEHAVIORAL TREATMENT

Modifying Precipitating Factors

Factors which may be triggering the chain of events resulting in a headache may be identified through the careful scrutiny of the headache monitoring data. The list of potential precipitating factors is quite long. Its length emphasizes the importance of having the patient monitor more than just the frequency, intensity, and duration of headaches. If precipitating factors are identified, the first line of treatment is to eliminate those that can be eliminated; for example, altering diets, sleep patterns, use of medications, and use of alcohol. Collaborating with the patient's physician may be necessary if prescribed reserpine or histamine is suspected of triggering migraine headaches. As mentioned previously, ergot derivatives, that are often prescribed to abort migraines, may produce "rebound headaches" if taken on even two consecutive days, and may need to be withdrawn (Friedman, 1978; Saper, 1987).

The analysis of posture during prolonged activities, possibly through a job analysis or during activities that require the patient to assume their "normal" posture for these activities, may reveal the need for postural corrections. A licensed physical therapist is helpful for identifying postural problems. One recent study found that providing EMG biofeedback to a patient, with a seventeen-year history of tension headaches, while he was walking, reduced headache activity significantly (Ahles, et al., 1984).

Modifying the environment in order to eliminate or avoid stressful circumstances has, more recently, become a component of cognitive–behavioral treatment approaches for chronic headaches (Mitchell and White, 1976, 1977; Holroyd and

Andrasik, 1982; Sorbi and Tellegen, 1984). Most of these treatments direct their influence at altering an individual's cognitive, behavioral, and physiological reactions (after the fact) to "triggering" events, and will be discussed in more detail below under the heading of "maintaining factors." The approach for treating triggering stressors is to prevent them from occurring in the first place. If stress is identified as being associated with an individual's headaches, it is also important to ask the patient to monitor his or her interpretations and judgments of the "stressfulness" of the events, because these are likely to determine the individual's ultimate reactions to them (Holroyd and Andrasik, 1982; Lazarus and Folkman, 1982; Beck, 1984). Beck (1984) believes that even an individual's self-demands, self-nagging, and self-reproaches, what he calls "internal" stressors, which may not have referents to environmental events, may actually "mobilize" the autonomic nervous system and musculoskeletal responses to produce psychosomatic disorders such as headaches. A patient may be taught to eliminate stress-producing self-statements through thought-stopping or possibly shifting cognitive sets; for example, attending to music or the scenery rather than to how fast the traffic is moving while driving (Beck, 1984). Time-management instructions may be helpful in order to avoid overloading a daily schedule. Lastly, a patient might be instructed to take a bus or carpool to work, or eat with different people in different places, in order to reduce the stress associated with driving to work every day or being exposed to others who bring up unwanted conversational topics. When avoidance of an activity or situation is not feasible, however, shifting the focus of treatment to address maintaining factors may be more appropriate.

Modifying Maintaining Factors

This category includes those factors that may prevent patients from neutralizing the effects of exposure to precipitating factors, particularly stress. Prolonged exposure to stress is thought to keep patients in the physiologically aroused state that will eventually lead to a headache (Mathew, Weinman, and

Largen, 1982). There is some evidence, however, that both migraine and tension headache sufferers may have more difficulty recovering from the effects of stress (Williamson, 1981; Passchier et al., 1984). Although no studies have addressed the reasons for this, some theorists have proposed that an autonomic regulatory dysfunction may be the reason that headaches may eventually become autonomous from triggering factors (Bakal, 1975; Bakal and Kaganov, 1979). Others have suggested that headache sufferers may not have adequate cognitive, behavioral, and physiological self-regulatory skills to cope with stress (Holroyd and Andrasik, 1982; Budzynski and Stoyva, 1984).

Relaxation and Biofeedback Training. The bulk of the psychological treatment literature focusing on headache disorders has investigated methods for modifying or interrupting the pathophysiologic precursors to headaches. The two most investigated procedures have been relaxation training and biofeedback. Relaxation training is by far the most often prescribed and easily provided treatment strategy for migraine, tension, and mixed headache disorders. Generally, patients are taught a modified version of Jacobson's (1938) procedure or some variant such as that of Bernstein and Borkovec (1973). In these procedures, patients are trained, usually on an individual basis, to alternately tense then relax various muscle groups throughout the entire body. In research protocols, biofeedback and relaxation training are usually provided in eight to twelve sessions spread over six to ten weeks. Patients are often provided an audiotaped version of relaxation to allow home practice in addition to the clinic training.

Forehead–frontal EMG biofeedback is recognized as the standard biofeedback treatment for tension headaches and skin temperature biofeedback, usually from an index finger, is recognized as the standard biofeedback treatment for migraine headaches by the Biofeedback Society of America (Andrasik and Blanchard, 1987; Blanchard and Andrasik, 1987). There is, as yet, no standard biofeedback procedure recognized by this society for combined headaches.

Recent reviews concur that relaxation training is effective

for reducing both migraine and tension headaches (Williamson, 1981; Blanchard and Andrasik, 1982). Further, both relaxation and biofeedback treatments for chronic headaches have been endorsed by the American Association for the Study of Headache (Board of Directors, 1978). Comparisons between relaxation training alone, EMG biofeedback alone, and the two procedures combined suggest that they are equally efficacious and can benefit greater than 50 percent of migraine and combined headache sufferers and approximately 75 percent of tension headache sufferers (Silver and Blanchard, 1978; Adams et al., 1980; Williamson, 1981). More recent data suggest, however, that some treatments are more effective than others for the treatment of different headache types. For example, Blanchard et al. (1982) found that over one-half of their tension headache patients but only about one-fourth of their patients with vascular headaches were "much improved" (greater than a 50 percent reduction in headache activity parameters) after a course of relaxation, whereas nearly 80 percent of combined and 50 percent of migraine headache sufferers, who did not respond to relaxation alone, showed additional improvement from adding a course of thermal biofeedback. In addition, they found that an additional 50 percent of the tension headache patients who did not respond to relaxation alone, responded to a subsequent course of EMG biofeedback. The findings of other recent studies also suggest that more tension headache patients receive benefits from relaxation training, and that biofeedback may be more beneficial to migraine patients and less beneficial to tension headache patients, with combined headache sufferers falling somewhere in the middle (Billings et al., 1984; Diamond and Montrose, 1984; Blanchard, Andrasik, Evans, Neff, Appelbaum, and Rodichok, 1985).

Because of the vascular nature of migraine headache symptoms, an additional biofeedback treatment approach, besides skin temperature biofeedback, has been to teach patients to constrict their temporal arteries in an attempt to prevent the painful rebound vasodilation phase. Although much less data are available on this technique, it has been shown to produce comparable benefits to patients as with thermal biofeedback (Friar and Beatty, 1976; Bild and Adams, 1980; Elmore and

Tursky, 1981). Direct comparisons between skin temperature and vasomotor biofeedback have not found one to be superior to the other (Elmore and Tursky, 1981; Gauthier, LaCroix, Cote, Doyon, and Drolet, 1985).

There is some controversy regarding the advantage of combining biofeedback with relaxation training, as in autogenic feedback training (Sargent, Green, and Walters, 1973), versus providing only one or the other. Some researchers believe they are equally efficacious (Williamson, 1981; Sorbi and Tellegen, 1984; Sargent, Solbach, Coyne, Spohn, and Segerson, 1986). Others suggest that if they are used sequentially, rather than concurrently, biofeedback may help a significant additional number of patients (Blanchard et al., 1982). In addition, when Blanchard and Andrasik (1982) compared the results of twenty-four treatment studies for migraine headaches, with a meta-analytic procedure, they concluded that autogenic feedback training provided benefits comparable to relaxation training alone but was superior to biofeedback alone. In conclusion, the current data suggest that a significant number of migraine, combined, and tension headache sufferers will benefit from an initial course of relaxation training and that adding biofeedback may be particularly beneficial to patients who have headaches with a vascular component.

Cognitive and Behavioral Approaches. Cognitive coping-skills training is increasingly becoming a part of the treatment armamentarium for chronic headaches. The typical treatment protocol involves: (1) helping the patient identify situations or cues that trigger tension and anxiety; (2) identifying how the patient behaviorally responds when anxious (e.g., passive, confrontative, aggressive, impulsive); (3) helping the patient identify self-thoughts (e.g., self-reproaches, catastrophizing) prior to becoming aware of anxiety, while anxious, and following the awareness of anxiety; (4) identifying the way in which the patient's cognitions appear to contribute to tension and headaches; and (5) teaching the patient to interrupt the sequence of events that lead to tension, at the earliest possible moment (Holroyd and Andrasik, 1978; Holroyd, Andrasik, and Westbrook, 1977). Working with tension headache sufferers, Holroyd, Andrasik, and associates (1977, 1978) found that up to 80 percent of their subjects showed at least a 50 percent reduction in headache symptoms from eight sessions of cognitive therapy and that adding relaxation training did not improve the results over cognitive therapy alone.

Most other investigations of the effectiveness of cognitive therapy for the treatment of chronic headaches have combined cognitive therapy techniques with relaxation, biofeedback, and with a variety of other behavioral techniques (Mitchell and White, 1977; Lake, Rainey, and Papsdorf, 1979; Steger and Harper, 1980; Bakal, Demjen, and Kaganov, 1981). These treatment approaches are typically provided over eight to twelve sessions, in these studies, and may provide the patient with a variety of strategies such as thought-stopping, relaxation training, flooding, in-vivo desensitization, assertion training, self-instructions training, imagery production, problem-solving skills training, rational–emotive therapy, biofeedback, and marital therapy. A clear distinction between what is considered strictly cognitive therapy and what is considered behavioral therapy is not made in these treatment regimens. Consequently, they have been called cognitive–behavioral treatment or stress-coping skills training. Results of studies suggest that these multimodal approaches may be at least as effective as relaxation and biofeedback approaches (Mitchell and White, 1977; Bakal et al., 1981; Sorbi and Tellegen, 1984) and that they may be particularly useful for increasing the endurance of treatment effects (Holroyd and Andrasik, 1982). Holroyd and Andrasik (1982) have suggested that cognitive–behavioral therapy may be the treatment of choice when headaches are accompanied by depression because depression reduces the effects of biofeedback or relaxation training and because cognitive-behavioral treatment strategies are effective for both depression and headaches.

Modifying Consequences Maintaining Symptoms of Headache

As previously mentioned, headache symptoms may include more than just the patient's verbal report that a headache is being experienced. A host of other symptoms indicative of pain (e.g., rubbing the head, facial grimaces, decreased activity, medication intake, moaning, and heavy sighing) may also be displayed, the consequences of which may be reinforced through increased attention from a significant other or an increase in the patient's ability to control or avoid some unpleasant activity or situation; for example, the "I have a headache" phenomenon (Roy, 1984). Such mechanisms leading to increased displays of pain by chronic pain patients have been exquisitely described by Fordyce (1976). Although the likelihood of reinforcement contributing to complaints of headache is considered to be perpetuating the problem in only a small number of patients (Blanchard and Andrasik, 1985), and reports of the effects of treatments addressing this issue with headache sufferers are nonexistent, it seems worth addressing for those patients who are unresponsive to other psychological interventions.

Another consequence of headache is the emotional or affective response of the patient who comes to believe that he or she is helpless to control the relentless headaches and becomes depressed as a result of headaches. This is the view of many theorists who believe that patients' aberrant scores on psychological tests (e.g., MMPI) are the result of headaches rather than the cause (Philips, 1976; Sternbach et al., 1980; Andrasik, Blanchard, Arena, Teders, Teevan, and Rodichok, 1982; Dalessio, 1987). The inability to engage in previously reinforcing activities because of the disabling effects of constant head pain also fits well with some theories of the causes of depression. To complete the cycle, depression is also thought to cause headaches (Diamond and Dalessio, 1986) and both may need to be addressed in treatment.

Emerging Trends in Treatment

The therapeutic efficacy of relaxation and biofeedback for the treatment of migraine, tension, and combined migraine and tension headaches is well established and there appears to be no need for further comparative efficacy studies alone (Blanchard and Andrasik, 1982). The more recent literature is beginning to investigate methods for increasing the cost-effectiveness of the delivery of these two methods. The main methods for the delivery of biofeedback and relaxation that have appeared in the literature are minimal therapist contact procedures (Jurish, Blanchard, Andrasik, Teders, Neff, and Arena, 1983; Teders, Blanchard, Andrasik, Jurish, Neff, and Arena, 1984; Williamson Monguillot, Jarrell, Cohen, Pratt, and Blouin, 1984; Blanchard et al., 1985; Attanasio, Andrasik, and Blanchard, 1987), self-help procedures (Steger and Harper, 1980; Kohlenberg and Cahn, 1981), and group treatment (Holroyd and Andrasik, 1978). In general, the minimal therapist contact approaches appear to be as efficacious as therapist-delivered procedures, rendering them more cost-effective, whereas the results of investigations using self-help manuals (with no contact or only mail or telephone contacts with therapists) have been less consistent. Holroyd and Andrasik (1978) found the cognitive therapy developed and applied individually in an earlier study (Holroyd, Andrasik, and Westbrook, 1977), yielded comparable benefits to patients when provided in a group modality.

A second trend in the treatment of chronic headaches is an extension of the multidimensional model of treatment and follows the concepts of "wellness" and "health promotion" (Simons, Solbach, Sargent, and Malone, 1986). The Wellness Program developed at the Menninger Foundation (Simons et al., 1986) includes providing patients with the modalities of stress management, aerobic exercise, nutritional counseling, work on self-esteem, and the patients' "sense of family, community, and environment," and appropriate pharmacological therapy; a consistent emphasis is changing maladaptive life-style habits. The results of this treatment program indicate that although patients initially started making positive life-style changes, these changes were not maintained following discharge. Unfortunately, data regarding change in headache parameters were not presented.

Researchers have come to realize that the headache problems of some patients are exceedingly difficult to treat effectively in the traditional outpatient format (an office visit for an hour or so, once or twice per week). This has led to exploration of brief, time-limited hospitalizations, followed by outpatient aftercare. Researchers at several clinics (Diamond, Freitag, and Maliszewski, 1986; Lake et al., 1986) have developed inpatient programs that can provide detoxification, relaxation, and bio-feedback, both group and individual psychotherapy, drug therapy, stress management, exercise classes, physical therapy, art therapy, leisure therapy, and dietary instructions "in an atmosphere that promotes positive social interactions" (Diamond et al., 1986). These programs list strict criteria for admission and accept only those patients who have been refractory to previous multiple attempts at managing their headaches and who have coexisting medical conditions that complicate the patient's treatment. Outcome data from one such clinic (Diamond et al., 1986) indicate that more than 50 percent of all patients, with the one exception of posttraumatic headache patients, showed more than a 50 percent reduction in headache symptoms upon discharge. These results are quite impressive when considering the difficult population of headache sufferers being treated.

Because severe and chronic headaches often have multiple determinants, these multidimensional treatment programs may be particularly beneficial to patients who do not respond to less comprehensive approaches. As Diamond et al. (1986) comment, however, the current trend of limiting health care costs will require meticulous efforts to select only those patients who may not respond to less costly outpatient treatment. Toward this end, Rose (1986) has suggested that inpatient facilities may be most appropriate for the population of headache disorders for which there are diagnostic problems, intractable headaches, symptomatic cases, and psychiatric disorders.

References

Ad Hoc Committee on Classification of Headache (1962), Classification of headache. *J. Amer. Med. Assn.*, 179:717–718.

Adams, H. E., Feuerstein, M., & Fowler, J. L. (1980), Migraine headache: Review of parameters, etiology, and intervention. *Psycholog. Bull.*, 87:217–237.

Ahles, T. A., King, A., & Martin, J. E. (1984), EMG biofeedback during dynamic movement as a treatment for tension headache. *Headache*, 24:41–44.

354 CHRONIC PAIN

Alexander, F. (1950), *Psychosomatic Medicine: Its Principles and Applications*. New York: W. W. Norton.

Anderson, C. D., & Fanks, R. D. (1981), Migraine and tension headache: Is there a physiological difference? *Headache*, 21:63–71.

Andrasik, F., & Baskin, S. (1987), Headache. In: *Medical Factors and Psychological Disorders: A Handbook for Psychologists*, eds. R. L. Morrison & A. S. Bellack, New York: Plenum, pp. 325–349.

———Blanchard, E. B. (1987), The biofeedback treatment of tension headache. In: *Biofeedback: Studies in clinical efficacy* eds. J. P. Hatch, J. G. Fisher, & J. D. Rugh. New York: Plenum, pp. 281–363.

——— ——— Arena, J. G., Saunders, N. L., & Barron, K. D. (1982), Psychophysiology of recurrent headache: Methodological issues and new empirical findings. *Behav. Ther.*, 13:407–429.

——— ——— ——— Teders, S. J., & Rodichok, L. D. (1982), A cross-validation of the Kudrow-Sutkus classification system for diagnosing headache type. *Headache*, 22:2–5.

——— ——— ——— ——— Teevan, R. C., & Rodichok, L. D. (1982), Psychological functioning in headache sufferers. *Psychosom. Med.*, 44:171–182.

——— Holroyd, K. A. (1980a), Physiologic and self-report differences between tension and nontension headache sufferers. *J. Behav. Med.*, 2:135–141.

——— ——— (1980b), Reliability and concurrent validity of headache questionnaire data. *Headache*, 20:44–46.

——— ——— (1980c), A test of specific and nonspecific effects in the biofeedback treatment of tension headache. *J. Consult. & Clin. Psychol.*, 48:575–586.

Anthony, M., Hinterberger, H., & Lance, J. W. (1967), Plasma serotonin in migraine and stress. *Arch. Neurol.*, 16:544–552.

Appenzeller, O. (1969), Vasomotor function in migraine. *Headache*, 9:147–155.

——— (1976), Monoamines, headache, & behavior. In: *Pathogenesis and Treatment of Headache*, 2nd ed., ed. Appenzeller, O. New York: Spectrum, pp. 43–48.

——— Becker, W. J., & Ragaz, A. (1981), Cluster headache. Ultrastructural aspects and pathogenetic mechanisms. *Arch. Neurol.*, 38:302–306.

——— Feldman, R. G., & Friedman, A. P. (1979), Migraine, headache, and related conditions: Panel 7. *Arch. Neurol.*, 36:784–805.

Attanasio, V., Andrasik, F., & Blanchard, E. B. (1987), Cognitive therapy and relaxation training in muscle contraction headache: Efficacy and cost-effectiveness. *Headache*, 27:254–260.

Bakal, D. A. (1975), Headache: A psychobiological perspective. *Psycholog. Bull.*, 82:369–382.

——— (1982), *The Psychobiology of Chronic Headache*. New York: Springer.

——— Demjen, S., & Kaganov, J. A. (1981), Cognitive behavioral treatment of chronic headache. *Headache*, 21:81–86.

——— Kaganov, J. A. (1977), Muscle contraction and migraine headache: Psychophysiologic comparison. *Headache*, 17:208–214.

——— ——— (1979), Symptom characteristics of chronic and nonchronic headache sufferers. *Headache*, 19:285–289.

Beck, A. T. (1984), Cognitive approaches to stress. In: *Principles and Practice of Stress Management*, eds. R. Woolfolk & P. Lehner. New York: Guilford Press, pp. 255–305.

Belar, C. D. (1979), A comment on Silver and Blanchard's (1978) review of the treatment of tension headaches by EMG feedback and relaxation training. *J. Behav. Med.*, 2:215–220.

Bernstein, D. A., & Borkovec, T. D. (1973), *Progressive Relaxation Training*. Champaign, IL: Research Press.

Bild, R., & Adams, H. E. (1980), Modification of migraine headaches by cephalic blood volume pulse and EMG biofeedback. *J. Consult. & Clin. Psychol.*, 48:51–57.

Billings, R. F., Thomas, M. R., Rapp, M. S., Reyes, E., & Leith, M. (1984), Differential efficacy of biofeedback in headache. *Headache*, 24:211–215.

Blanchard, E. B., & Andrasik, F. (1982), Psychological assessment and treatment of headache: Recent developments and emerging issues. *J. Consult. & Clin. Psychol.*, 50:859–879.

——— ——— (1985), *Management of Chronic Headaches: A Psychological Approach*. New York: Pergamon Press.

——— ——— (1987), Biofeedback treatment of vascular headache. In: *Biofeedback: Studies in Clinical Efficacy*, eds. J. P. Hatch, J. G. Fisher, & J. D. Rugh. New York: Plenum, pp. 1–79.

——— ——— Arena, J. G., Neff, D. F., Jurish, S. E., Teders, S. J., Barron, K. D., & Rodichok, L. D. (1983), Nonpharmacologic treatment of chronic headache: Prediction of outcome. *Neurol.*, 33:1596–1603.

——— ——— ——— Neff, D. F., Jurish, S. E., Teders, S. J., Saunders, N. L., Pallmeyer, T. P., Dudek, B. C., & Rodichok, L. D. (1984), A bio-psycho-social investigation of headache activity in a chronic headache population. *Headache*, 24:79–87.

——— ——— ——— ———Saunders, N. L., Jurish, S. E., Teders, S. J., & Rodichok, L. D. (1983), Psychophysiological responses as predictors of response to behavioral treatment of chronic headache. *Behav. Ther.*, 14:357–374.

——— ——— Evans, D. D., Neff, D. F., Appelbaum, K. A., & Rodichok, L. D. (1985), Behavioral treatment of 250 chronic headache patients: A clinical replication series. *Behav. Ther.*, 16:308–327.

——— ——— Neff, D. F., Arena, J. G., Ahles, T. A., Jurish, S. E., Pallmeyer, T. P., Saunders, N. L., Teders, S. J., Barron, K. D., & Rodichok, L. D. (1982), Biofeedback and relaxation training with three kinds of headache: Treatment effects and their prediction. *J. Consult. & Clin. Psychol.*, 50:562–575.

Blau, J. N. (1971), Migraine research. *Brit. Med. J.*, 2:751–754.

——— Diamond, S. (1985), Dietary factors in migraine precipitation: The physicians' view. *Headache*, 25:185–187.

Board of Directors (1978), American Association for the Study of Headache: Biofeedback therapy. *Headache*, 18:107.

Botney, M. (1981), An inquiry into the genesis of migraine headache. *Headache*, 21:179–185.

Brantley, P. J. (1980), *Headache: The Role of Environmental and Emotional Stress*. Unpublished doctoral dissertation, University of Georgia, Athens, GA.

———Waggoner, C. D., Jones, G. N., & Rappaport, N. B. (1987), A daily stress inventory: Development, reliability, and validity. *J. Behav. Med.* 10:61–74.

Bruhn, P., Olesen, J., & Melgaard, B. (1979), Controlled trial of EMG feedback in muscle contraction headache. *Ann. Neurol.*, 6:34–36.

Budzynski, T., & Stoyva, J. (1984), Biofeedback methods in the treatment of anxiety and stress. In: *Principles and Practice of Stress Management*, eds. R. Woolfolk & P. Lehrer. New York: Guilford Press, pp. 188–219.

——— ——— Adler, C. S. (1970), Feedback-induced muscle relaxation: Application to tension headache. *J. Behav. Ther. & Experiment. Psychiat.* 1:205–211.

Burnstock, G. (1981), Pathophysiology of migraine: A new hypothesis. *Lancet*, 7:1397–1399.

Cahn, T., & Cram. J. R. (1980), Changing measurement instrument at follow-up: A potential source of error. *Biofeedback & Self-Reg.*, 5:265–273.

Carroll, J. D. (1971), Migraine: General management. *Brit. Med. J.* 2:756–757.

Cinciripini, P. M., Williamson, D. A., & Epstein, L. H. (1980), Behavioral treatment of migraine headaches. In: *The Comprehensive Handbook of Behavioral Medicine: Syndromes and Special Areas*, Vol. 2, eds. J. M. Ferguson & C. B. Taylor. New York: Spectrum, pp. 207–227.

Cleary, P. J. (1980), A checklist for life event research. *J. Psychosom. Res.*, 24:199–207.

Cohen, R. A., Rickles, W. H., & McArthur, D. L. (1978), Evidence for physiological response stereotypy in migraine headache. *Psychosom. Med.*, 40:344–354.

——— Williamson, D. A., Monguillot, J. E., Hutchinson, P. C., Gottlieb, J., & Waters, W. F. (1983), Physiological response patterns in vascular and muscle-contraction headaches. *J. Behav. Med.*, 6:93–107.

Dalessio, D. J. (1978), Mechanisms of headache. *Med. Clin. N. Amer.*, 62:430–442.

——— ed. (1987), *Wolff's Headache and Other Head Pain*, 5th ed. New York: Oxford University Press.

Dalsgaard-Nielsen, T. (1965), Migraine and heredity. *Acta Neurol. Scand.*, 41:287–300.

DeLongis, A., Coyne, J. C., Folkman, S., & Lazarus, R. S. (1982), Relationship of daily hassles, uplifts, and major life events to health status. *Health Psychol.*, 1:119–136.

Delozier, J. E., & Gagnon, R. O. (1975), *National Ambulatory Care Survey: 1973 summary, United States* (DHEW Publication No. HRA 76-1772). Washington, DC: U. S. Government Printing Office.

Demjen, S., & Bakal, D. (1981), Illness behavior and chronic headache. *Pain*, 10:221–229.

Diamond, S., & Dalessio, D. J., eds. (1986), *The Practicing Physician's Approach to Headache*, 5th ed. Baltimore, MD: Williams & Wilkins.

——— Diamond-Falk, J., & DeVeno, T. (1978), Biofeedback in the treatment of vascular headache. *Biofeedback & Self-Reg.*, 3:385–408.

——— Freitag, F. G., & Maliszewski, M. (1986), Inpatient treatment of headache: Long-term results. *Headache*, 26:343–352.

——— Montrose, D. (1984), The value of biofeedback in the treatment of chronic headache: A four-year retrospective study. *Headache*, 24:5–18.

Drummond, P. D. (1983), Predisposing, precipitating and relieving factors in different categories of headache. *Headache*, 23:16–22.

——— Lance, J. W. (1984), Clinical diagnosis of headache symptoms. *J. Neurol. Neurosurg. & Psychiat.*, 47:128–133.

Dunbar, F. (1954), *Emotions and Bodily Changes*. New York: Columbia University Press.

Editorial (1983), Biofeedback. *J. Amer. Med. Assn.*, 250:2381.

Elmore, A. M., & Tursky, B. (1981), A comparison of two psychophysiological approaches to the treatment of migraine. *Headache*, 21:93–101.

Engel, G. L., Ferris, E. B., & Romano, J. (1945), Focal electroencephalographic changes during the scotomatas of migraine. *Amer. J. Med. Sci.*, 209:650–656.

Epstein, L. H., & Able, G. G. (1977), An analysis of biofeedback training effects for tension headache patients. *Behav. Ther.*, 8:37–47.

——— Cinciripini, P. M. (1981), Behavioral control of tension headache. In: *The Comprehensive Handbook of Behavioral Medicine: Syndromes and Special Areas*, Vol. 2, eds. J. M. Ferguson & C. B. Taylor. New York: Spectrum, pp 229–240.

Feuerstein, M., Bush, C., & Corbisiero, R. (1982), Stress and chronic headache: A psychophysiological analysis of mechanisms. *J. Psychosom. Res.*, 26:319–324.

Fordyce, W. E. (1976), *Behavioral Methods For Chronic Pain and Illness*. St. Louis, MO: C. V. Mosby.

Friar, L. R., & Beatty, J. (1976), Migraine: Management by trained control of vasoconstriction. *J. Consult. & Clin. Psychol.*, 44:46–53.

Friedman, A. P. (1963). Studies in pharmacotherapy of headache. *Neurol.*, 13:27–33.

—— (1978), Migraine. *Med. Clin. N. Amer.*, 62:481–494.

—— (1979), Characteristics of tension headache: A profile of 1,420 cases. *Psychosomat.*, 20:451–461.

—— von Storch, T. J., & Merritt, H. H. (1954), Migraine and tension headaches: A clinical study of two thousand cases. *Neurol.*, 4:773–788.

Fromm-Reichmann, F. (1937), Contributions to the psychogenesis of migraine. *Psychoanal. Rev.*, 24:26–30.

Gannon, L. R., Haynes, S. N., Safranek, R., & Hamilton, J. (1981), A psychophysiological investigation of muscle-contraction and migraine headache. *J. Psychosom. Res.*, 25:271–280.

Gauthier, J., LaCroix, R., Cote, A., Doyon, J., & Drolet, M. (1985), Biofeedback control of migraine headaches: A comparison of two approaches. *Biofeedback & Self-Reg.*, 10:139–159.

Haber, J. D., Kuczmierczyk, A. R., & Adams, H. E. (1985), Tension headaches: Muscle overactivity or psychogenic pain. *Headache*, 25:23–29.

Harrison, R. (1975), Psychological testing in headache: A review. *Headache*, 15:177–185.

Hart, J. D., & Chichanski, K. A. (1981), A comparison of frontal EMG biofeedback and neck EMG biofeedback in the treatment of muscle-contraction headache. *Biofeedback & Self-Reg.*, 6:63–74.

Haynes, S. N., Griffin, P., Mooney, D., & Parise, M. (1975), Electomyographic biofeedback and relaxation instructions in the treatment of muscle contraction headaches. *Behav. Ther.* 6:672–678.

Henryk-Gutt, R., & Rees, W. L. (1973), Psychological aspects of migraine. *J. Psychosom. Res.*, 17:141–153.

Holmes, T. H., & Rahe, R. H. (1967), The Social Readjustment Rating Scale. *J. Psychosom. Res.*, 11:213–218.

Holroyd, K. A., & Andrasik, F. (1978), Coping and the self-control of chronic tension headache. *J. Consult. & Clin. Psychol.*, 5:1036–1045.

—— —— (1982a), Do the effects of cognitive therapy endure? A two-year follow-up of tension headache sufferers treated with cognitive therapy or biofeedback. *Cog. Ther. & Res.*, 6:325–334.

—— —— (1982b), A cognitive–behavioral approach to recurrent tension and migraine headache. In: *Advances in Cognitive-Behavioral Research and Therapy*, Vol. 1, ed. P. C. Kendall. New York: Academic Press, pp. 275–320.

—— —— Westbrook, T. (1977), Cognitive control of tension headache. *Cog. Ther. & Res.*, 1:121–133.

Horton, B. (1956), Histaminic cephalgia: Differential diagnosis and treatment. *Proc. Mayo Clin.*, 31:325–330.

Howarth, E. (1965), Headache, personality and stress. *Brit. J. Psychiat.*, 119:1193.

Jacobson, E. (1938), *Progressive Relaxation*. Chicago: University of Chicago Press.

Johnson, E. S. (1978), A basis for migraine therapy—The autonomic theory reappraised. *Grad. Med. J.*, 54:231–242.

Jurish, S. E., Blanchard, E. B., Andrasik, F., Teders, S. J., Neff, D. F., & Arena, J. G. (1983), Home versus clinic-based treatment of vascular headache. *J. Consult. & Clin. Psychol.*, 51:743–751.

Kanner, A. D., Coyne, J. C., Schaefer, C., & Lazarus, R. S. (1981), Comparison of two modes of stress measurement: Daily hassles and uplifts versus major life-events. *J. Behav. Med.*, 4:1–39.

Kewman, D., & Roberts, A. H. (1980), Skin temperature biofeedback and migraine headaches. *Biofeedback & Self-Reg.*, 5:327–45.

Klein, S. H. (1983), Perception of stimulus intensity by migraine and non-migraine subjects. *Headache*, 23:158–161.

Kohlenberg, R. J., & Cahn, T. (1981), Self-help treatment for migraine headaches: A controlled outcome study. *Headache*, 21:196–200.

Kudrow, L. (1975), The relationship of headache frequency to hormone use in migraine. *Headache*, 15:36–40.

—— (1978), Current aspects of migraine headache. *Psychosomat.*, 19:48–57.

—— Sutkus, B. J. (1979), MMPI pattern specificity in primary headache disorders. *Headache*, 19:18–24.

Kunkle, E. C. (1959), Acetylcholine in the mechanism of headache of the migraine type. *Arch. Neurol. & Psychiat.*, 81:135.

Lacey, J. I., & Lacey, B. C. (1958), Verification and extension of the principle of autonomic response stereotypy. *Amer. J. Psychiat.*, 71:50–73.

Lake, A., Rainey, J., & Papsdorf, J. D. (1979), Biofeedback and rational motive therapy in the management of migraine headache. *J. Appl. Behav. Anal.*, 12:127–140.

Lake, A. E., III, Yeglic, E., & Saper, J. R. (1986), Comprehensive treatment planning in an inpatient headache unit (abstract). *Headache*, 26:324.

Lance, J. W., & Anthony, M. (1966), Some clinical aspects of migraine: A prospective survey of 500 patients. *Arch. Neurol.*, 15:356–361.

Lazarus, R. S., & Folkman, S. (1982), Coping and adaptation. In: *The Handbook of Behavioral Medicine*, ed. W. D. Gentry. New York: Guilford Press, pp. 282–325.

Leviton, A. (1978), Epidemiology of headache. In: *Advances in Neurology*, Vol. 19, New York: Raven Press, pp. 43–50.

Levor, R. M., Cohen, M. J., Naliboff, B. D., McArthur, D., & Heuser, G. (1986), Psychosocial precursors and correlates of migraine headache. *J. Consult. & Clin. Psychol.*, 54:347–353.

Lucas, R. M. (1977), Migraine in twins. *J. Psychosom. Res.*, 20:147–156.

Malmo, R., & Shagass, C. (1949), Physiologic study of symptom mechanisms in psychiatric patients under stress. *Psychosom. Med.*, 11:25–29.

Martin, M. J. (1966), Tension headache, a psychiatric study. *Headache*, 6:47–54.

—— (1983), Muscle-contraction (tension) headache. *Psychosom.*, 24:319–324.

—— Mathews, A. M. (1978), Tension headaches: Psychophysiological investigation and treatment. *J. Psychosom. Res.*, 22:389–399.

Masland, W. S. (1978), Electroencephalography and electromyography in the diagnosis of headache. *Med. Clin. N. Amer.*, 62:571–584.

Mathew, R. G., Weinman, M. L., & Largen, J. W. (1982), Sympathetic-adrenomedullary activation and migraine. *Headache*, 22:13–19.

Maxwell, H. (1966), *Migraine: Background and Treatment.* Baltimore, MD: J. Wright, Bristol.

Miller, T. W. (1988), Advances in understanding the impact of stressful life events on health. *Hospi. & Commun. Psychiat.*, 39:615–622.

Mitchell, K. R., & White, R. G. (1976), Self-management of tension headaches: A case study. *J. Behav. Ther. Experiment. Psychiat.*, 7:387–389.

——— White, R. G. (1977), Behavioral self-management: An application to the problem of migraine headaches. *Behav. Ther.*, 8:213–221.

Moskowitz, M. A., Reinhard, J. F., Romero, J., Melamed, E., & Pettibone, D. J. (1979), Neurotransmitters and the fifth cranial nerve: Is there a relation to the headache phase of migraine? *Lancet*, 5:883–885.

Moss, R. A., Lombardo, T., Villarosa, G., Cooley, J., & Gramling, S. (1987), The role of sleep in depression in classic migraine headaches. *J. Craniomandibular Pract.*, 5:137–142.

Ostfeld, A. M. (1962), *The Common Headache Syndromes: Biochemistry, Pathophysiology, Therapy.* Champaign, IL: Charles C. Thomas.

——— Reis, D. J., & Wolff, H. G. (1957), Studies on headache: Bulbar conjunctival ischemia and muscle-contraction headache. *Arch. Neurol. & Psychiat.*, 77:113–119.

Parnell, P., & Cooperstock, R. (1979), Tranquilizers and mood elevators in the treatment of migraine: An analysis of the Migraine Foundation Questionnaire. *Headache*, 19:78–86.

Passchier, J., van der Helm-Hylkema, H., & Orlebeke, J. F. (1984), Psychophysiological characteristics of migraine and tension headache patients: Differential effects of sex and pain state. *Headache*, 24:131–139.

Philips, C. (1976), Headache and personality. *J. Psychosom. Res.*, 20:535–542.

——— (1977), The modification of tension headache pain using EMG biofeedback. *Behav. Res. & Ther.*, 15:119–129.

——— (1978), Tension headache: Theoretical problems. *Behav. Res. & Ther.*, 16:249–261.

——— Hunter, M. (1981), Pain behavior in headache sufferers. *Behav. Anal. & Mod.*, 4:257–266.

Pozniak-Patewicz, E. (1976), Cephalic spasm of head and neck muscles. *Headache*, 16:261–266.

Pratt, J., Williamson, D., Cohen, R., Granberry, S., & Jarrel, P. (unpublished), *Psychological Differences Among Headache Populations: Stress, Depression, Anxiety and Locus of Control*, 1982. Louisiana State University, Baton Rouge, LA.

Rabkin, J. G., & Streuning, E. L. (1976), Life events, stress, and illness. *Science*, 194:1013–1020.

Rose, F. C. (1986), Headache clinics: Their role in health care systems and science. *Headache*, 26:112–116.

Roy, R. (1984), The phenomenon of "I have a headache": Functions of pain in marriage. *Internat. J. Fam. Ther.*, 6:165–176.

Sacks, O. W. (1970), *Migraine.* Berkeley, CA: University of California Press.

Sakai, F., & Meyer, J. S. (1978), Regional cerebral haemodynamics during migraine and cluster headaches measured by the xenon inhalation method. *Headache*, 18:122–132.

Saper, J. R. (1978), Migraine II: Treatment. *J. Amer. Med. Assn.*, 239:2480–2484.

——— (1987), Ergotamine dependency: A review. *Headache*, 27:435–438.

Sarason, I. G., Johnson, J. H., & Seigel, J. M. (1978), Assessing the impact of life changes: Development of the Life Experiences Survey. *J. Consult. & Clin. Psychol.*, 40:932–946.

Sargent, J. D., Greene, E. E., & Walters, E. D. (1973), Preliminary report on the use of autogenic feedback training in the treatment of migraine and tension headaches. *Psychosom. Med.*, 35:129–135.

——— Solbach, P., Coyne, L., Spohn, H., & Segerson, J. (1986), Results of a controlled, experimental, outcome study of nondrug treatments for the control of migraine headaches. *J. Behav. Med.*, 9:291–323.

——— Walters, E. D., & Greene, E. E. (1973), Psychosomatic self-regulation of migraine headache. *Sem. in Psychiat.*, 65:415–428.

Selby, G., & Lance, J. W. (1960), Observations on 500 cases of migraine and allied vascular headache. *J. Neurol. Neurosurg. & Psychiat.*, 23:230–232.

Sicuteri, F. (1959), Prophylactic and therapeutic properties of methyl lysurgic acid butanolamide in migraine. *Internat. Arch. Allergy*, 15:300.

Silver, B. V., & Blanchard, E. B. (1978), Biofeedback and relaxation training in the treatment of psychophysiologic disorders: Or, are the machines really necessary? *J. Behav. Med.*, 1:217–239.

Simons, A., Solbach, P., Sargent, J., & Malone, L. (1986), A wellness program in the treatment of headache. *Headache*, 26:184–187.

Skinhoj, E. (1973), Haemodynamic studies within the brain during migraine. *Arch. Neurol.*, 29:95–98.

Somerville, B. W. (1972), The influence of progesterone and estradiol upon migraine. *Headache*, 12:93–102.

Sorbi, M., & Tellegen, B. (1984), Multimodal migraine treatment: Does thermal feedback add to the outcome? *Headache*, 24:249–255.

Sovak, M., Kunzel, M., Sternbach, R., & Dalessio, D. (1981), Mechanism of the biofeedback therapy of migraine: Volitional manipulation of the psychophysiological background. *Headache*, 21:89–92.

Steger, J. C., & Harper, R. G. (1980), Comprehensive biofeedback versus self-monitored relaxation in the treatment of tension headache. *Headache*, 20:137–142.

Steiner, T. J., Guha, P., Capildeo, R., & Rose, F. C. (1980), Migraine in patients attending a migraine clinic: An analysis by computer of age, sex, and family history. *Headache*, 20:190–195.

Sternbach, R. A., Dalessio, D. J., Kunzel, M., & Bowman, G. E. (1980), MMPI patterns in common headache disorders. *Headache*, 20:311–315.

Strauss, H., & Selinsky, H. (1941), EEG findings in patients with migrainous syndrome. *Trans Amer. Neurolog. Assn.*, 67:250–254.

Teders, S. J., Blanchard, E. B., Andrasik, F., Jurish, S. E., Neff, D. F., & Arena, J. G. (1984), Relaxation training for tension headache: Comparative efficacy and cost-effectiveness of a minimal therapist contact versus a therapist delivered procedure. *Behav. Ther.*, 15:59–70.

Tunis, M. M., & Wolff, H. G. (1952), Analysis of cranial artery pulse waves in patients with vascular headache of the migraine type. *Amer. J. Med. Sci.*, 224:565–568.

——— ——— (1953), Studies on Headache: Long term observations of the reactivity the cranial arteries in subjects with vascular headaches of the migraine type. *Arch. Neurol. & Psychiat.*, 70:551–557.

——— ——— (1954), Studies on headache: Cranial artery vasoconstriction and muscle contraction headache. *Arch. Neurol. & Psychiat.*, 71:425–434.

van Boxtel, A., & van der Ven, J. R. (1978), Differential EMG activity in subjects with muscle-contraction headaches related to mental effort. *Headache*, 18:233–237.

Vaughn, R., Pall, M. L., & Haynes, S. N. (1977), Frontalis EMG responses to stress in subjects with frequent muscle-contraction headaches. *Headache*, 17:313–317.

Waggoner, C. D. (1986), *The Relation Among Stressful Life-Events, Affective Responses, and Headaches*. Unpublished doctoral dissertation, Louisiana State University, Baton Rouge, LA.

Waters, W. E. (1971), Migraine: Intelligence, social class, and familial prevalence. *Brit. Med. J.*, 2:77–78.

——— O'Connor, P. J. (1971), Epidemiology of headache and migraine in women. *J. Neurol. Neurosurg. & Psychiat.*, 54:148–153.

——— ——— (1975), Prevalence of migraine. *J. Neurol. Neurosurg. & Psychiat.*, 38:613–616.

Watson, D. (1982), Neurotic tendencies among chronic pain patients: An MMPI item analysis. *Pain*, 14:365–385.

Weeks, R., Baskin, S., Rapoport, A., Sheftell, F., & Arrowsmith, F. (1983), A comparison of MMPI personality data and frontalis electomyographic readings in migraine and combination headache patients. *Headache*, 23:75–82.

Werder, D. S., Sargent, J. D., & Coyne, L. (1981), MMPI profiles of headache patients using self-regulation to control headache activity. Paper presented at the American Association of Biofeedback Clinicians, Kansas City, October.

Whitehouse, D., Pappas, J. A., Escala, P. H., & Livingston, S. (1967), Electroencephalographic changes in children with migraine. *New Eng. J. Med.*, 276:33.

Williamson, D. A., (1981), Behavioral treatment of migraine and muscle contraction headaches: Outcome and theoretical explanations. *Prog. in Behav. Mod.*, 2:163–201.

——— Monguillot, J., Jarrell, P., Cohen, R., Pratt, M., & Blouin, D. (1984), Relaxation treatment of headache: Controlled evaluation of two group programs. *Behav. Mod.*, 8:407–424.

Wolff, H. G. (1963), *Headache and Other Head Pain.* New York: Oxford University Press.

Ziegler, D. K. (1978), Tension headache. *Med. Clin. N. Amer.* 62:495–505.

——— (1979), Headache syndromes: Problems of definition. *Psychosom.*, 20:443–447.